Urological Care for the Transgender Patient

AF290232

Dmitriy Nikolavsky · Stephen A. Blakely
Editors

Urological Care for the Transgender Patient

A Comprehensive Guide

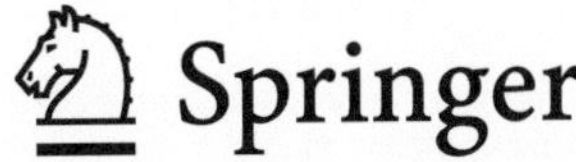

Springer

Editors
Dmitriy Nikolavsky
Urology Department
SUNY Upstate Medical University
Syracuse, NY
USA

Stephen A. Blakely
Urology Department
SUNY Upstate Medical University
Syracuse, NY
USA

ISBN 978-3-030-18535-0   ISBN 978-3-030-18533-6   (eBook)
https://doi.org/10.1007/978-3-030-18533-6

© Springer Nature Switzerland AG 2021
This work is subject to copyright. All rights are reserved by the Publisher, whether the whole or part of the material is concerned, specifically the rights of translation, reprinting, reuse of illustrations, recitation, broadcasting, reproduction on microfilms or in any other physical way, and transmission or information storage and retrieval, electronic adaptation, computer software, or by similar or dissimilar methodology now known or hereafter developed.
The use of general descriptive names, registered names, trademarks, service marks, etc. in this publication does not imply, even in the absence of a specific statement, that such names are exempt from the relevant protective laws and regulations and therefore free for general use.
The publisher, the authors and the editors are safe to assume that the advice and information in this book are believed to be true and accurate at the date of publication. Neither the publisher nor the authors or the editors give a warranty, expressed or implied, with respect to the material contained herein or for any errors or omissions that may have been made. The publisher remains neutral with regard to jurisdictional claims in published maps and institutional affiliations.

This Springer imprint is published by the registered company Springer Nature Switzerland AG
The registered company address is: Gewerbestrasse 11, 6330 Cham, Switzerland

Preface

in regione caecorum rex est luscus (in the land of the blind, one-eyed man is a king)
attributed to Desiderius Erasmus, 1500 AD

We must admit, when we encountered our first patient with post-phalloplasty complications in 2013, we panicked. Our lack of knowledge about transgender anatomy, care, and complications was a bit embarrassing. In an attempt to feign competence, we were frantically searching PubMed, Google, and UpToDate to figure out what kinds of questions to ask. This topic was omitted through our years of training in medical school, residency, and even reconstructive urology fellowship. At that point, the medical literature was outpaced by the growing public interest and, more importantly, growing population of transgender patients in need. We couldn't find helpful review papers, textbooks, or online courses. Our first thought, guided by the mantra "do no harm," was to admit our deficit and refer the patient to someone else with sound experience. Fortunately, the patient put the problem in perspective. "You ARE the reconstructive guys. That is why I am here." Thanks to this patient's trust and the infinite patience of our mentors and good friends in reconstructive community who taught us phalloplasty anatomy over the phone that day (trying to protect their identity, but Curtis Crane, you know who you are), we were able to identify the problem and eventually help this and many other patients. This book is intended to spare the reader the embarrassment that we suffered that day, and to significantly shorten the learning curve of the trial-and-error learning. We hope it will help physicians to run transgender-friendly general urology clinics, even without specialized reconstructive training. We hope it will help transgender patients to get established with a urologist for long-term care, even if there are no urological complications after gender affirmation.

The aim of this book, with the general urologist as the audience, is to provide a comprehensive guide on a variety of topics related to the care of transgender and gender nonconforming individuals. Furthermore, we aim to help providers understand the medical needs of transgender patients, clarify surgical steps and changes after gender affirmation, and educate and counsel patients regarding available medical and surgical treatments options. We will also discuss the importance of a multidisciplinary approach in providing these services for transgender patients via a multispecialist, team care program.

Further chapters will describe urologically relevant surgical anatomy of both feminizing and masculinizing gender-affirming procedures, including vaginoplasty, orchiectomy, hysterectomy, vaginectomy, phalloplasty, metoidioplasty, and prosthetics. We will also explore diagnosis and management of common complications of genital-related gender-affirming surgery in addition to a separate discussion on postsurgical incontinence.

We provide detailed discussions of endocrinological care and options for fertility preservation. Surgical, endourologic, and oncologic considerations with respect to reconstructed genitourinary anatomy and physiologic changes related to hormone therapy— a vital knowledge for the practicing general urologist—will be discussed. Future directions, including the use of robotics in gender-affirming surgery and the history of transgender healthcare, will be discussed in the last two chapters.

We hope this first book on the urological care for transgender patients will be a helpful resource for our general and reconstructive urology colleagues alike. We also hope that this is just one of the initial steps on a path toward making a care for transgender patients a part of routine urological practice.

Syracuse, NY, USA   Dmitriy Nikolavsky
Syracuse, NY, USA   Stephen A. Blakely

Contents

Part IV Perioperative Care and Follow Up

Part V Special Topics—Regrets, Robotics, and History

Contributors

Jens Berli, MD Division of Plastic Surgery, Oregon Health & Science University, Portland, OR, USA

Jasmine Bhinder, MD Department of Surgery, SUNY Upstate Medical University, Syracuse, NY, USA

Marta Bizic, MD, PhD Belgrade Center for Urogenital Reconstructive Surgery, School of Medicine, University of Belgrade, Belgrade, Serbia

Stephen Blakely, MD Department of Urology, SUNY Upstate Medical University, Syracuse, NY, USA

Rachel Bluebond-Langner, MD NYU Langone Health, New York, NY, USA

Gennady Bratslavsky, MD Department of Urology, Upstate University Hospital, SUNY Upstate Medical University, Syracuse, NY, USA

Jillian Cardinali, PT, DPT, Upstate University Hospital, SUNY Upstate Medical University, Syracuse, NY, USA

Olivia H. Chang, MD, MPH Cleveland Clinic Foundation, Section of Female Pelvic Medicine and Reconstructive Surgery, Department of Obstetrics and Gynecology, Cleveland, OH, USA

Amanda C. Chi, MD Urology Department, Kaiser Permanente West Los Angeles Medical Center, Los Angeles, CA, USA

Nim Christopher University College London Hospital, London, UK
St Peters Andrology Centre, London, UK

Miroslav L. Djordjevic, MD, PhD Belgrade Center for Urogenital Reconstructive Surgery, School of Medicine, University of Belgrade, Belgrade, Serbia

James J. Drinane, DO Albany Medical College, Albany, NY, USA

Daniel Dugi, MD FACS Department of Urology, Oregon Health & Science University, Portland, OR, USA

Geolani W. Dy NYU Langone Health, New York, NY, USA

Alexander R. Facque, MD Gender Confirmation Center of San Francisco, Morton, IL, USA

Cecile A. Ferrando, MD, MPH Cleveland Clinic Foundation, Section of Female Pelvic Medicine and Reconstructive Surgery, Department of Obstetrics and Gynecology, Cleveland, OH, USA

Elizabeth Ferry, MD Department of Urology, Upstate University Hospital, SUNY Upstate Medical University, Syracuse, NY, USA

Maurice M. Garcia, MD, MAS Division of Urology, Department of Surgery, Cedars-Sinai Medical Center Los Angeles, Los Angeles, CA, USA

Cedars-Sinai Transgender Surgery and Health Program, Cedars-Sinai Medical Center, Los Angeles, CA, USA

Department of Urology, University of California San Francisco, San Francisco, CA, USA

Department of Anatomy, University of California San Francisco, San Francisco, CA, USA

Natasha Ginzburg, MD Upstate Urology, Syracuse, NY, USA

Rachel Hopkins, MD SUNY Upstate Medical University, Department of Medicine, Division of Endocrinology, Syracuse, NY, USA

Michael Hughes, MD Department of Urology, SUNY Upstate Medical University, Syracuse, NY, USA

Matthew Katz, MD NYU Langone, New York, NY, USA

Darryl Manzer, PT, DPT, Upstate University Hospital, SUNY Upstate Medical University, Syracuse, NY, USA

Lei Lei Min, MD SUNY Upstate Medical University, Department of Medicine, Division of Endocrinology, Syracuse, NY, USA

Dmitriy Nikolavsky, MD Urology Department, SUNY Upstate Medical University, Syracuse, NY, USA

Ian T. Nolan New York University School of Medicine, New York, NY, USA

Michael Owyong University of Miami Miller School of Medicine, Miami, FL, USA

Amy Penkin, LCSW Transgender Health Program, Oregon Health & Science University, Portland, OR, USA

Melissa M. Poh, MD Department of Plastic Surgery, Kaiser Permanente West Los Angeles Medical Center, Los Angeles, CA, USA

Ranjith Ramasamy University of Miami Miller School of Medicine, Miami, FL, USA

Polina Reyblat, MD Urology Department, Kaiser Permanente Los Angeles Medical Center, Los Angeles, CA, USA

Richard A. Santucci, MD, FACS, HON FC Urol(SA) Brownstein-Crane Surgical Services, Austin, TX, USA

Jessica Schardein, MD, MS Department of Urology, SUNY Upstate Medical University, Syracuse, NY, USA

Loren S. Schechter, MD Clinical Professor of Surgery, The University of Illinois at Chicago Attending Surgeon Rush University, Director, The Center for Gender Confirmation Surgery Weiss Memorial Hospital, Morton, IL, USA

Kathryn Scott, MD Department of Urology, SUNY Upstate Medical Center, Syracuse, NY, USA

Nabeel A. Shakir Department of Urology, University of Texas Southwestern Medical Center, Dallas, TX, USA

Borko Stojanovic, MD Belgrade Center for Urogenital Reconstructive Surgery, School of Medicine, University of Belgrade, Belgrade, Serbia

Prashant Upadhyaya, MD Department of Surgery, SUNY Upstate Medical University, Syracuse, NY, USA

Lee C. Zhao NYU Langone Health, New York, NY, USA

Part I

Overview, Decision Making, Endocrinological Care, and Pre-operative Considerations

The Current State of Transgender Care

Michael Hughes, Stephen Blakely, and Dmitriy Nikolavsky

A Changing Landscape for Patients and Physicians

At the time of creating this text, attitudes toward lesbian, gay, bisexual, transgender, and queer (LGBTQ) issues have shifted dramatically in the United States in recent years. Highly publicized media attention given to transgender figures has helped raise awareness of societal and political issues effecting the transgender population. The Public Religion Research Institute (PRRI), an American nonprofit and nonpartisan research organization which examines the intersection of political issues and religious values, conducted a population survey to assess how Americans view transgender issues. The survey uncovered that 62% of Americans reported they had become more supportive of transgender rights compared to their views five years previous. Sixty-three percent of Americans also reported they would be comfortable having a close friend come out to them as transgender [1].

According to survey data published by the Williams Institute in 2016, an estimated 1.4 million adults (0.6%) in the United States identify as transgender. This study conducted a phone survey, in 19 anonymous states, asking subjects if they identified as transgender "male-to-female, female-to-male, or gender nonconforming." When compared to the same group's 2011 findings, this figure had doubled. The authors explain that the increasing visibility and acceptance of transgender people may contribute to the increase in self-reporting. State-level estimates of transgender-identifying adults ranged from 0.3% in North Dakota to 0.8% in Hawaii. The survey also found that young adults (18–24 years of age; 0.7%) were more likely than older adults (65+; 0.5%) to identify as transgender [2]. Furthermore, in the largest population-based survey, including ten states and nine urban school districts, the Centers for Disease Control (CDC) reported 1.8% of high school students identified as transgender [1]. This is significantly higher than any other age group. If this is accurate, we can expect to see a much greater number of transgender patients throughout our healthcare system for years to come as this group ages.

The healthcare industry has already seen a significant uptick in the number of transgender patients seeking care. A recently published study evaluating national temporal trends in gender-affirming surgery for transgender patients in the United States found a threefold increase in Medicare and Medicaid coverage of gender-affirming surgery from 25% in 2012–2013 to 70% in 2014. The proportion of genital surgery in

M. Hughes (✉) · S. Blakely
Department of Urology, SUNY Upstate Medical University, Syracuse, NY, USA
e-mail: hughesmi@upstate.edu

D. Nikolavsky
Urology Department, SUNY Upstate Medical University, Syracuse, NY, USA

© Springer Nature Switzerland AG 2021
D. Nikolavsky, S. A. Blakely (eds.), *Urological Care for the Transgender Patient*,
https://doi.org/10.1007/978-3-030-18533-6_1

gender-affirming procedures was also noted to increase from 72% in 2000–2005 to 83.9% in 2006–2011. The study also found an increasing trend in reporting gender identity information in electronic health records [3].

We have noted an increase in patients presenting to the clinic seeking care and advice in preparation for gender-affirming surgeries or postsurgical patients with a variety of urologic needs from treatment of complications, catheter management, hormone therapy, incontinence, nephrolithiasis, and beyond. In speaking to our colleagues, we have found that this is not unique to our practice or region. These trends underscore the importance of physician education and familiarity with health issues afflicting this population.

Disparities and the Road to Healthcare Equality

Despite progress in the twenty-first century, our transgender patients are members of a vulnerable population. The 2015 US Transgender Survey conducted by the National Center for Transgender Equality collected 27,715 respondents from all 50 states. The study, using an online questionnaire (>300 items), reported on adults aiming to shed light on the transgender experience on a variety of topics ranging from education, healthcare, family life, and interactions with the criminal justice system. The findings illustrated the disparities effecting the transgender community particularly in regard to access to healthcare and health insurance. The survey found 25% of respondents experienced an issue with health insurance coverage including denial of coverage for gender transition care and upward of 55% of respondents had been denied coverage for transition-related surgery. A significant proportion (25%) of respondents was unwilling to seek medical treatment for fear of mistreatment. A third of respondents reported having at least one negative experience related to gender including refusal of treatment, harassment, and assault [4]. Transgender patients are also at increased risk for self-prescription of hormonal therapy. Mepham et al. reported a quarter of patients referred to a gender clinic over a one-year period had self-

prescribed hormonal therapy, 70% of which were obtained from the internet [5]. Similarly, a study by De Haan et al. reported ~50% of 215 transgender women had taken hormones not prescribed by a physician. This behavior was seen more frequently in patients who had previously experienced verbal abuse due to their gender identity [6].

Transgender minors face an uphill healthcare battle as well. A 2018 population-based study reports that transgender and gender-nonconforming students reported significantly poorer health, lower rates of preventive health checkups, and more nurse office visits than cisgender youth.

A study published in 2007 reported more than a fourth of self-identifying transgender adolescents had attempted suicide, all of which cited reasons related to being transgender [7]. Data collected from the National Violent Death Reporting System between 2013 and 2015 revealed that LGBT minors are overwhelmingly more likely to die from violent causes than their non-LGBT classmates. LGBT minors accounted for twenty-five percent of violence-related deaths between the ages of 12 and 14 [8]. Another study demonstrated transgender youth report significant discrimination compared to their cisgender peers, with higher rates of suicidal ideation and self-harm than their heterosexual and cisgender peers [9]. The CDC survey also found transgender youths were at increased risk for violence victimization, substance abuse, and suicide risk. They were also more likely to report having been tested for human immunodeficiency virus [10].

There have been recent legislative efforts to improve transgender persons' access to healthcare. The Affordable Care Act (ACA) introduced under President Obama in 2014 has prohibited discrimination by healthcare providers based on gender in addition to preventing insurance companies from denying coverage on basis of gender identity [11]. Since 1981, gender-affirming surgery was excluded to Centers for Medicare and Medicaid beneficiaries citing "surgical procedures and attendant therapies for transsexualism" as "experimental" with "high rates of serious complications." However, in 2014, the US

Department of Health and Human Services ended this policy citing consensus medical literature demonstrating the efficacy and safety of gender affirmation care, effectively leaving the decision to local coverage determinations on case-specific basis [12]. Despite this progress, private insurance coverage is often regulated at a state level, resulting in variations in coverage by both state and employer [13]. In June of 2016, the Department of Defense lifted a preexisting ban which prohibited transgender individuals from joining the armed services. In September of 2016, TRICARE, the health benefit program for active-duty military personnel, their dependents, and retirees, released a new policy allowing for the nonsurgical treatment of gender dysphoria. Although the policy covers hormone therapy and psychological counseling for gender dysphoric patients, surgical treatment remains uncovered except in cases where an active-duty service member is granted a waiver by a medical provider deeming the surgery necessary [14].

Medical Education

The World Professional Association for Transgender Health (WPATH), formerly known as the Harry Benjamin International Gender Dysphoria Association, is a nonprofit interdisciplinary organization which endorses high standards of healthcare for the transsexual, transgender, and gender-nonconforming individuals through evidence-based medicine. WPATH has published the standards of care (SOC) and ethical guidelines which provide a comprehensive multidisciplinary overview of the SOC in the realm of psychiatric, medical, and surgical treatment for transgender and gender-nonconforming patients. The original SOC were published in 1979; the most recent seventh edition was published in 2011.

The SOC have not made it into medical education uniformly. Exposure to transgender and gender-nonconforming patients during urologic residency and fellowship training varies by institution. In a 2016 survey of 289 urology residents, only 54% of trainees reported any experience with transgender patient care. Education regarding the psychological, medical, and surgical care of these patients was also limited ranging from 6% to 11% of respondents reporting having didactic teaching on these topics. Significantly more female respondents placed greater priority on gender-affirming surgical training than did their male colleagues (91% vs 70%); however, the majority of residents agreed transgender-related surgical training should be offered as a fellowship focus [15]. Even small efforts to integrate transgender health topics into medical school curriculum, e.g., didactic lectures and small group discussions, have been shown to improve medical students' attitudes and knowledge of health issues affecting transgender patients as evidenced by pre- and post-educational surveys [16].

With the increasing visibility of the transgender and gender-nonconforming population and these patients appropriately having increasing access to care, it is vital that the practicing urologist is well-acquainted with the appropriate and sensitive management of these individuals. As many care pathways and genital-affirming procedures were developed by gynecologists and plastic surgeons, urologists were not extensively involved in this field. However, urologic organizations are beginning to recognize the importance of the inclusion of transgender-oriented care in urologic education. The American Urological Association first offered an update series on genital gender-affirming surgery for transgender patients in 2017 with the goal of teaching appropriate terminology, surgical options, complications, and care pathways of surgical patients. Today, a variety of courses, lectures, and workshops on these topics including genital-affirming surgery and transgender care exist in the *AUA University* Core Curriculum. The American Urogynecologic Society (AUGS), European Association of Urology (EAU), Society of Urodynamics, Female Pelvic Medicine and Urogenital Reconstruction (SUFU), and Société Internationale d'Urologie (SIU) have followed suit in their inclusion of educational courses and material regarding transgender health topics.

In summary, all healthcare workers are likely to experience an increase in interactions with transgender patients. This is due to a growing and aging transgender population as well as improved access to healthcare for this patient population. It is critical that we all keep in mind that there are disparities and challenges faced by our transgender patients. One aspect of this disparity that we can all improve is the care we provide when given the opportunity. We can create and utilize educational material to ensure that we are most suitably equipped to be healthcare providers to all.

Take-Home Points
- Visibility and recognition of the transgender population are growing, as well as the societal and cultural adversity the transgender community faces.
- Transgender patients commonly meet adversity in access to proper healthcare, including issues with medical insurance coverage and mistreatment from providers.
- Formal medical education regarding transgender health is currently limited; however, there are ongoing movements within medical education and various medical societies worldwide to address this gap.
- It is important that all healthcare providers, particularly the practicing urologist, have a well-rounded knowledge of common medical issues and treatments unique to the transgender patient population.

References

1. Jones RP, Jackson N, Najle M, Bola O, Greenberg D. America's growing support for transgender rights. PRRI. 2019;6:10.
2. Flores AR. How many adults identify as transgender in the United States? Los Angeles: The Williams Institute; 2016.
3. Canner JK, Harfouch O, Kodadek LM. Temporal trends in gender-affirming surgery among transgender patients in the United States. JAMA Surg. 2018;153(7):609–16.
4. James SE, Herman JL, Rankin S, Keisling M, Mottet L, Anafi M. Executive summary of the report of the 2015 U.S. Transgender Survey. Washington, DC: National Center for Transgender Equality; 2016.
5. Mepham N, et al. People with gender dysphoria who self-prescribe cross-sex hormones: prevalence, sources, and side effects knowledge. J Sex Med. 2014;11:2995–3001.
6. De Haan G, et al. Non-prescribed hormone use and barriers to care for transgender women in San Francisco. LGBT Health. 2015;2:313–23.
7. Grossman AH, D'Augelli AR. Transgender youth and life-threatening behaviors. Suicide Life Threat Behav. 2007;37(5):527–37.
8. Ream GL. What's unique about lesbian, gay, bisexual, and transgender (LGBT) youth and young adult suicides? Findings from the National Violent Death Reporting System. J Adolesc Health. 2018;64(5):602–7.
9. Almeida J, Johnson R, Corliss H, Molnar B, Azrael D. Emotional distress among LGBT youth: the influence of perceived discrimination based on sexual orientation. J Youth Adolesc. 2009;38(7):1001–14.
10. Johns MM, Lowry R, Andrzejewski J, et al. Transgender identity and experiences of violence victimization, substance use, suicide risk, and sexual risk behaviors among high school students — 19 states and large urban school districts, 2017. MMWR Morb Mortal Wkly Rep 2019;68:67–71. http://dx.doi.org/10.15585/mmwr.mm6803a3.
11. OCR. U.S. Department of Health and Human Services (HHS): office for civil rights. Nondiscrimination in health programs and activities proposed rule - Section 1557 of the Affordable Care Act; 2015.
12. Stroumsa D. The state of transgender health care: policy, law, and medical frameworks. Am J Public Health. 2014;104(3):e31–e38. https://doi.org/10.2105/AJPH.2013.301789.
13. Deutsch MB, editor. Guidelines for the primary and gender-affirming care of transgender and gender nonbinary people. 2nd ed. San Francisco: Prod. Department of Family and Community Medicine, University of California San Francisco, Center of Excellence for Transgender Health; 2016.
14. Gender dysphoria. TRICARE policy manual chapter 7, section 1.2 gender dysphoria, 2016, chapter 7, section 1.2.
15. Dy GW, et al. Exposure to and attitudes regarding transgender education among urology residents. J Sex Med. 2016;13:1466–72.
16. Click IA, Mann AK, Buda M, Rahimi-Saber A, Schultz A, Shelton KM, Johnson L. Transgender health education for medical students. Clin Teach. 2020;17:190–4. https://doi.org/10.1111/tct.13074.

Decision-Making in Masculinizing Surgery and Feminizing Surgery

2

Maurice M. Garcia

The goal of genital gender affirming surgery (gGAS) is to create genitalia that align with the gender that the given patient identifies with [1]. For most transgender people, and to varying degrees for patients whose gender is non-binary, this includes elimination of the presence and/or visibility of their *birth-sex* genitalia *and* creation of the *feminine* or *masculine* genitalia that align with their gender. Different patients may have very different attitudes toward the multitude of surgical options available to them [2, 3]. Surgical risks and risk of postsurgery complications (short and long-term) should always be discussed when surgical options are reviewed with patients.

If the care goal of a gender affirming reconstructive *surgeon* is to help the patient identify what surgical option(s) best meet their needs (whatever these may be), then it is clear that what would serve patients *best* is to be able to grasp *all* available options, and what each of these "costs" with respect to risks, advantages, and disadvantages to (specifically) them. (Here, "surgical options" encompass all options available to patients in general and not only what the particular surgeon offers.) [2] The gGAS surgeon should be sufficiently *familiar with* all available reconstructive genital surgery options to be able to describe them (even if only in general terms) and discuss the risks and benefits of each. For those options that the surgeon *does not* offer, she/he should give patients the option to be referred to a provider *who does* offer what the patient identifies as what best meets their needs, goals, and tolerance for the risk of short- and long-term complications or to accept what options the given surgeon *does* offer which might also meet some of their needs and goals. However, for the surgeon to not inform patients about the spectrum of surgical options available to them is out of line with key aspects of gender affirming care as described by the WPATH Standards of Care guidelines – that care should be based on the *individual* and that it should be *patient-centered* [1, 4, 5]. To approach discussion about surgery based on *assumptions* about what the patient wants is not in line with care-quality goals and does not serve patients. The recommended approach of covering all options with patients is based on the perspective that every transgender and gender non-binary patient is an individual whose needs and goals may differ from other patients [1, 3, 6].

M. M. Garcia (✉)
Division of Urology, Department of Surgery, Cedars-Sinai Medical Center, Los Angeles, CA, USA

Cedars-Sinai Transgender Surgery and Health Program, Cedars-Sinai Medical Center, Los Angeles, CA, USA

Department of Urology, University of California San Francisco, San Francisco, CA, USA

Department of Anatomy, University of California San Francisco, San Francisco, CA, USA
e-mail: Maurice.Garcia@csmc.edu

© Springer Nature Switzerland AG 2021
D. Nikolavsky, S. A. Blakely (eds.), *Urological Care for the Transgender Patient*,
https://doi.org/10.1007/978-3-030-18533-6_2

Masculinizing Genital Gender Affirming Surgery

Transgender men and patients who identify as gender non-binary who seek masculinizing genital gender affirming surgery have a wide variety of surgical options.

For the purposes of initiating the process of review and discussion of options, the discussion can perhaps most easily be framed around the two phallus options patients can choose from: *metoidioplasty* – creation of a "small penis" using the patient's own *current* penis (the virilized clitoris) [7–9], or alternatively, *phalloplasty* – creation of a *full (adult)-sized* penis using skin harvested from elsewhere on the patient's body (forearm: radial artery forearm free flap phalloplasty (RAP); anterior thigh: anterior lateral thigh (ALT) pedicle or free flap phalloplasty; groin or suprapubic skin: groin or suprapubic (SP) pedicle flaps) [3, 10–14]. Both of these options include, separately, the option to undergo urethral lengthening, such that the patient can void from the tip of their penis [11, 15–17]. We emphasize to patients that the principal source of complications related to masculinizing surgery is associated with urethral lengthening (urethral strictures and their sequelae including fistulae, obstructive lower urinary tract symptoms) and the relatively high risk for need for additional future surgeries and interventions associated with choice for urethral lengthening [18–23].

Both metoidioplasty and phalloplasty *can* be combined with additional gender affirming surgical procedures, including urethral lengthening, vaginectomy, creation of a scrotum, and implant of testicle prostheses [3, 14].

Both options can also be performed with the option to preserve the uterus and vaginal canal. Patients who elect preservation of the vaginal canal should be advised that, while it is possible to undergo urethral lengthening *with* preservation of the vaginal canal, doing so is associated with a significantly higher rate of urethral related complications (neo-urethral stricture and fistulae) [24].

Only phalloplasty affords the option to achieve erection by implant of an erectile device [3].

Metoidioplasty has the following potential *advantages and disadvantages* [3].

Advantages include the following:

1. Creation of a penis of normal shape and appearance.
2. Maximal preservation of erogenous sensation localized to their phallus.
3. Absence of a non-local surgical donor site scar (such as for the skin flaps needed to create the phallus or urethral lengthening with phalloplasty).
4. Decreased to no risk of loss of phallus viability, in contrast to phalloplasty, where part or all of the phallus can potentially become nonviable if blood supply is compromised.
5. Patients who undergo metoidioplasty *can* undergo *phalloplasty* later if they wish.

Disadvantages include the following:

1. Phallus length that is below the mean length of an adult male phallus – a metoidioplasty phallus typically has a dorsal length of only 2–5 cm.
2. Lack of commercially available implantable penile prosthetic devices to allow rigid erection .

Phalloplasty has the following potential *advantages and disadvantages* [3]:

Advantages include the following:

1. Affords creation of a phallus whose dimensions and appearance are more in alignment with a cis-gender adult penis.
2. Erogenous sensation of a phallus made from either a radial-artery forearm flap or an anterior lateral thigh flap (ALT) *can* be achieved.
3. Erection is possible after implant of a penile prosthesis (inflatable 2 or 3-piece penile prosthesis or malleable penile prosthesis).
4. It is possible to *eliminate the visibility* of the native clitoris while preserving its function to yield erogenous sensation capable of producing orgasm. The clitoris glans and shaft are de-epithelized and then transposed to the base of the phallus, thereby preserving the

erogenous sensation of the clitoris while eliminating the clitoris from view.

5. Glansplasty of the distal phallus affords the appearance of a natural glans shape.
6. Testicle and penile prosthetics are an option with any phalloplasty approach.

Disadvantages include the following:

1. Phalloplasty, in comparison to metoidioplasty, is a more extensive, and thereby potentially morbid, surgery.
2. Presence of a scar at the tissue donor site and the possibility of decreased function of the donor site. The most common concern patients who consider phalloplasty report is the presence of a donor site scar and fear of losing or developing limited function at their donor site, particularly of the arm with RAP. Many patients also report concern that scarring at the donor site reveals that they have undergone phalloplasty.
3. Risk of loss of viability of some (focal necrosis) or all of the phalluses, resulting in compromised cosmesis and/or function.

Choice for Phalloplasty Donor Site

In our experience, the radial artery forearm flap is superior to the ALT and suprapubic and groin skin donor sites for the following reasons:

1. Suprapubic and groin-flap donor sites do not yield flaps that have sensory innervation along the shaft of the phallus [25].
2. The *sensory innervation* of the arm is, anatomically, more extensive than for the skin of the anterior lateral thigh. The medial and lateral antebrachial cutaneous nerves of the forearm provide sensory innervation to all areas of the flap, and when these nerve ends are anastomosed to the proximal end of the clitoral nerve, the result is erogenous sensation to the phallus that is on average *superior to what*, in our experience, is achieved with an ALT flap. The sensory innervation of an ALT flap is based on the *lateral femoral cutaneous* nerve, which can vary in size and location (and hence the nerve itself may not be included within the flap, which would preclude anastomosis to the clitoral nerve to achieve erogenous sensory sensation directly from the flap's sensory nerves) [3, 25].

3. A radial artery forearm flap yields a flap whose final tubularized girth is generally 10–12 cm. This size is height/size appropriate for an average man. With an ALT flap, it is often a challenge to make the final flap girth *less than* 13–15 cm *maximum* because the thickness of an ALT flap is significantly greater than the thickness of a radial artery forearm flap. During surgery, it is clear that an ALT flap will yield an overly thick phallus; the surgeon is faced with the decision to either attempt to thin the flap (i.e., cut away excess adipose tissue within Scarpa's fascia, which risks injury to important perforator vessels and, if interrupted, results in loss of viability of some or all of the flap) or, to proceed and then risk the patient being dissatisfied with the resulting excess girth. As Isaacson et al. reported previously [26, 27], phallus girth greater than 13–15 cm is likely to cause discomfort with insertion into the receptive partner (Fig. 2.1).
4. Anatomic variability of the vessels and nerves is much more constant and their location/anatomy is more reliable with a forearm flap as compared to an ALT flap. The net *number of* perforator vessels and the exact location of their take off from the femoral vessels, which the ALT flap depends on, can vary. Such variability makes it possible that at the time of surgery, it may not be possible to utilize the ALT flap. Alternatively, if the perforator vessels of an ALT flap are located aberrantly, it may be necessary to alter the location of the flap on the patient's thigh, which necessitates that a larger-than-needed area of the anterior thigh be permanently cleared of hair growth in anticipation of possibly needing to relocate the flap harvest site. This is not a challenge faced with radial artery forearm flaps.

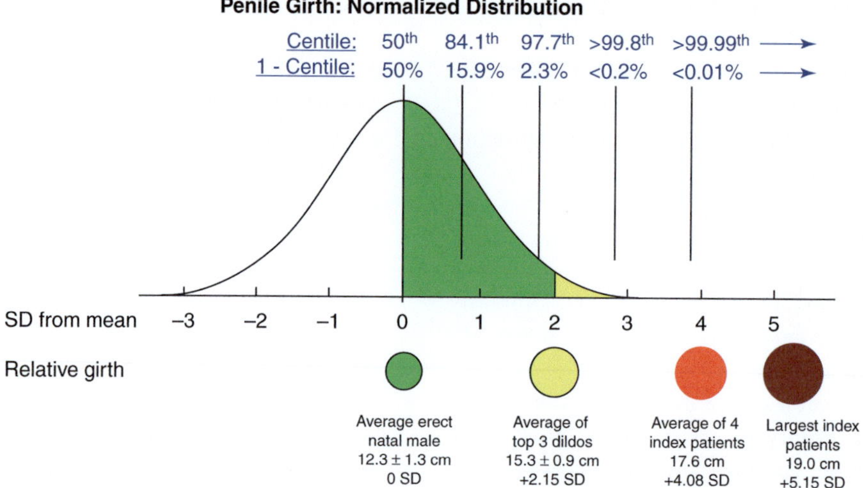

Fig. 2.1 Graphic showing data from *How big is too big? The girth of bestselling insertive sex toys to guide maximal neophallus dimensions*, by Isaacson & Garcia et al (*Journal of Sexual Medicine*, Vol. 14, Issue 11, November 2014). In this work, we compared the mean girth of four index patients who had undergone phalloplasty at an outside hospital, and complained that their phallus girth exceeded what they could insert into their partners during intercourse. This work sought to estimate the upper limit of acceptable penis girth by using the girth of the largest best-selling dildos as a proxy. The average erect penis girth among adult men of all ages was reported to be 12.3 cm, while the average girth of the three largest topselling dildos was found by our group to be 15.1 cm. (± 0.9 cm) (equals +2.15 standard deviations (SD), which is >95% of all men). The mean girth of the four index patients in this series was 17.6 cm, which is just over 4 SD. We concluded that to help ensure that a phallus a surgeon creates is insertable into patient's partners, final phallus length should likely not exceed 13–15 cm

Phallus Length

Decision-making related to phallus length is very important, as the desired length of the phallus defines the final length of the urethral and phallus portions of the flap, and satisfaction regarding the final dimensions of the phallus is an important driver of overall satisfaction [2, 28]. Effective management of patient expectations in this context is especially important.

Desired Length and Appearance

Beginning during discussions in clinic, we suggest that patients consider what phallus length they desire. We explain that the average *erect* penile length for cis-gender men is 12.89 ± 2.91 cm (i.e., 5.01 inches) [29], while flaccid mean flaccid length is only 8.85 ± 2.38 cm (i.e., ~3.5 inches), which is significantly shorter. We also address a common assumption by patients that if they undergo insertion of an erectile device, their phallus will become longer and thicker: it will not [28]. Hence, the length that the patient ultimately chooses will be the length that their phallus exists in continuously. We suggest that patients consider day to day comfort when choosing what size phallus to request. We encourage patients to initiate discussion about phallus size goals with their surgeon, as well to ensure not only that the end result is as close to their goal as is feasible and safe but also to help ensure that it is not significantly longer or shorter than they desire.

Desired Length and Surgical Outcomes

Other phallus size-related considerations include *excess* length risks compromising perfusion to the distal and proximal ends of the phallus (as these areas are furthest from the pedicle's vessels).

Desired Length and Future Penile Prosthesis Placement

An excessively long phallus will be especially *heavy* and that excess weight could possibly cause it to migrate more posteriorly on the patient's pelvis, resulting in an overly posteriorly located phallus, which can result in discomfort and can make implant of the penile prosthesis technically challenging [2].

Decision-Making Aids

We *show* patients penis models of 3.5–6 inches to help them consider which length they most prefer in light of all of the aforementioned considerations. Use of penis models in clinic is especially useful, as many patients have reported to us that, for example, 5 ¼ inches when viewed as a penis model is substantially "larger appearing" than when considered using just a ruler, where proportional width and girth are not visualized.

Erogenous Sensation

Erogenous sensation of a phallus made from either a radial-artery forearm flap *or* an anterior lateral thigh flap (ALT) *can* be achieved by one or both of the following two methods [3, 10, 11, 28]: (1) the sensory nerves of the flap (medial and lateral antebrachial cutaneous nerves of the radial artery forearm flap and the lateral femoral cutaneous nerves of the ALT flap) will be anastomosed to the proximal transected end of one of the two clitoral nerves (2) the sensory nerve distribution of the *lateral* antebrachial cutaneous nerve will be corresponded to the portion of the flap that is destined to be the phallus *shaft* skin, whereas the portion of the flap innervated by the *medial* antebrachial cutaneous nerve is destined to be the *urethra* portion of the phallus (Fig. 2.2) and (3) transposition of the native clitoris glans and shaft to a sub-cutaneous location at the ventral base of the phallus, where the clitoral structures can be easily stimulated with either masturbation or with insertive intercourse. Previous work by our group found that patients who underwent transposition of the clitoris to the base of the phallus reported *no decrease* in sensation from the native clitoris at its new location [28]. By these two strategies, it is possible for patients who have undergone phalloplasty to achieve orgasm from their penis with insertive intercourse.

Genitourinary Prosthetics

Decision-making about genitourinary (GU) prosthetics is important because complications regarding these are especially morbid [2, 23, 30]. The most feared adverse event regarding prosthetics is infection of the prosthetic, which invariably requires explant of the prosthetic. Salvage surgeries, wherein a new, sterile device is used, are *not* recommended, as the host tissue prosthesis site does not have compartmentalized anatomy that might otherwise help protect the device from collaterally located infection (e.g., a neophallus does not have the tunica-defined compartment of the corpora cavernosa as in a cis-gender penis or the protective tunica and dartos layers of a cis-gender scrotum). Also, in a phallus, there is no anatomic barrier from the neourethra, which means that any fistula or local infection stemming from the urinary tract risks infection of the penile prosthesis [2, 3, 30].

Furthermore, the tissues of a neophallus or neoscrotum are not as well perfused (and thereby protected by the immune system or presumably by systemic antibiotics) as a cis-gender penis.

Testicle Prosthesis Size

We advise patients to elect implant of testicle prostheses of a size *small enough* that allows for a competent three-layer wound closure. Not uncommonly, the neoscrotum is not sufficiently capacious to allow for implant of one or two large-size (20 cc) testicle prostheses. In such cases, we advise implant of the largest testicle prosthesis that will *easily* fit, with a plan to

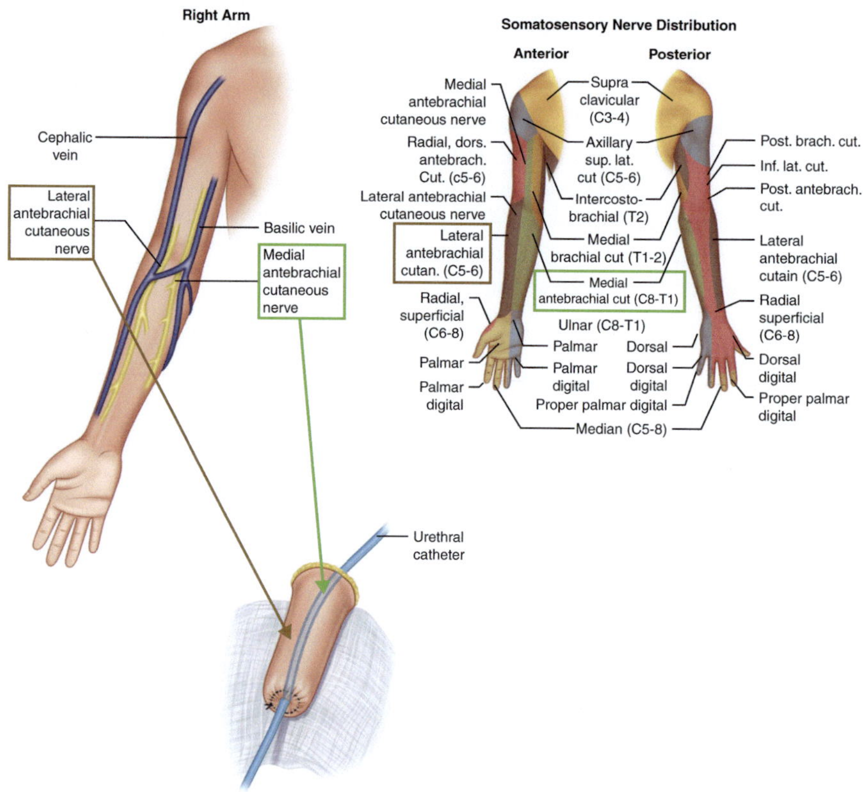

Fig. 2.2 (*Top-left*) Tactile and erogenous sensation of the phallus are achieved by anastomosing the sensory nerves from the radial artery forearm flap (medial and lateral antebrachial cutaneous nerves) to one of the two clitoral nerves. Only one clitoral nerve (in our practice, the clitoral nerve ipsilateral to the phallus deep inferior epigastric artery/veins vascular pedicle) is dissected and *partially* transected so that the flaps' sensory nerves can be anastomosed to the proximal end of the clitoral nerve in an end-to-side anastomosis using three single 9-0 nylon sutures. (*Top-right*) The *medial antebrachial cutaneous nerve* provides sensory innervation to the skin of the ventral medial forearm (green), which will be used to construct the neo-urethra. The *lateral antebrachial cutaneous nerve* provides sensory innervation to the forearm skin of the ventral lateral (and dorsal) forearm, which will constitute the phallus shaft skin. (*Bottom figure*) Ultimately, the *medial antebrachial cutaneous nerve* provides tactile and erogenous sensation to the neo-urethra, while the *lateral antebrachial cutaneous nerve* provides tactile and erogenous sensation to the phallus shaft and glans (i.e., all externally located flap skin)

allow the operative site to heal adequately before upsizing the testicle prostheses (typically at least 3–4 months later) with larger testicle prosthesis [2].

Inflatable Penile Prosthesis Type and Size

Current penile prosthesis options for transgender men are limited to devices designed and manufactured for cis-gender male anatomy. These include inflatable penile prosthesis (IPP) devices (2-piece and 3-piece devices) and malleable devices.

Regardless of what penile prosthesis type is used, any implanted penile prosthesis must be anchored to the patient's body to prevent the device from migrating and eroding through the walls of the phallus or into the neourethra [23, 30, 31]. We use inflatable devices exclusively (almost always only *single* cylinder) and we anchor the cylinder to the anteromedial aspect of the obturator ramus (just medial and posterior to the insertion of the *adductor longus* tendon) by securing the proximal end of the cylinder within a Dacron "boot" and then suturing this boot to the flat surface of the bone of the obturator ramus using non-absorbable Ethibond suture or bone screws connected to non-absorbable monofilament suture.

We believe that use of inflatable penile prostheses is superior to use of malleable devices and affords better clinical long-term outcomes. This is so for two important reasons [2, 3]:

1. An inflatable device is in the flaccid state (which means that majority of the time the device remains inside the patient), is softer, and occupies significantly less volume than a malleable cylinder, thereby reducing local pressure-related ischemic necrosis of the adipose tissue that comprises nearly all of the interior of the phallus. With semi-rigid malleable devices, any position that the patient assumes in the awake or sleeping state compresses the phallus tissues against the cylinder, thereby accelerating ischemic pressure necrosis of the interior of the phallus. Over time such ischemic necrosis results in a flabby phallus. The more "flabby" the phallus is, the less tissue support there is for the cylinder, and, therefore, the more likely it is that the end of the semi-rigid cylinder will erode through the (typically distal end) phallus.
2. However, a malleable penile prosthesis is anchored to the patient's body, and the net vector force of the device *onto* the phallus is directed to the dorsal aspect of the phallus. This, combined with the fact that the phallus "hangs" on the penile prosthesis cylinder, results in *increased risk of erosion of the cylinder* through the *dorsal aspect* of the phallus, most especially where the tip of the cylinder is located – at the distal end of the phallus.

Number of Cylinders

Penile prosthesis placement in a cis-gender penis always includes implant of two cylinders into the interior of each corpora cavernosa, which is defined and enveloped by the thick tunica of the corpora, which not only eliminate lateral-wise movement and sheer-stress of the device but also serve to protect the urethra from the cylinders by excluding the dorsally located cylinders from the ventrally located urethra. With any neophallus, the interior of the phallus has *no* internal compartments, and the cylinder will directly abut the somewhat centrally located neourethra and its pedicle. Unless the girth of a phallus is especially great, there is relatively little room for two cylinders, and implant of two cylinders risks impingement of the cylinders upon the urethra and its vascular pedicle. Furthermore, the presence of two cylinders versus one amplifies the effect of phallus adipose tissue ischemic necrosis as described above.

We have found that use of a single inflatable cylinder yields sufficient on-demand rigidity to afford penetration while minimizing risk of injury/compression to the urethra and adipose tissue necrosis-related loss of girth/fullness.

Feminizing Genital Gender Affirming Surgery

Vaginoplasty

With *vaginoplasty* surgery, a female vulva (the *medical* term for the external female genitalia) is created by a combination of removal of male structures (testes, penile shaft and penile urethra, a majority of the glans penis, and nearly all of the scrotum) and reconstruction of the residual genital tissues to create the key structures of a vulva and vagina.

Vaginoplasty surgery can be offered either *with creation of a vaginal canal* (to afford vaginal-receptive intercourse, referred to as *"full depth vaginoplasty"* / *"vaginoplasty with a vaginal canal"*) or ***without*** a vaginal canal (which *we* term *shallow-depth vaginoplasty* and also sometimes referred to as *"zero-depth vaginoplasty," "vaginoplasty without canal,"* and *"vulvoplasty"*) [14].

Vaginoplasty with creation of a vaginal canal *absolutely requires* that the patient regularly perform vaginal dilation and douching on a regular basis for variable duration in order to maintain patency and hygiene of the vaginal canal. Unfortunately, there is no evidence-based data to guide recommendations for *how long* and *how frequently* patients should dilate and douche. Interruption of the vaginal dilation regimen likely significantly increases the risk of vaginal stenosis and loss of vaginal function. This is also especially so during the first 1–2 years postsurgery. If vaginal stenosis occurs, it may result in the inability to engage in vaginal-receptive intercourse and severe stenosis may also result in retention of vaginal epithelial discharge (dead skin cell debris, sweat, skin oils, and other debris colonized with bacteria). When local infection develops, it results in inflammation, pain, foul discharge, and foul smell [3]. It is certainly possible that the stenosis may *not* always result in the aforementioned symptoms, but it is our opinion that this is likely the exception rather than the rule. In our experience, cessation of dilation is more likely to result in stenosis sufficient to cause infection and pain when it occurs during the first 1–2 years after surgery.

Patients should be discouraged from deciding to undergo creation of a vaginal canal based on the assumption that they have the option, whenever they wish, to simply stop dilation and douching activities, without consequence. Rather, patients should be encouraged to proceed with the creation of a vaginal canal *only* if they feel that they can commit to the dilation and douching schedule that their surgeon recommends. We relay that they should consider this a lifelong process [2]. During the decision-making process it is helpful for the surgeon to provide clear information about what vaginoplasty with, and vaginoplasty without creation of a vaginal canal requires re. post-operative care and maintenance. In our experience, the patients most likely to cease dilating their vaginal canal regularly are those that did not anticipate using it for intercourse even before surgery.

Weighing the Relative Advantages and Disadvantages Associated with a Vaginal Canal

Both full-depth and shallow-depth options should *always* be reviewed when discussing surgery options, as each has important potential advantages and disadvantages depending on the patient's needs with respect to the following five important domains:

1. *Option to have vaginal-receptive intercourse.* For patients who are or who plan to be sexually active and engage in vaginal-receptive intercourse (with men *or* women), a vaginal canal is necessary. For patients whose partners are exclusively female, having a vaginal canal *may* play a less important role with sexual intimacy, though this cannot be assumed and should be discussed with each patient. Some patients, regardless of their sexuality preferences, may find it very unlikely that they will be sexually active after genital surgery (e.g., personal preference, lack of partner, advancing age) and, therefore, have no reason to maintaining a vaginal canal that they will not use.

2. *Ability and commitment to perform vaginal dilation and douching.* Some patients may have physical limitations (e.g., obesity, limited neck and back range of motion, neuromuscular disorders that compromise manual dexterity, and blindness) that prevent them from being able to perform vaginal dilation and douching. Other patients may not be able to commit to being sufficiently *reliable* to perform essential vaginal dilation and douching tasks on a regular basis. Mental health conditions that may render a patient unable to care for themselves can also limit a patient's ability to perform dilation and douching.

3. *Access to necessary supplies (vaginal dilators and a douche) and a safe environment in which to perform vaginal dilation and douching.* Patients with very marginal income may not be able to afford (or replace) their essential self-care supplies (vaginal dilators and douche kit). Patients who are marginally housed or homeless will not be able to reliably perform vaginal dilation and douching tasks owing to lack of space (douching should ideally be done in a tub, in a recumbent or supine position) or a safe and private environment in which to perform these activities. Patients who are incarcerated or institutionalized are

especially vulnerable to these challenges, as they may not be given access to the necessary supplies and/or environment.

4. *Tolerance for risk of complications*: Vaginoplasty *with* creation of a vaginal canal is associated with a larger number of potential complications, and thereby higher overall risk of postoperative complications, as compared to vaginoplasty without creation of a vaginal canal. For example, creation of a vaginal canal carries the added risk of a rectal and/or urethral injury during creation of the vaginal canal space. A vaginal canal is subject to risk of prolapse, loss of viability of the epithelial lining of the canal, stenosis (loss of canal girth and depth), granulation tissue, pain associated with dilation, and infection. Management of these complications almost always necessitates close contact with, ideally, the surgeon who performed the surgery or another surgeon with vaginoplasty surgery experience, and, at a minimum, a provider with specialized knowledge about care and management of post-vaginoplasty complications – to provide care to the patient in the event that they suffer such complications.

   For some patients, *access to care* in the event of complications may be a mitigating factor in their decision to elect to undergo creation of a vaginal canal. Access to care can be a limiting factor based on availability of providers close to where the patient lives, affordability of care, and/or transportation to providers. Incarcerated or institutionalized patients, and patients who live especially far from comprehensive healthcare services, are especially vulnerable to these limitations.

   Some patients may simply have a lower (or higher) "risk-tolerance" than others and make their decision regarding surgery options without due consideration of the nature of the risks. A thorough discussion about perioperative and postoperative risks is helpful to patients to decide what surgery options best suit their expectations, abilities, resources, and risk-tolerance [2].

5. *Perceptions of appearance of the vagina and the importance of a vaginal canal:* Patients who elect vaginoplasty *without* creation of a vaginal canal (what we refer to as "shallow-depth vaginoplasty") can be divided into two groups: (1) those who are familiar with this surgical option, have had time to consider it, and are confident that this is the most suitable option for them, and (2) patients who have never heard of this option, but who, during surgery discussion, find that it could well meet their needs. In other words, patients often "do not know what they do not know," and simply learning about shallow-depth vaginoplasty and the requirements associated with full-depth vaginoplasty makes it easy for them to choose the best option for themselves. For these reasons, we believe that all patients should be offered vaginoplasty with and without canal.

Underlying reasons for why many patients choose shallow-depth vaginoplasty and to forego creation of a vaginal canal include the following: no plan to be sexually active (at all or specifically with vaginal-receptive intercourse) after surgery; no interest in intercourse with men (e.g., partners are exclusively female), vaginal-receptive intercourse is not sufficiently "important" for them to warrant the lifelong commitment to dilation and douching, physical inability to perform dilation (e.g., limited manual dexterity, back pain that precludes arching back to insert the dilators), and simply finding the need to dilate/douche too burdensome to do reliably.

General Concerns Related to Feminizing gGAS that Many Patients Share

Some of our patients who present for vaginoplasty (with or without creation of a vaginal canal) have the following three concerns:

1. To be "correct" or "real," their vagina should have a particular appearance. Patients considering vaginoplasty *without* creation of a vaginal canal have also reported struggling with doubts about:

2. Whether the absence of a vaginal canal will be visible and obvious to others.

3. Whether or not a vagina without a canal is a "real vagina," and therefore within the context of the *gender affirming* nature of their surgery, whether a vagina without a canal would make them less "female."

Development of a Feminizing gGAS Discussion Aid

We developed a teaching/discussion aid to use with patients when discussing the options of vaginoplasty *with* and *without* a vaginal canal (Fig. 2.3) [32]. This teaching aid speaks to 3 common concerns that patients considering vaginoplasty without creation of a vaginal canal might struggle with.

In this figure we show a panel of 40 plaster casts of cis-gender women's vaginas. These casts are from a series of 400 plaster casts made by a UK artist Jamie McCartney (https://jamiemccartney.com/portfolio/the-great-wall-of-vagina/).

The *first* of the three common concerns patients sometimes struggle with concerns is the feeling that their vagina must look a certain way to be "normal". This concern is addressed by explaining to patients that all vaginas are different from one another in appearance and that no two are identical. In our experience, the majority of patients mostly want anatomy that is *normal*. We emphasize that *normal* is a *spectrum* and that therefore there is no "gold standard" appearance for a vagina. Anyone used to seeing vaginas knows that each different one will be at a minimum slightly different from the next. Labia, for example, may be *more* or *less* prominent from person to person, and while both are well within the spectrum of normal, we explain that with vaginoplasty the final appearance of the vagina is, to a large degree, a function of what tissues are available locally for the construction of the vagina. Hence, for example, exaggerated long and thin pendulous labia, as

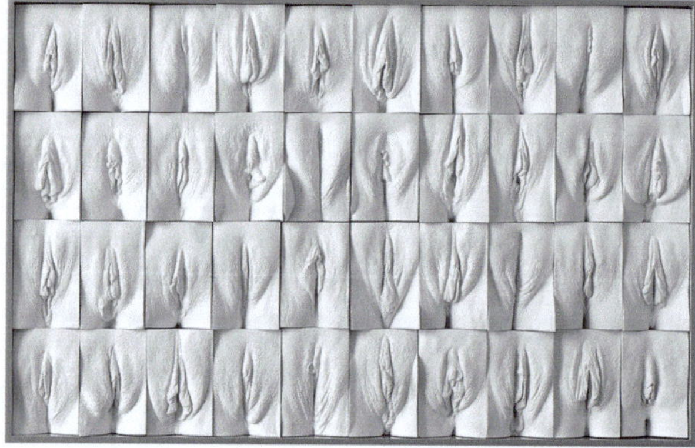

Forty plaster casts of cisgender women's vaginas. This is one panel from a series of 400 casts titled "The Great Wall of Vagina," a sculpture by UK artist Jamie McCartney

1. **All vaginas are different** → No gold standard. All vaginas are different; *normal* is a wide spectrum
2. **Limited tissue available for reconstruction** → Less prominent Labia are part of spectrum of normal
3. **The vaginal canal (and a vagina's depth) are <u>not</u> visible** → With or without a canal, we still call what we see a "*vagina*"
4. **Reminder to use patient-centered, normative language, when possible** → Though the correct medical term for what we see is "vulva", most people (including the artist) refer to what is shown above as a "*vagina*"

Fig. 2.3 Vaginoplasty: Pre-surgery teaching and discussion aid. (1) *All vaginas are different* → no gold standard. All vaginas are different; *normal* is a wide spectrum. (2) *Limited tissue available for reconstruction* → less prominent labia are part of spectrum of normal. (3) *The vaginal canal (and a vagina's depth) are not visible* → with or without a canal, we still call what we see a "*vagina*." (4) *Reminder to use patient-centered, normative language, when possible* → though the correct medical term for what we see is "vulva," lay-people (like the artist and most of our patients) refer to what we see above as a "*vagina*." (Forty plaster casts of cisgender women's vaginas. This is one panel from a series of 400 casts titled "The Great Wall of Vagina," a sculpture by UK artist Jamie McCartney)

some women have, are not possible to create (as tissues similar to this are not already present in this region of the patient's body), but their labia will instead be *less* exaggerated (labia majora less pendulous and labia minora slightly more fold-like) – but these features too are entirely *normal*.

The *second* of these concerns is that a vagina without a vaginal canal will look abnormal, and that other people will easily be able to tell if the patient either doesnt have a vaginal canal, or that they lack an especially deep vaginal canal. These concerns are addressed by explaining that the vaginal canal of any vagina is **never** visible by external view. A close look at the plaster casts of vaginas shown in Fig. 2.3 confirms that the vaginal canal is never visible by external view. It follows too that vaginal depth is not visible either.

The *third* of these concerns is that a vagina without a vaginal canal is "not a real vagina". We address this concern by *asking patients a series of questions* exactly as described below [32]. We start by asking the patient what word/term they use for what each of the casts displays in Fig. 2.3 shows. (In order to not bias patients, we do not show them the title of the artwork; we show them only the image of the plaster casts). Most patients refer to what is shown in Fig. 2.3 as "vaginas." Then, we ask patients whether or not they can *see* the vaginal canal in any of the casts (correct answer is no). We ask whether they can tell which vagina has the longer or shorter vaginal canal (correct answer is no). When patients respond that they cannot see the canal or tell how deep it is, we emphasize that because the canal is not visible, whether or not there is a vaginal canal does not determine whether what is shown is or is not a "vagina". What we see is still clearly a "vagina." We also point out that the artist who made the artwork also referred to them as "vaginas".

Decision-Making and Vaginal Depth

Patients who elect vaginoplasty *with* creation of a vaginal canal must have a suitable source of epithelium-lined tissue to line the canal. The depth of the vaginal canal space itself is generally not a limiting factor to achieve satisfactory depth, as the space can (barring an anatomic abnormality) be dissected to achieve a canal of up to ~6.5–7 inches.

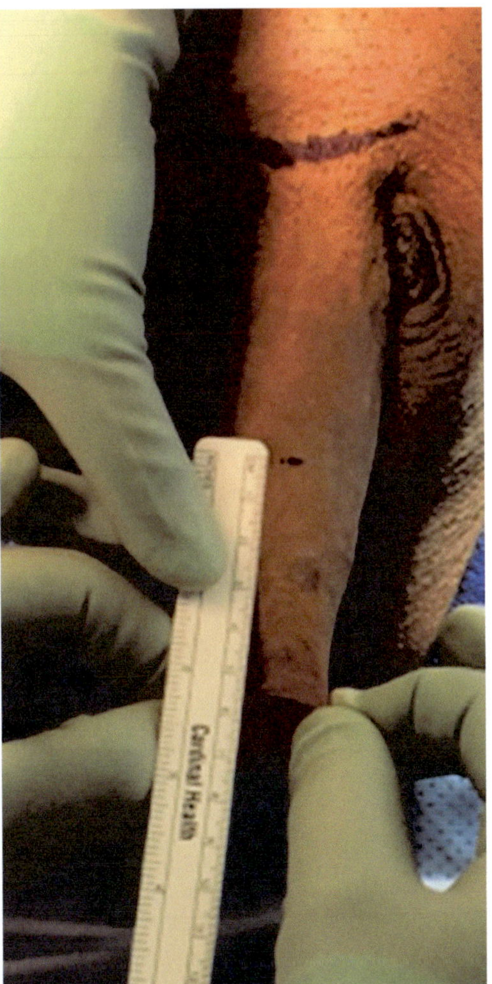

Fig. 2.4 The skin of the penile shaft, including the foreskin, is left intact in a tube-shape, and the distal end of the skin tube is over-sewn and then *inverted* so that, upon delivery into the vaginal canal space, the skin surface of the tube faces inward. This tube of penile shaft skin is a pedicle flap because it remains intact at what previously corresponded to the base of the penile shaft

For patients who are uncircumcised *and* have healthy penile skin[1], this generally poses little challenge because with the *penile inversion* technique (Fig. 2.4), the uncircumcised penis almost

---

[1] Penile foreskin that is tight owing to phimosis, or which is of poor quality due to chronic inflammation, is often unusable for use to line the vaginal canal space. In such cases, the surgeon should explain to the patient that, in order to achieve satisfactory vaginal depth, the surgeon will likely need to harvest skin or other epithelium from an additional source to line the vaginal canal (e.g., full-thickness or pedicled scrotal skin grafts or peritoneal local advancement or rotational flaps) and achieve satisfactory vaginal depth.

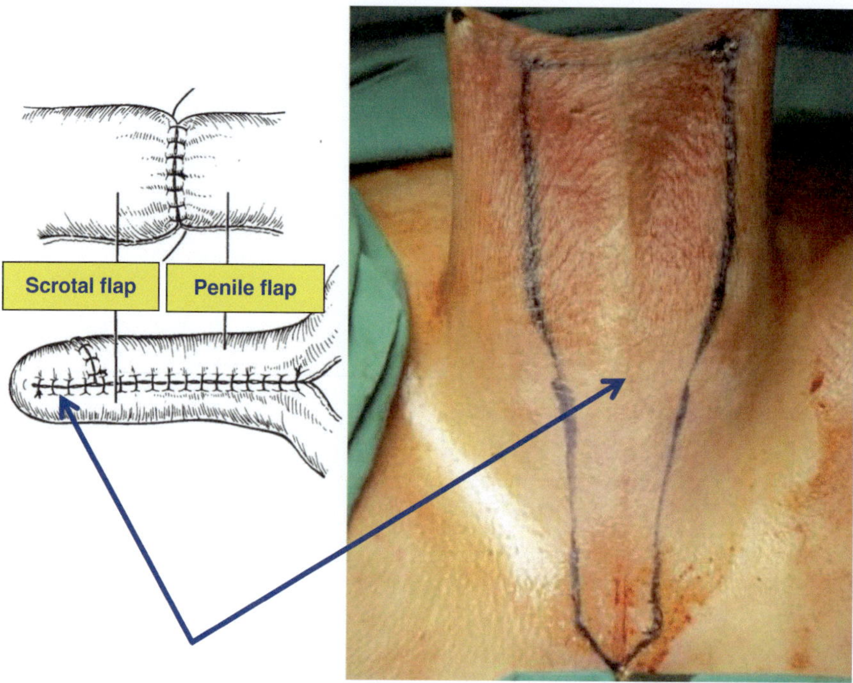

Fig. 2.5 The pedicle segment of scrotal skin will be anastomosed to the intact penile shaft skin (tube). The scrotal segment will comprise the ventral aspect of the vaginal canal skin lining, in addition to a portion of the dorsal aspect of the canal

always provides sufficient skin with which to create vaginal depth of at least 5 inches, as the intact foreskin yields a tubular-shaped segment of skin longer than the penis itself.

For circumcised patients, however, creation of a vaginal canal will absolutely require *augmentation* of the intact segment of tube-shaped penile skin with skin from elsewhere on the body. It is our experience that, after penile shaft skin, *scrotal skin* is the *next best* source of skin for lining the vaginal canal.

Scrotal skin can be used as a free pedicle flap (Fig. 2.5) *or* a free full-thickness (free) skin graft (Fig. 2.6). The scrotum often yields a segment of skin that is about 19–22 cm long and 10–14 cm wide.

A favorable feature of a scrotal skin pedicle flap is that it has a pedicle of tissue that supplies blood to it, which makes its viability more reliable than a skin *graft*. Despite this, a challenge with using a pedicle scrotal skin graft is that if the penile skin tube is especially short, the scrotal skin pedicle flap must be especially long in order to yield sufficient vaginal depth. This is because, when the penile skin portion is short, the pedicle flap must comprise not only the ventral aspect of the vaginal canal lining but also a portion of the dorsal aspect of the vaginal canal lining. Unless the scrotal skin is especially long and pendulous, the length of the pedicled scrotal skin flap may be insufficient. In such cases, use of scrotal skin as a *full-thickness free skin graft* is the next best option. For this, skin from the entire scrotum is harvested, defatted on the back table to the level of dermis, and sutured into a tube shape which is then sutured to the distal end of the native penile skin tube.

When scrotal skin is used as a *full-thickness skin graft* there is almost always sufficient to yield

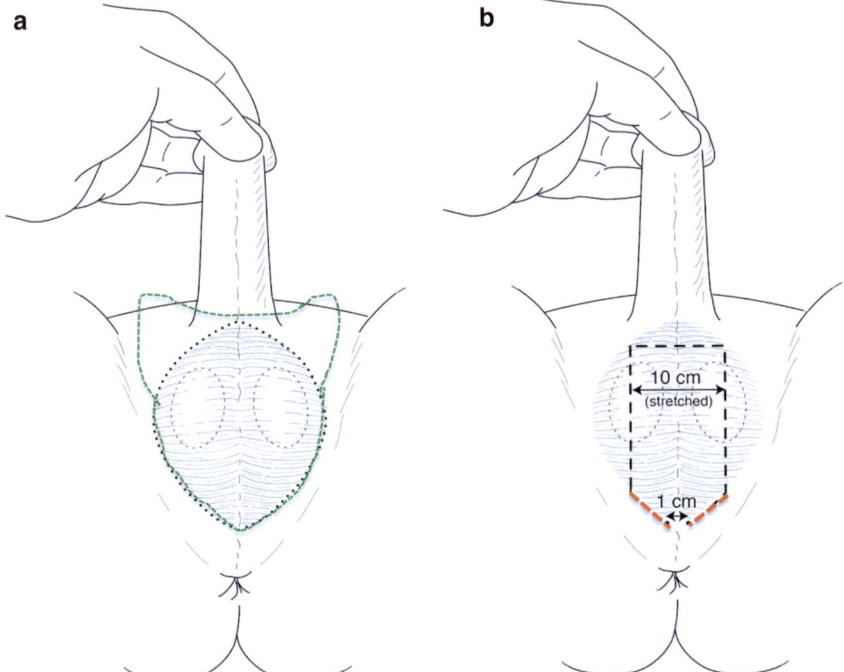

Fig. 2.6 Scrotal skin can be harvested as a free (full thickness) skin graft (**a**), using either only some of the scrotal skin (*black hatched line*), or the graft area can be extended anteriorly to immediately lateral to the base of the penis (*green hatched line*). When used as a free graft, the deep surface of the scrotal skin graft must be de-fatted to the level of dermis to optimize likelihood of graft "take." Alternatively, a midline segment of scrotal skin can be harvested as a pedicle flap (**b**); the skin is incised along the dotted lines shown, but remains ***intact*** at its ~1 cm-wide base (*orange hatched lines*). The blood supply to the pedicle flap reaches the flap via this ~1 cm-wide base that remains intact. When scrotal skin is used as a pedicle flap, its deep surface is not de-fatted, as it carries the skin's blood supply. The scrotal skin flap will comprise the *posterior* aspect of the vaginal canal lining, whereas the de-tubularized penile shaft-skin flap will comprise the *anterior* face of the vaginal canal lining. For this reason, either flap need be only 6–10 cm wide

vaginal depth of 5–7 inches. It is important, to explain to patients that use of full-thickness scrotal skin grafts (versus a pedicle scrotal skin flap) carries an increased and non-zero risk that the scrotal skin graft portion could not "take" and ultimately sloughed-off. (The relative risks for flap loss among pedicle flap and free scrotal skin grafts is not well defined in the literature.)

Discussion with patients about surgical options should always include the *choice* of whether or not to pursue alternative surgical options to garner additional skin to line the vaginal canal and augment vaginal depth. Discussion should include the surgeon's estimation of the added risks associated with use of scrotal skin grafts .

Conclusions

The decision-making process with gGAS should be individualized, patient-centered, and comprehensive. Choice of surgery is a delicate balance of form, function, and risk considerations. A review of all surgical options is essential. The decision-making process is highly nuanced for both patient and surgeon. The patient's needs, concerns, and limitations must be ascertained by the surgeon, while the patient must be helped to understand their options, all risks associated with each option, and what outcomes are reasonable (and not reasonable) to expect. Management of expectations is a key driver of short- and long-term patient satisfaction with outcomes and with their surgeon.

Take-Home Points

1. Patients can have not only very different sexual practices, but they can also have different needs regarding sexual function and gGAS. It is incumbent on the surgeon to understand what these needs are, and highlight how they may or may not be met by different gGAS options.
2. Patients do not know what they do not know about gGAS. Alternatively, some may believe that they are well informed about a specific surgery or what options exist, but their knowledge base may in fact be lacking. Therefore, it is in the patient's interest for the surgeon to cover and contrast all options whenever possible.
3. Each and every surgical option has different advantages and disadvantages, with respect to surgical morbidity and surgical risks (short and long term), the functionality it offers, cosmesis, what other surgical options it can or cannot be combined with, and self-care requirements.
4. Specific surgical options can make possible, or preclude, additional surgical options.
5. Surgeons be able to knowledgably discuss all surgical options with patients, and refer the patient to another surgeon who offers options that they themselves do not offer.

References

1. Coleman E, Bockting W, Botzer M, et al. Standards of care for the health of transsexual, transgender, and gender-nonconforming people, version 7. Int J Transgender. 2012;13(4):165–232.
2. Garcia MM. Men's health and transgender surgery: a urologist's perspective. Transl Androl Urol. 2016;5(2):225–7.
3. Garcia MM, Christopher NA, Thomas P, Ralph DJ. AUA updates series lesson 5: genital gender affirming surgeries for transgender patient. AUA Updates. 2017.
4. Bockting W, Coleman E, De Cuypere G. Care of transsexual persons. N Engl J Med. 2011;364(26):2559–60; author reply 2560
5. Bockting WO, Knudson G, Goldberg JM. Counseling and mental health care for transgender adults and loved ones. Int J Transgender. 2006;9:35–82.
6. Gardner IS, Joshua D. Progress on the road to better medical care for transgender patients. Curr Opin Endocrinol Diabet Obes. 2013;20(6):553–8.
7. Djordjevic ML, Stanojevic D, Bizic M, et al. Metoidioplasty as a single stage sex reassignment surgery in female transsexuals: Belgrade experience. J Sex Med. 2009;6(5):1306–13.
8. Djordjevic ML, Stojanovic B, Bizic M. Metoidioplasty: techniques and outcomes. Transl Androl Urol. 2019;8(3):248–53.
9. Lin-Brande M, Clennon E, Sajadi KP, Djordjevic ML, Dy GW, Dugi D. Metoidioplasty with urethral lengthening: a stepwise approach. Urology. 2020;S0090–4295(20)31152–3. https://doi.org/10.1016/j.urology.2020.09.013.
10. Garaffa G, Christopher NA, Ralph DJ. Total phallic reconstruction in female-to-male transsexuals. Eur Urol. 2010;57(4):715–22.
11. Monstrey S, Hoebeke P, Selvaggi G, et al. Penile reconstruction: is the radial forearm flap really the standard technique? Plast Reconstr Surg. 2009;124(2):510–8.
12. Monstrey SJ, Ceulemans P, Hoebeke P. Sex reassignment surgery in the female-to-male transsexual. Semin Plast Surg. 2011;25(3):229–44.
13. Rubino C, Figus A, Dessy LA, et al. Innervated island pedicled anterolateral thigh flap for neo-phallic reconstruction in female-to-male transsexuals. J Plast Reconstr Aesthet Surg. 2009;62(3):e45–9.
14. Chen ML, Reyblat P, Poh MM, Chi AC. Overview of surgical techniques in gender-affirming genital surgery. Transl Androl Urol. 2019;8(3):191–208.
15. Djordjevic ML, Bizic M, Stanojevic D, et al. Urethral lengthening in metoidioplasty (female-to-male sex reassignment surgery) by combined buccal mucosa graft and labia minora flap. Urology. 2009;74(2):349–53.
16. Djordjevic ML, Bizic MR. Comparison of two different methods for urethral lengthening in female to male (metoidioplasty) surgery. J Sex Med. 2013;10(5):1431–8.
17. van der Sluis WB, Smit JM, Pigot GLS, et al. Double flap phalloplasty in transgender men: surgical technique and outcome of pedicled anterolateral thigh flap phalloplasty combined with radial forearm free flap urethral reconstruction. Microsurgery. 2017;37(8):917–23.
18. Nikolavsky D, Hughes M, Zhao LC. Urologic complications after phalloplasty or metoidioplasty. Clin Plast Surg. 2018;45(3):425–35.
19. Neuville P, Morel-Journel N, Maucourt-Boulch D, Ruffion A, Paparel P, Terrier JE. Surgical outcomes of erectile implants after phalloplasty:

retrospective analysis of 95 procedures. J Sex Med. 2016;13(11):1758–64.

20. Santucci RA. Urethral complications after transgender phalloplasty: strategies to treat them and minimize their occurrence. Clin Anat. 2018;31(2):187–90.

21. Esmonde N, Bluebond-Langner R, Berli JU. Phalloplasty flap-related complication. Clin Plast Surg. 2018;45(3):415–24.

22. Hoebeke P, Selvaggi G, Ceulemans P, et al. Impact of sex reassignment surgery on lower urinary tract function. Eur Urol. 2005;47(3):398–402.

23. Hoebeke PB, Decaestecker K, Beysens M, Opdenakker Y, Lumen N, Monstrey SM. Erectile implants in female-to-male transsexuals: our experience in 129 patients. Eur Urol. 2010;57(2):334–40.

24. Al-Tamimi M, Pigot GL, van der Sluis WB, et al. Colpectomy significantly reduces the risk of urethral fistula formation after urethral lengthening in transgender men undergoing genital gender affirming surgery. J Urol. 2018;200(6):1315–22.

25. Garcia MCN, Thomas P, Ralph D. Genital gender affirming surgery for transgender patients. American Urologic Association. 2017; AUA Update Series 2017.

26. Isaacson D, Aghili R, Wongwittavas N, Garcia M. How big is too big? The girth of bestselling insertive sex toys to guide maximal neophallus dimensions. J Sex Med. 2017;14(11):1455–61.

27. Garcia MM. Decision-making challenges for patients and surgeons regarding genital gender affirming surgery. In: Nikolavsky D, Blakely SA, editors. Urological care for the transgender patient. Switzerland: Springer Nature; 2020.

28. Garcia MM, Christopher NA, De Luca F, Spilotros M, Ralph DJ. Overall satisfaction, sexual function, and the durability of neophallus dimensions following staged female to male genital gender confirming surgery: the Institute of Urology, London U.K. experience. Transl Androl Urol. 2014;3(2):156–62.

29. Wessells H, Lue TF, McAninch JW. Penile length in the flaccid and erect states: guidelines for penile augmentation. J Urol. 1996;156(3):995–7.

30. Falcone M, Garaffa G, Gillo A, Dente D, Christopher AN, Ralph DJ. Outcomes of inflatable penile prosthesis insertion in 247 patients completing female to male gender reassignment surgery. BJU Int. 2018;121(1):139–44.

31. Pigot GLS, Al-Tamimi M, Ronkes B, et al. Surgical outcomes of neoscrotal augmentation with testicular prostheses in transgender men. J Sex Med. 2019;16(10):1664–71.

32. Garcia MM. Sexual function after shallow and full-depth vaginoplasty: challenges, clinical findings, and treatment strategies – urologic perspectives. Clin Plast Surg. 2018;45(3):437–46.

Endocrinological Care for Patients Undergoing Gender Affirmation (Including Risk of Thromboembolic Events)

Lei Lei Min and Rachel Hopkins

Abbreviations

DHT	Dihydrotestosterone
DSM	Diagnostic and Statistical Manual of Mental Disorders
EE	Ethinyl estradiol
GD	Gender dysphoria
GnRH	Gonadotrophin-releasing hormone
Hct	Hematocrit
HDL	High-density lipoprotein
ICD	International Classification of Disease
LDL	Low-density lipoprotein
QoL	Quality of life
VTE	Venous thromboembolism
WPATH	World Professional Association for Transgender Health

Introduction to the Role of Hormonal Therapy

Transgender hormone therapy (also called cross-sex hormone therapy) is a form of hormonal therapy in which the administration of exogenous sex hormones is used to induce secondary sex characteristics consistent with self-identified gender while suppressing endogenous hormone levels.

L. L. Min · R. Hopkins (✉)
SUNY Upstate Medical University, Department of Medicine, Division of Endocrinology,
Syracuse, NY, USA
e-mail: hopkinra@upstate.edu

In transgender women, this is often called feminizing hormone therapy; in transgender men, masculinizing or virilizing hormone therapy is a common term. Gender dysphoria (GD) refers to distress caused by a conflict between a person's assigned gender and experienced gender. Hormone therapy may be part of treatment aimed at reducing negative symptoms of GD. Many transgender people who undergo hormone therapy desire or proceed with gender affirmation surgery. Some are satisfied with the physical and mental health changes achieved through hormone therapy alone, although it is unclear at this time what percentage of transgender people fall into that category. A large national survey of transgender and gender-nonconforming people found that 35% of transgender men did not want to undergo phalloplasty while 12% of transgender women were not interested in having vaginoplasty or labiaplasty [1]. It is not clear in the report whether these respondents were satisfied with hormone transition alone or had other reasons for not wanting the surgeries. It is also important to note that many people encounter barriers to obtaining surgery [1].

The decision to proceed with hormone therapy is first and foremost an individual choice made by the transgender person. The provision of medical care for transgender persons has been improved over the years by the availability of guidelines from both the World Professional Association for Transgender

© Springer Nature Switzerland AG 2021
D. Nikolavsky, S. A. Blakely (eds.), *Urological Care for the Transgender Patient*,
https://doi.org/10.1007/978-3-030-18533-6_3

Box 3.1 Criteria for Gender-Affirming Hormone Therapy for Adults

1. Persistent, well-documented gender dysphoria.
2. Capacity to make a fully informed decision and to consent for treatment.
3. Age of majority in a given country (if younger, follow the standards of care (SOC) for children and adolescents).
4. If significant medical or mental concerns are present, they must be reasonably well controlled.

Reference: WPATH [1]

Box 3.2 ICD-10 Criteria for Transsexualism

Transsexualism (F64.0) has three criteria:

1. The desire to live and be accepted as a member of the opposite sex, usually accompanied by the wish to make his or her body as congruent as possible with the preferred sex through surgery and hormone treatments.
2. The transsexual identity has been present persistently for at least 2 years.
3. The disorder is not a symptom of another mental disorder or a genetic, DSD, or chromosomal abnormality.

Health (WPATH) and more recently by the Endocrine Society [2, 3].

Transgender hormone therapy requires the use of prescription medications and should be administered under the supervision of an experienced licensed medical provider. Recommended criteria to be met prior to initiation of hormone therapy in adults include persistent symptoms of gender dysphoria, capacity to make informed decisions and give informed consent, and reasonable control of any mental health comorbidities (Box 3.1).

Many prescribing medical providers require a statement or a "letter" from a qualified mental health provider (MHP) confirming the diagnosis of GD before initiation of hormone therapy. The MHP also assists in evaluating the transgender person's readiness to undergo hormonal transition and can help confirm that any comorbid mental health issues are reasonably stable [4, 5]. Some specialized transgender clinics in the United States use an "informed consent" model that does not require evaluation by a mental health professional prior to initiation of hormone therapy. This model requires experienced non-mental health providers who are comfortable making a diagnosis of GD and evaluating for a capacity to provide an informed consent. In both routes to supervised hormone therapy, the clinician should assess and diagnose GD by using the most current criteria of the Diagnostic and Statistical Manual of Mental Disorders V (DSM-V) [6] or International Classification of Disease-10 (ICD 10) as described in Box 3.2.

Not all transgender patients desire gender-affirming surgeries, but many who desire surgery have not had access to it. In the large national US survey mentioned previously, 55% of respondents who sought insurance coverage for transition-related surgery were denied such coverage [1]. In the United States, as compared to Europe, fewer patients have had access to surgical interventions, and therefore, many have remained on hormone therapy without undergoing these procedures. Therefore, it is important to look at the quality of life (QoL) in those who have hormonal therapy alone. The existing literature has generally found a positive patient-reported response to hormone therapy and a positive impact on QoL (social, emotional, and mental). Two European studies reported that transgender patients on hormone therapy experience improvements in psychological functioning such as reduction in depression, somatization, interpersonal sensitivity, anxiety, phobic anxiety, and hostility after initiation of hormone therapy [7, 8]. Improvement in general QoL has been identified in hormone-treated transgender populations [9]. In a cross-sectional study, transgender patients on hormone therapy had a higher mental health score (79.4 vs 73.4, $P = 0.02$) and general health score (79.4 vs 69.5, $P = 0.001$) compared with non-hormone-treated individuals [10]. A recent systematic review reported an overall positive effect of hormone therapy on psychological functioning but noted a lack of prospective controlled trials investigating this area [11]. Since it might not be ethically feasible to conduct placebo-controlled studies in this setting, it may be necessary to rely on uncontrolled studies.

Hormone Therapy for Transgender Women

The goal of feminizing hormone therapy is to induce female secondary sex characteristics and suppress male secondary sex characteristics. This is usually achieved through a combination of estrogen and anti-androgen therapy. The goal is to maintain serum estrogen and testosterone levels in the normal physiologic range established for assigned female at birth (AFAB) people. Combination therapy allows for the use of a lower dose of estrogen, thus minimizing its side effects, and is more effective than estrogen therapy alone in suppressing testosterone [12–16].

Hormone therapy should be initiated and adjusted according to the individual's gender transition goals and the presence of underlying medical conditions. Availability and cost of specific medications may also affect therapy choices.

Estrogens

Several routes of administration for estrogens are available as shown in Table 3.1. There are no good comparison studies to determine the best form of estrogen to be used in transgender care, so the choice among these is based on patient preference, cost, and safety profile. Variations in safety among the routes of administration will be discussed in the section on risks of therapy. For reasons that will be discussed below, it is recommended that ethinyl estradiol (EE) not be used for the treatment of transgender women. There is also concern about the safety of conjugated equine estrogens; therefore, these preparations are used much less often.

Injectable estradiol valerate and cypionate are long-acting estrogens that are less frequently used in transgender women. Our empirical experience is that use of injectable estrogens results in wide variability in serum estradiol levels that can

Table 3.1 Hormone regimens in transgender females

Medications[a]	Dosage
Estrogen	
Oral: estradiol	2.0–6.0 mg/d
Transdermal: estradiol transdermal patch (new patch placed every 3–5 days)	0.025–0.2 mg/d
Parenteral: estradiol valerate or cypionate	5–30 mg IM every 2weeks 2–10 mg IM every week
Anti-androgens	
Spironolactone	100–300 mg/d
Cyproterone acetate[b]	25–50 mg/d
GnRH agonist	3.75 mg SQ (SC) monthly 11.25 mg SQ (SC) 3-monthly

Reference: Endocrine treatment of gender-dysphoric/gender-incongruent persons: an endocrine society clinical practice guideline [2]

Abbreviations: *IM* intramuscularly, *SQ* sequentially, *SC* subcutaneously

[a]Estrogens used with or without anti-androgens or GnRH agonist

[b]Not available in the United States

make monitoring difficult. Although there is no evidence that this variability actually increases risk, caution must be used to avoid supraphysiologic doses when using injectable estradiol.

Estrogen therapy is contraindicated in patients with prior history of venous thromboembolism (VTE) with an underlying hypercoagulable state (unless patients are on lifelong anticoagulation therapy), estrogen-sensitive neoplasm, and chronic liver disease.

Anti-androgens

Anti-androgen therapy is used to inhibit androgen secretion or to block its action on the peripheral tissue, thereby suppressing male secondary sex characteristics. Spironolactone, an androgen receptor antagonist, is the most commonly used and most affordable anti-androgen in the United States. It suppresses testosterone synthesis by inhibiting steroidogenesis and blocks the action of testosterone at the receptor level [17]. Since spironolactone is also a potent antimineralocorticoid, the main concern with the use of spironolactone is hyperkalemia.

In some cases, serum testosterone levels are resistant to suppression despite the combination of estrogen and anti-androgen. In such circumstances, GnRH agonists can be used with a low incidence of side effects [18]. They suppress gonadotrophin secretion resulting in decreased testosterone production. The drawback of these medications is high cost, and as a result, they are rarely used in the adult transgender population in the United States.

In patients who are not able to tolerate or have contraindication to spironolactone, the less potent anti-androgens finasteride or dutasteride might be considered. Their anti-androgenic effect is via inhibition of 5-alpha reductase, an enzyme responsible for the conversion of testosterone to dihydrotestosterone (DHT). DHT is the more potent androgen required for many aspects of virilization in males. Finasteride can be used in the dose of 1–5 mg per day, and dutasteride can be used at 0.5 mg per day.

Cyproterone acetate, a progestogen with strong anti-androgen activity, is commonly used in Europe but is not available in the United States.

Progesterone and Progestins

Some clinicians use progesterone or progestins with the aim of augmenting breast development and improving mood and libido [19]. This approach is not supported by current evidence and theoretically questionable, but a recent published literature review concluded that the overall low quality of available studies prevents a definitive recommendation in this area [20]. In our clinical experience, most patients do well without addition of progesterone or progestins to their regimen, but some patients have subjective positive responses to these agents. Medroxyprogesterone and micronized progesterone are the agents most often used for this purpose.

Expected Effects of Feminizing Hormone Therapy

Physical changes that are expected to occur with feminizing hormone therapy and the usual time course are outlined in Table 3.2. Many changes, including redistribution of body fat, decreased spontaneous erections, decreased muscle mass, skin softening, decreased oiliness, and decreased sexual desire, are usually seen within the first few months of therapy. Signs of breast development are seen within 3–6 months of initiation of hormonal therapy, and breasts reach maximum development after 2–3 years of treatment. This expected timeline can inform plans for breast augmentation surgery. It is important to note that virilized vocal cords do not change with feminizing hormone therapy and many patients pursue

Table 3.2 Feminizing effects in transgender females

Effect	Onset	Maximum
Redistribution of body fat	3–6 months	2–3 years
Decrease in muscle mass and strength	3–6 months	1–2 years
Softening of the skin/decreased oiliness	3–6 months	Unknown
Decreased sexual desire	1–3 months	3–6 months
Decreased spontaneous erections	1–3 months	3–6 months
Male sexual dysfunction	Variable	Variable
Breast growth	3–6 months	2–3 years
Decreased testicular volume	3–6 months	2–3 years
Decreased sperm production	Unknown	>3 years
Decreased terminal hair growth	6–12 months	>3 years (a)
Scalp hair	Variable	(b)
Voice changes	None	(c)

Reference: Endocrine treatment of gender-dysphoric/gender-incongruent persons: an endocrine society clinical practice guideline [2]

(a) Complete removal of male sexual hair requires electrolysis or laser treatment or both

(b) Familial scalp hair loss may occur if estrogens are stopped

(c) Treatment by speech pathologist for voice training is more effective

additional training with a speech therapist to achieve a more feminine voice.

Risks of Feminizing Hormone Therapy

Venous Thromboembolism

There are no randomized prospective studies available on the risk of VTE in transgender females on estrogen. There are some established and theoretical differences in the level of risk among the available forms and routes of administration of estrogen [21]. Oral estrogen preparations have the highest risk of VTE and are thought to induce more thrombogenic effect compared with non-oral preparation due to the "first pass" effect of liver metabolism [22].

Several retrospective studies have provided insight into the risk of VTE in transgender women. An early study showed a 45-fold increase in VTE (incidence: 6.3%, 142/10,000 user years) compared to a population reference group [23, 24]. The transgender women in this study population were almost all being treated with oral EE and cyproterone acetate, and the risk of VTE was markedly higher in those women over the age of 40 [23]. Following the publication of this study in 1989, the use of EE in feminizing hormone therapy decreased significantly. A larger 1997 study (an extension of the 1989 study using the same clinic population) included data from transgender women on EE but also transgender women on several other forms of estrogen and found a lower VTE incidence of 5.5% (58/10,000 user years) [24, 25] but still a 20-fold increase in transgender women using EE compared to the general cisgender male population. In that study, only one VTE event was found in patients using transdermal estradiol [25]. A more recent cross-sectional study by Wierckx et al. found an incidence of VTE of 5.1% [26]. This study looked at a European population in which most patients were using cyproterone acetate as their anti-androgen [26]. Close examination of those who suffered VTE showed that several patients were smokers,

had undergone periods of prolonged immobilization, or had underlying clotting disorders.

Among anti-androgens, cyproterone acetate may increase the risk of VTE compared to other agents. There is some evidence for a thrombogenic effect of this medication. A case-control study of men with prostate cancer showed that VTE risk in patients on cyproterone acetate was significantly higher than those who were on LHRH analogue or who had had an orchidectomy (adjusted odd ratio 5.23, 95% CI 3.12–8.79), although cofounding effect of disease severity may have been present [27]. A systematic review and meta-analysis found that combined oral contraceptives (COCs) containing cyproterone acetate carried a higher risk of VTE than COCs containing lower-risk progestogens [28].

A 2013 review of the topic of VTE in transgender women concluded that the prevalence and incidence of VTE in transgender women have decreased over the past several decades and attributes this decrease to the cessation of EE use and improved perioperative thrombosis prophylaxis [24]. A recent study looking at patients on a regimen more typically used in the United States – oral estradiol and spironolactone – showed a very low incidence of VTE (7.8 events per 10,000 patient-years). It is especially notable that this population included patients with risk factors for VTE including smoking and obesity [29].

Transdermal estrogen appears to be safer in terms of VTE risk especially in patients over 40 years old. In a phase II study of 24 men with prostate cancer, homeostatic factors did not change with the application of transdermal estrogen (0.6 mg per 24 hours) [30]. A meta-analysis of postmenopausal women showed a pooled risk ratio of VTE was 1.9 with oral estrogen and 1.0 with transdermal estrogen [31]. A retrospective study indicated that use of transdermal hormone has a low risk of VTE even when combined with cyproterone acetate. In the 162 transgender women studied, none of the patients developed VTE during a mean of 52.5 months of follow-up despite the fact that 8% were also found to have thrombophilic defects [32].

In previous studies, the incidence of VTE has been highest in the first year of treatment and decreased after that [23, 24, 25]. However in a large 2018 cohort study done within one health system in the United States, the overall incidence rate for VTE was 5.5% in transgender women, but the higher incidence was seen only after 2 years on treatment and continued to rise for several years after that [33]. The reason for this discrepancy is unclear and needs to be investigated further.

Taken in total, the above information indicates that there is most likely some increased risk of VTE in any patient taking exogenous estradiol at the relatively high doses used for gender affirmation. The exact risk on regimens currently used in the United States is unknown and likely lower than indicated by earlier European studies. The safest regimens seem to be those using either transdermal estradiol or oral estradiol, and it is likely that use of spironolactone as an antiandrogen reduces the risk compared to use of cyproterone acetate.

Cardiovascular Disease

Studies have indicated an increased risk of cardiovascular disease in transgender females compared with cisgender females and comparable to that of cisgender males [26, 39]. This is surprising because the incidence of cardiovascular disease is known to be higher in cisgender men compared to cisgender women until the age of 75 years when the risk for women increases. This risk differential has been attributed at least in part to the hormonal milieu and specifically to a protective effect of higher estrogen in cisgender women.

Data on the impact of feminizing therapy on cardiovascular risk factors have not adequately explained the increased cardiovascular risk. Studies have shown increased triglyceride levels in hormone-treated transgender women compared to cisgender men and women but no difference in other lipid levels [34, 35]. Route of estrogen delivery does not seem to affect the impact on lipid levels when comparing oral with transdermal estrogen [36]. Elevations in both systolic and diastolic blood pressure have been found in transgender women taking cross-sex hormone therapy [37, 38].

Increased risk of cardiovascular disease has been seen in several retrospective studies. In a case-control study of 214 transgender women on various estrogen preparations, the prevalence of myocardial infarction in transgender women was significantly greater than in cisgender women (18 vs 0, $P = 0.001$) and similar to cisgender men. Additionally, in the study, transgender women had a higher prevalence of cerebrovascular events than cisgender men (23.4 vs 9.4, $P = 0.03$) but similar to cisgender women [26]. In another recent cohort study, the incidence of myocardial infarction in transgender women was higher than cisgender women (adjusted hazard ratio 1.8), but not significantly different from that of cisgender men [33]. Lastly, in another European study, transgender women aged 40–64 years had higher mortality due to ischemic heart disease (standardized mortality ratio 1.64) and stroke (standardized mortality ratio 2.11) with a median follow-up of more than 18 years [39].

Risk has been shown to increase with advancing age, current use of EE, and presence of other cardiovascular risk factors such as smoking. Because some of the above studies included transgender women who were on EE and many who smoked as well, there is still uncertainty about the risk for cardiovascular disease in transgender women on current hormone regimens with lower rates of smoking. At this point, it seems wise to exercise increased vigilance for cardiovascular disease in transgender women. Further studies are needed to explore the correlation between feminizing therapy and cardiovascular risk.

Liver and Gallstones

Estrogen therapy is known to increase the risk of gallbladder disease. A large prospective cohort study of postmenopausal women following hysterectomy found that those on hormone replacement therapy had a higher risk of gallbladder disease than those who had never been on hormones (relative risk 1.64, 95% CI 1.58–1.69). The risk was lower with transdermal therapy than oral therapy (RR 1.17, CI 1.10 to 1.24 vs 1.74, CI 1.68 to 1.80) [40]. Mild elevation of liver function tests was reported in one study of a transwomen population [25]. However, in a 2013 study of 55 transgender women with a median age of 45 years, no difference in aspartate aminotransferase and alanine aminotransferase levels among cisgender male, cisgender female, and transgender females was reported. Alkaline phosphatase levels of transgender women resembled cisgender male values [34].

Prolactin

Estrogen is a stimulant of prolactin secretion from the anterior pituitary, and hyperprolactinemia has been reported in transgender women. A few cases of prolactinomas have been reported in transgender women on estrogen therapy [41, 42], but these seem to be rare occurrences, and it is not clear whether causation can be attributed to estradiol use. Recently published data suggest no significant rise in prolactin levels when transgender women are treated with estrogen, with spironolactone as the adjunct anti-androgen as opposed to cyproterone acetate [43]. However, current guidelines still recommend annual monitoring of prolactin levels in transgender women on hormone therapy.

Prostate Cancer

Given the decreased androgen levels in transgender women, it would be expected that the rate of prostate cancer might be lower in this population than in cisgender men. However, cases of prostate cancer have been reported in transgender women on feminizing hormone therapy [25, 44, 45]. A study of 2306 orchiectomized transgender females from Amsterdam reported that the overall incidence of prostate cancer in this population is 0.04%. The incidence was higher (0.13%) in

patients who started hormonal therapy at 40 years of age or older [46]. The risk may be underestimated by decreased screening rates in the transgender population. Therefore, the Endocrine Society suggests routine screening for prostate cancer in transgender women following current guidelines for cisgender men [2].

Breast Cancer

Studies have not shown an increased risk of breast cancer in transgender women compared with the general female population. In a European study of 2307 transgender women, the estimated incidence of breast cancer in transwomen was reported to be 4.1/100,000 person-years which is lower than the expected rate for cisgender female breast cancer and comparable to rates for cisgender male breast cancer [47]. In a retrospective study of 3556 transgender women followed in the Veterans Administration healthcare system, three cases of late-stage breast cancer were found, but the risk was lower than for the general female population [48]. It is recommended that breast cancer screening follows current guidelines for cisgender women [2].

Monitoring Feminizing Hormone Therapy

Patients should be evaluated clinically every 3 months in the first year and then every 6–12 months to monitor for appropriate signs of feminization, development of adverse effects, measurement of serum hormonal level, and the patient's subjective experience of and response to changes.

During the first year of therapy, serum testosterone and estradiol level should be measured every 3 months until they reach the normal range for cisgender females (testosterone: <50 ng/dl, estradiol: 100–200 pg/ml). Serum electrolytes should be monitored every 3 months in the first year and then every 12 months thereafter when patients are on spironolactone [2].

Hormone Therapy for Transgender Men

The goal of virilizing hormone therapy is to induce male secondary sex characteristics and suppress female secondary sex characteristics. This is accomplished by administration of exogenous testosterone with a goal of maintaining serum testosterone levels in the normal physiologic range for cisgender males. Within that range, hormone therapy should be individualized based on a patient's goals and preferences and the presence of underlying medical conditions and availability and cost of medications.

Testosterone Regimens

Different preparations of testosterone are available: transdermal, parenteral, buccal, and implantable. Table 3.3 includes the most commonly used testosterone methods and doses. Oral testosterone is not recommended because of a high risk of damage to the liver. In our practice, we most commonly prescribe testosterone via subcutaneous injection, usually given once weekly at doses of 60–100 mg weekly. This is a method supported by recent studies and seems to offer less fluctuation in serum testosterone levels and less discomfort than intramuscular injections [49, 50, 51, 52].

Testosterone therapy is contraindicated in patients who are pregnant, with unstable coronary artery disease or hematocrit (Hct) > 54%.

Adjuvant Therapies

Some providers prescribe depot medroxyprogesterone or GnRH agonist therapies to achieve the cessation of menses before starting testosterone therapy. This practice is at the discretion of the provider and patient and may not be necessary as testosterone alone is often quite effective in achieving this goal.

Expected Effects of Virilizing Hormone Therapy

Physical changes that are expected to occur with testosterone therapy are outlined in Table 3.4. Many transgender men report that menstrual bleeding exacerbates dysphoria. Cessation of menses usually occurs within 1–6 months of initiation of therapy. Increased skin oiliness, beard growth, body hair growth, voice deepening, change in body habitus, weight gain, and clitoral

Table 3.3 Hormone regimens in transgender males

Medications	Dosage
Testosterone	
Parenteral: testosterone enanthate or cypionate	100–200 mg SQ (IM) every 2 weeks or SQ (SC) 50% per week
Testosterone undecanoate (a)	1000 mg every 12 weeks
Transdermal: testosterone gel 1.6% (b)	50–100 mg/d 2.5–7.5 mg/d
Testosterone transdermal patch	

Endocrine treatment of gender-dysphoric/gender-incongruent persons: an endocrine society clinical practice guideline [2]

Abbreviations: *IM* intramuscularly, *SQ* sequentially, *SC* subcutaneously

(a) One thousand milligrams initially followed by an injection at 6 weeks and then at 12 weeks intervals

(b) Avoid cutaneous transfer to other individuals

Table 3.4 Masculinizing effects in transgender males

Effects	Onset	Maximum
Skin oiliness/acne	1–6 months	1–2 years
Facial/body hair growth	6–12 months	4–5 years
Scalp hair loss	6–12 months	(a)
Increased muscle mass/strength	6–12 months	2–5 years
Fat redistribution	1–6 months	2–5 years
Cessation of menses	1–6 months	(b)
Clitoral enlargement	1–6 months	1–2 years
Vaginal atrophy	1–6 months	1–2 years
Deepening of voice	6–12 months	1–2 years

Reference: Endocrine treatment of gender-dysphoric/gender-incongruent persons: an endocrine society clinical practice guideline [2]

(a) Prevention and treatment as recommended for biological men

(b) Menorrhagia requires diagnosis and treatment by a gynecologist

enlargement are usually seen within the first 6 months of therapy and continue to develop over the next few years.

Risks of Virilizing Hormone Therapy

Polycythemia

Androgens have an erythrogenic effect [53] which is thought to be due to either direct or indirect effect on bone marrow erythropoiesis or a combination of both. Polycythemia correlates with dose and serum testosterone levels [54, 55], but not with duration of therapy in hypogonadal men who are treated with testosterone [55]. The risk is highest in the first 6 months of therapy and then plateaus. Polycythemia may be reversible with lowering of testosterone dose or withdrawal of therapy. Current guidelines for treatment of hypogonadism in cisgender males recommend discontinuation of therapy if Hct is >54%; however, no clear parameters exist for safe Hct levels in transgender males. In our practice, we generally respond to Hct levels higher than the upper limit of the normal range in our laboratory with reduction of testosterone dose followed by measurement of Hct on the lower dose. If significant erythrocytosis occurs, patients should be evaluated for contributing or causative factors such as smoking, sleep apnea, obesity hypoventilation syndrome, or hematologic disorders.

Venous Thromboembolism

Testosterone-induced VTE is thought to be due to peripheral aromatization of testosterone to estrogen which can induce a prothrombotic state. Erythrocytosis as described above is an additional risk factor for thrombogenesis.

Studies have shown mixed results on the association between testosterone therapy and risk of VTE. Although a large UK-population-based case-control study demonstrated a positive correlation of VTE with testosterone treatment in hypogonadal cisgender men [56], a recent retrospective cohort study conducted using data from the Veterans Administration database did not detect an association between testosterone use and thrombotic risk in adult cisgender men [57].

Available data from several retrospective studies show no increase in thrombotic risk in testosterone-treated transgender men [26, 32, 58, 59, 60]. The presence of thrombophilic disorders has been shown to increase the risk of VTE in cisgender men on testosterone and to increase resistance to anticoagulation therapy after a thrombotic event [61]. However, in a study looking at thrombophilia and VTE in transgender patients, no VTE was seen in 89 transgender men followed for almost 48 months despite five patients being shown to have a thrombophilic defect [32].

The Food and Drug Administration (FDA) currently requires that testosterone package inserts include a warning that the drug may increase the risk of VTE. Despite the lack of evidence for this risk in transgender men, clinicians should discuss this issue with patients and encourage patients to report any potential symptoms of VTE without delay.

Cardiovascular Risk

Testosterone therapy does seem to increase some known cardiovascular risk factors in transgender men but with some contradictory findings. A retrospective observational study of 81 transgender men (mean age of 37 years), comparing before and after initiation of testosterone therapy, found a small but statistically significant decrease in HDL, increase in LDL, decrease in blood pressure, and no significant change in triglyceride and total cholesterol levels [62]. A 2008 study looking at arterial stiffness in transgender men found higher systolic blood pressure, diastolic blood pressure, mean arterial blood pressure, total cholesterol, and triglyceride levels and increased arterial stiffness as well as lower HDL among testosterone-treated compared with non-treated transgender men [63]. In a small study of 12 transgender individuals, followed for 12 months, no significant change in mean arterial blood pressure and lipid parameters with the exception of decreased HDL was detected [64].

Available data from retrospective studies of risk in transgender hormone therapy have not shown an increased rate of cardiovascular disease or cardiovascular mortality among testosterone-treated transgender men compared with cisgender women or cisgender men [26, 33, 39, 58]. However, it is important to note that transgender male subjects in these studies have mostly been a relatively young population and data in transgender men over age 65 years are limited.

Skin and Hair

Testosterone stimulates facial and body hair. However, androgenic alopecia may develop after long periods of testosterone therapy. Acne is a common side effect as well. The severity increases during first year of treatment and declines thereafter [65] but can persist [66]. Although the former study reported that acne severity does not correlate with serum testosterone level, reduction of testosterone dose can result in improvement in symptom. If acne does not resolve or is severe, patients should be referred to a specialist for treatment.

Perioperative Hormone Management

Discontinuation of Estrogen Before Surgery

The incidence of VTE with the use of estrogen during the perioperative period is unknown. The incidence of DVT has been reported to be 0.69% in general surgery [67]. It may be higher in patients who have additional risk factors for VTE that would reasonably be considered to include those taking exogenous estrogen.

There is no consensus available regarding the exact details of the management of hormonal therapy in transgender women during the perioperative period. Little is known about the risk of perioperative estrogen therapy in transgender women. Much of the available data comes from the use of oral contraceptives and postmenopausal hormone therapy in cisgender women and is not rooted in the types or doses of estrogens commonly used in transgender women [69]. Female gender affirmation surgery is a complex and extensive procedure that requires a relatively prolonged period of immobilization. It is therefore common practice to discontinue estrogen therapy two to four weeks before surgery. Given the nature of the surgery, patients should be given appropriate DVT prophylaxis with subcutaneous heparin or enoxaparin together with sequential compression device during the perioperative period [68].

It has been suggested that in cisgender women using estrogen therapies after menopause or as birth control, transdermal estrogen may be continued during the perioperative period without VTE prophylaxis and cessation of oral estrogen therapy may not be required with an appropriate prophylactic regimen [70]. However, given the higher estrogen doses used in transgender women and the extensive nature of vaginoplasty, we do not recommend this approach until more studies are produced to support it.

Temporary discontinuation of estradiol therapy can have potential adverse effects in patients, and very little is known about the risks of short-term discontinuation of treatment. For some patients, there is a return of gender dysphoria, although this might be mitigated by anticipation of the upcoming surgery. In the relatively brief period of time recommended, it is unlikely that any significant increase in virilization would occur although there could be some recurrence of hirsutism and unwanted erections. Patients should be warned about these possible effects. Further study is required to determine the optimal management of hormone therapy in transgender women in the perioperative period.

Estrogen therapy is usually held during the postoperative period until full mobilization has been regained – usually 2–4 weeks.

Anti-androgens are generally not needed in transgender women after gonadectomy. However, in some transgender women who continue to have significant hirsutism after gonadectomy, spironolactone therapy can be reinitiated.

Discontinuation of Testosterone Before Surgery

There is no consensus regarding cessation of testosterone perioperatively. Because the risk of VTE in exogenous testosterone therapy is poorly understood or quantified, it is difficult to know whether testosterone therapy should be interrupted for surgery, and there are no studies specifically looking at this question in transgender men. A recent systematic review did not find evidence of an increased risk of VTE or other complications with exogenous testosterone therapy during the surgical period [68]. In a small study, perioperative use of low-dose testosterone injections (in children with hypospadias) was not associated with VTE events [71]. These findings raise the possibility that low-dose testosterone therapy may continue in healthy transgender men during the perioperative period. The main concern of testosterone discontinuation is that the patient may experience testosterone withdrawal symptoms. Resumption of menses is a particular concern for transgender men.

Because the quantity and quality of available data are limited and some stages of phalloplasty may involve prolonged immobilization, we consider it safest to discontinue testosterone therapy prior to these specific steps. Therapy would need to be discontinued 1–2 weeks before surgery depending on the dosing regimen. For procedures that will not require prolonged immobilization, cessation of testosterone therapy might not be necessary. Patients should receive appropriate VTE prophylaxis measures with both mechanical and pharmacological methods during the perioperative period.

If the choice is made to discontinue testosterone therapy prior to surgery, it is usually recommended that it should be held until full mobilization is regained or 1 week after surgery, whichever is earlier.

Role of DHT Cream Prior to Metoidioplasty

DHT is a metabolite of testosterone that cannot be aromatized to estradiol. It is a more powerful androgen (3–6 times greater) than testosterone due to its binding affinity to the testosterone receptor. External virilization (external male genitalia development and maturation) is mediated by the androgenic effect of DHT.

External virilization in cisgender females, illustrated by females with virilizing forms of congenital adrenal hyperplasia, is associated with high DHT levels. In female patients with these conditions, androgen receptors in genital tissues are stimulated by the elevated DHT levels causing clitoromegaly.

So far, there are no available studies examining the effects of topical DHT on clitoral growth in transgender males. However, some centers recommend using topical DHT 10%, three times daily [72] to maximize genital growth prior to and after surgery. This practice extrapolates from the available data on the treatment of children with microphallus [73].

> **Take-Home Points**
> - Hormone therapy can play an important role in gender affirmation therapy and is generally safe and effective.
> - Transgender hormone therapy has been shown to improve quality of life for transgender individuals.
> - Medical therapy for transgender females includes estrogen therapy and usually anti-androgens. The most concerning risk of this therapy is development of venous thromboembolism.
> - Medical therapy for transgender males includes testosterone therapy, the main risk of which is development of erythrocytosis.
> - It is generally recommended that estradiol therapy be stopped temporarily

before gender affirmation surgeries or other major surgical interventions.

- It is not clear whether it is necessary to hold testosterone therapy prior to surgery.
- Usual thromboprophylaxis measures are recommended for any gender-affirming surgeries that require extensive surgery and prolonged immobilization.

References

1. James SE, Herman JL, Rankin S, Keisling M, Mottet L, Anafi M. The report of the 2015 U.S. transgender survey. Washington DC: The National Center for Transgender Equality; 2016. http://www.ustranssurvey.org.
2. World Professional Association for Transgender Health (WPATH). Standards of care 7th version; 2012.
3. Hembree WC, Cohen-Kettenis PT, Gooren L, Hannema SE, Meyer WJ, Murad MH, Rosenthal SM, Safer JD, Tangpricha V, T'Sjoen GG. Endocrine treatment of gender-dysphoric/gender-incongruent persons: an endocrine society clinical practice guideline. J Clin Endocrinol Metabol. 2017;102(11):3869–903.
4. Wallien MSC, Swaab H, Cohen-Kettenis PT. Psychiatric comorbidity among children with gender identity disorder. J Am Acad Child Adolesc Psychiatry. 2007;46(10):1307–14.
5. Hepp U, Kraemer B, Schnyder U, Miller N, Delsignore A. Psychiatric comorbidity in gender identity disorder. J Psychosom Res. 2005;58(3):259–61.
6. American Psychiatric Association. Diagnostic and statistical manual of mental disorders. 5th ed. Arlington: American Psychiatric Association; 2013.
7. Colizzi M, Costa R, Todarello O. Transsexual patients' psychiatric comorbidity and positive effect of cross-sex hormonal treatment on mental health: results from a longitudinal study. Psychoneuroendocrinology. 2014;39:65–73.
8. Heylens G, Verroken C, De Cock S, T'Sjoen G, De Cuypere G. Effects of different steps in gender reassignment therapy on psychopathology: a prospective study of persons with a gender identity disorder. J Sex Med. 2014;11(1):119–26.
9. Manieri C, Castellano C, Crespi C, Di Bisceglie C, Dell'Aquila C, Gualerzi A, Molo M. Medical treatment of subjects with gender identity disorder: the experience in an Italian public health center. Int J Transgenderism. 2014;15(2):53–65.
10. Gorin-Lazard A, Baumstarck K, Boyer L, Maquigneau A, Gebleux S, Penochet JC, Pringuey D, Albarel F, Morange I, Loundou A, Berbis J, Auquier P, Lançon C, Bonierbale M. Is hormonal therapy associated with better quality of life in transsexuals? A cross-sectional study. J Sex Med. 2011;9(2):531–41.
11. White Hughto JM, Reisner SL. A systematic review of the effects of hormone therapy on psychological functioning and quality of life in transgender individuals. Transgend Health. 2016;1(1):21–31.
12. Gooren L. Hormone treatment of the adult transsexual patient. Horm Res. 2005;64(suppl 2):31–6.
13. Levy A, Crown A, Reid R. Endocrine intervention for transsexuals. Clin Endocrinol (Oxf). 2003;59:409–18.
14. Gooren LJ, Bunck MC, Giltay EJ. Long-term treatment of transsexuals with cross-sex hormones: extensive personal experience. J Clin Endocrinol Metab. 2008;93(1):19–25.
15. Moore E, Wisniewski A, Dobs A. Endocrine treatment of transsexual people: a review of treatment regimens, outcomes, and adverse effects. J Clin Endocrinol Metabol. 2003;88(8):3467–73.
16. Prior JC, Vigna YM, Watson D. Spironolactone with physiological female steroids for presurgical therapy of male-to-female transsexualism. Arch Sex Behav. 1989;18(1):49–57.
17. Corvol P, Michaud A, Menard J, Freifeld M, Mahoudeau J. Antiandrogenic effect of spirolactones: mechanism of action. Endocrinology. 1975;97(1):52–8.
18. Dittrich R, Binder H, Cupistì S, Hoffmann I, Beckmann MW, Mueller A. Endocrine treatment of male-to-female transsexuals using gonadotropin-releasing hormone agonist. Exp Clin Endocrinol Diabetes. 2005;113(10):586–92.
19. Orentreich N, Durr NP. Proceedings: mammogenesis in transsexuals. J Invest Dermatol. 1974;63(1):142–6.
20. Wierckx K, Gooren L, T'Sjoen G. Clinical review: breast development in trans women receiving cross-sex hormones. J Sex Med. 2014;11(5):1240–7.
21. Laliberté F, Dea K, Sheng Duh M, Kahler K, Rolli M, Lefebvre P. Does the route of administration for estrogen hormone therapy impact the risk of venous thromboembolism? Estradiol transdermal system versus oral estrogen-only hormone therapy. Menopause (New York, NY). 2011;18(10):1052–9.
22. Rovinski D, Ramos RB, Fighera TM, Casanova GK, Spritzer PM. Risk of venous thromboembolism events in postmenopausal women using oral versus non-oral hormone therapy: a systematic review and meta-analysis. Thromb Res. 2018;168:83–95.
23. Asscheman H, Gooren L, Eklund PLE. Mortality and morbidity in trans patients with cross-gender treatment. Metab Clin Exp. 1989;38(9):869–73.
24. Asscheman H, T'Sjoen G, Lemaire A, Mas M, Meriggiola MC, Mueller A, Kuhn A, Dhejne C, Morel-Journel N, Gooren LJ. Venous thromboembolism as a complication of cross-sex hormone

treatment of male-to-female transsexual subjects: a review. Andrologia. 2013;46(7):791–5.

25. van Kesteren PJ, Asscheman H, Megens JA, Gooren LJ. Mortality and morbidity in transsexual subjects treated with cross-sex hormones. Clin Endocrinol (Oxf). 1997;47:337–42.

26. Wierckx K, Elaut E, Declercq E, Heylens G, De Cuypere G, Taes Y, Kaufman J, T'Sjoen G. Prevalence of cardiovascular disease and cancer during cross-sex hormone therapy in a large cohort of trans persons: a case–control study. Eur J Endocrinol. 2013;169(4):471–8.

27. Seaman HE, Langley SEM, Farmer RDT, de Vries CS. Venous thromboembolism and cyproterone acetate in men with prostate cancer: a study using the General Practice Research Database. BJU Int. 2007;99(6):1398–403.

28. Dragoman M, Tepper N, Fu R, Curtis K, Chou R, Gaffield M. A systematic review and meta-analysis of venous thrombosis risk among users of combined oral contraception. Int J Gynaecol Obstet. 2018;141(3):287–94.

29. Arnold JD, Eleanor PS, Coleman ME, Goldstein DA. Incidence of venous thromboembolism in transgender women receiving oral estradiol. J Sex Med. 2016;13(11):1773–7.

30. Bland LB, Garzotto M, Deloughery TG, Ryan CW, Schuff KG, Wersinger EM, Lemmon D, Beer TM. Phase II study of transdermal estradiol in androgen-independent prostate carcinoma. Cancer. 2005;103:717–23.

31. Olié V, Canonico M, Scarabin PY. Risk of venous thrombosis with oral versus transdermal estrogen therapy among postmenopausal women. Curr Opin Hematol. 2010;17(5):457–63.

32. Ott J, Kaufmann U, Bentz EK, Huber JC, Tempfer CB. Incidence of thrombophilia and venous thrombosis in transsexuals under cross-sex hormone therapy. Fertil Steril. 2010;93(4):1267–72.

33. Getahun D, Nash R, Flanders WD, Baird TC, Becerra-Culqui TA, Cromwell L, et al. Cross-sex hormones and acute cardiovascular events in transgender persons: a cohort study. Ann Intern Med. 2018;169(4):205–13.

34. Roberts T, Kraft C, French D, Wuyang J, Wu A, Tangpricha V, Fantz CR. Interpreting laboratory results in transgender patients on hormone therapy. Am J Med. 2014;127(2):159–62.

35. Maraka S, Singh Ospina N, Rodriguez-Gutierrez R, Davidge-Pitts CJ, Nippoldt TB, Prokop LJ, Murad MH. Sex steroids and cardiovascular outcomes in transgender individuals: a systematic review and meta-analysis. J Clin Endocrinol Metab. 2017;102(11):3914–23.

36. Wilson R, Spiers A, Ewan J, Johnson P, Jenkins C, Carr S. Effects of high dose oestrogen therapy on circulating inflammatory markers. Maturitas. 2009;62(3):281–6.

37. Quiros C, Patrascioiu I, Mora M, Aranda GB, Hanzu FA, Gomez-Gil E, Godas T, Halperin I. Effect of cross-sex hormone treatment on cardiovascular risk factors in transsexual individuals. Experience in a specialized unit in Catalonia. Endocrinol Nutr. 2015;62(5):210–6.

38. Colizzi M, Costa R, Scaramuzzi F, Palumbo C, Tyropani M, Pace V, Quagliarella L, Brescia F, Natilla LC, Giuseppe L, Todarello O. Concomitant psychiatric problems and hormonal treatment induced metabolic syndrome in gender dysphoria individuals: a 2year follow-up study. J Psychosom Res. 2015;78(4):399–406.

39. Asscheman H, Giltay E, Megens J, de Ronde W, van Trotsenburg M, Gooren L. A long-term follow-up study of mortality in transsexuals receiving treatment with cross-sex hormones. Eur J Endocrinol. 2001;164(4):635–42.

40. Lui B, Beral V, Balkwill A, Green J, Sweetland S, Reeves G. Gallbladder disease and use of transdermal versus oral hormone replacement therapy in postmenopausal women: prospective cohort study. BMJ. 2008;337:a386.

41. Cunha FS, Domenice S, Camara VL, Sircili MH, Gooren LJ, Mendonca BB, Costa EM. Diagnosis of prolactinoma in two male-to-female transsexual subjects following high-dose cross-sex hormone therapy. Andrologia. 2014;47(6):680–4.

42. Bunck M, Debono M, Giltay E, Verheijen A, Diamant M, Gooren L. Autonomous prolactin secretion in two male-to-female transgender patients using conventional estrogen dosages. BMJ Case Rep. 2009;2009:bcr0220091589.

43. Bisson JR, Chan KJ, Safer JD. Prolactin levels do not rise among transgender women treated with estradiol and spironolactone. Endocr Pract. 2018;24(7):646–51.

44. Turo R, Jallad S, Prescott S, Cross W. Metastatic prostate cancer in transsexual diagnosed after three decades of estrogen therapy. Can Urol Assoc J. 2013;7(7–8):E544–6.

45. Dorff T, Shazer R, Nepomuceno E, Tucker S. Successful treatment of metastatic androgen-independent prostate carcinoma in a transsexual patient. Clin Genitourin Cancer. 2007;5(5):344–6.

46. Gooren L, Morgentaler A. A prostate cancer incidence in orchidectomised male-to-female transsexual persons treated with oestrogens. Andrologia. 2013;46(10):1156–60.

47. Gooren LJ, van Trotsenburg MA, Giltay EJ, van Diest PJ. Breast cancer development in transsexual subjects receiving cross-sex hormone treatment. J Sex Med. 2013;10(12):3129–34.

48. Brown G, Jones K. Incidence of breast cancer in a cohort of 5,135 transgender veterans. Breast Cancer Res Treat. 2015;149(1):191–8.

49. Spratt DI, Stewart II, Savage C, Craig W, Spack NP, Chandler DW, Spratt LV, Eimicke T, Olshan JS. Subcutaneous injection of testosterone is an effective and preferred alternative to intramuscular injection: demonstration in female-to-male transgender patients. J Clin Endocrinol Metab. 2017;102(7):2349–55.

50. Wilson DM, Kiang TKL, Ensom MHH. Pharmacokinetics, safety, and patient acceptability of subcutaneous versus intramuscular testosterone injection for gender-affirming therapy: a pilot study. Am J Health Syst Pharm. 2018;75:351–8.

51. McFarland J, Craig W, Clarke NJ, Spratt DI. Serum testosterone concentrations remain stable between injections in patients receiving subcutaneous testosterone. JES. 2017;1(8):1095–103.

52. Olson J, Schrager SM, Clark LF, Dunlap SL, Belzer M. subcutaneous testosterone: an effective delivery mechanism for masculinizing young transgender men. LGBT Health. 2014;1(3):165–7.

53. Shahidi NT. Androgens and erythropoiesis. N Engl J Med. 1973;289(2):72–80.

54. Coviello AD, Kaplan B, Lakshman KM, Chen T, Singh AB, Bhasin S. Effects of graded doses of testosterone on erythropoiesis in healthy young and older men. J Clin Endocrinol Metab. 2007;93(3):914–9.

55. Ip FF, di Pierro I, Brown R, Cunningham I, Handelsman D, Liu P. Trough serum testosterone predicts the development of polycythemia in hypogonadal men treated for up to 21 years with subcutaneous testosterone pellets. Eur J Endocrinol. 2010;162(2):385–90.

56. Martinez C, Suissa S, Rietbrock S, Katholing A, Freedman B, Cohen AT, Handelsman DJ. Testosterone treatment and risk of venous thromboembolism: population based case-control study. BMJ (Clinical research ed). 2016;355:i5968.

57. Sharma R, Oni OA, Chen G, Sharma M, Dawn B, Sharma R, Parashara D, Savin VJ, Barua RS, Gupta K. Association between testosterone replacement therapy and the incidence of DVT and pulmonary embolism: a retrospective cohort study of the veterans administration database. Chest. 2016;150(3):563–71.

58. Wierckx K, Mueller S, Weyers S, Caenegem EV, Roef G, Heylens G, T'Sjoen G. Long term evaluation of cross-sex hormone treatment in transsexual persons. J Sex Med. 2012;9(10):2641–51.

59. Wierckx K, Van Caenegem E, Schreiner T, Haraldsen I, Fisher A, Toye K, Kaufmann JM, T'Sjoen G. Cross-sex hormone therapy in trans persons is safe and effective at short-time follow-up: results from the European network for the investigation of gender incongruence. J Sex Med. 2014;11(8):1999–2011.

60. Schlatterer K, Yassouridis A, von Werder K, Poland D, Kemper J, Stalla GK. A follow-up study for estimating the effectiveness of a cross-gender hormone substitution therapy on transsexual patients. Arch Sex Behav. 1998;27(5):475–92.

61. Glueck CJ, Prince M, Patel N, Patel J, Shah P, Mehta N, Wang P. Thrombophilia in 67 patients with thrombotic events after starting testosterone therapy. Clin Appl Thromb Hemost. 2015;22:548–53.

62. Giltay EJ, Toorians AW, Sarabdjitsingh AR, de Vries NA, Gooren LJ. Established risk factors for coronary heart disease are unrelated to androgen-induced baldness in female-to-male transsexuals. J Endocrinol. 2004;180(1):107–12.

63. Emi Y, Adachi M, Sasaki A, Nakamura Y, Nakatsuka M. Increased arterial stiffness in female-to-male transsexuals treated with androgen. J Obstet Gynaecol Res. 2008;34(5):890–7.

64. Chandra P, Basra SS, Chen TC, Tangpricha V. Alterations in lipids and adipocyte hormones in female-to-male transsexuals. Int J Endocrinol. 2010;2010:945053.

65. Wierckx K, Van de Peer F, Verhaeghe E, Dedecker D, Van Caenegem E, Toye K, Kaufman JM, T'Sjoen G. Short- and long-term clinical skin effects of testosterone treatment in trans men. J Sex Med. 2014;11(1):222–9.

66. Turrion-Merino L, Urech-García-de-la-Vega M, Miguel-Gomez L, Harto-Castaño A, Jaen-Olasolo P. Severe acne in female-to-male transgender patients. JAMA Dermatol. 2015;151(11):1260–1.

67. Aziz F, Patel M, Ortenzi G, Reed AB. Incidence of postoperative deep venous thrombosis is higher among cardiac and vascular surgery patients as compared with general surgery patients. Ann Vasc Surg. 2015;29(4):661–9.

68. Geerts WH, Bergqvist D, Pineo GF, Heit JA, Samama CM, Lassen MR, Colwell CW. Prevention of venous thromboembolism: American College of Chest Physicians evidence-based clinical practice guidelines (8th edition). Chest. 2008;133(6 Suppl):381S–453S.

69. Boskey ER, Taghinia AH, Ganor O. Association of surgical risk with exogenous hormone use in transgender patients: a systematic review. JAMA Surg. 2019;154:159–69.

70. Chalhoub V, Staiti G, Benhamou D, Edelman P. Oral contraception and hormone replacement therapy: management of their thromboembolic risk in the perioperative period. Annales Francaises d'Anesthesie et de Reanimation. 2008;27(5):405–15.

71. Heinrich UE, Bolkenius M. Supportive testosterone treatment in surgical repair of hypospadias. Eur J Pediatr Surg. 1982;37(9):20–2.

72. Cavanaugh T, Hopwood R, Gonzalez A, Thompson J. The medical care of transgender persons. Boston: Fenway Health; 2015. p. 38.

73. Xu D, Lu L, Xi L, Cheng R, Pei Z, Bi Y, Ruan S, Luo F. Efficacy and safety of percutaneous administration of dihydrotestosterone in children of different genetic backgrounds with micropenis. J Pediatr Endocrinol Metab. 2017;30(12):1285–91.

Preoperative Preparation and Perioperative Considerations for Gender-Affirming Genital Surgery

4

Amy Penkin, Jens Berli, and Daniel Dugi

Introduction

Preparation for gender-affirming surgery requires the usual presurgical evaluation for the patient, but ideally the health system should prepare as well. In this population, with many real and perceived barriers to care [1], making the health system more respectful and accommodating on multiple levels is critical.

Providing care for individuals suffering from gender dysphoria follows principles that apply to any field of medicine. While all the general medical principles hold true, there are unique aspects of which anyone providing care for this population should be aware. Transgender health has historically not been part of the curriculum at most medical schools and very few providers were exposed to this aspect of medicine in their training. Similarly, patients not only did not have access to healthcare they needed but were often

discriminated against when accessing even basic medical care. The healthcare landscape is fortunately changing, and since around 2014, access to care for transgender patients has dramatically improved in many regions of the United States. There is, however, still a lack of trained providers, and healthcare systems are not adequately prepared to take care of the volume of patients. In this chapter, we aim to illustrate some of the challenges in gender-affirming care and how we seek to overcome them.

Understanding Patient Desires and Expectations

Patients seeking care for gender dysphoria have diverse understandings of their gender identity, which means that there is not one pathway that works for each patient. It is a multidisciplinary field that includes mental health, medicine, and surgical subspecialties. Nothing is more dramatic in its aim to align the physical body and the internal identity than surgical therapy. It is not uncommon to hear from patients that they have been waiting for this moment for many decades. Furthermore, it may be the first time they have approached healthcare in months, years, or decades. Due to historically poor access to insurance, limited coverage for gender-affirming care, and legacies of mistrust in the healthcare system, those coming in to care may be experiencing

A. Penkin
Transgender Health Program, Oregon Health &
Science University, Portland, OR, USA
e-mail: penkin@ohsu.edu

J. Berli
Division of Plastic Surgery, Oregon Health & Science
University, Portland, OR, USA
e-mail: berli@ohsu.edu

D. Dugi (✉)
Department of Urology, Oregon Health & Science
University, Portland, OR, USA
e-mail: dugi@ohsu.edu

© Springer Nature Switzerland AG 2021
D. Nikolavsky, S. A. Blakely (eds.), *Urological Care for the Transgender Patient*,
https://doi.org/10.1007/978-3-030-18533-6_4

comorbid physical or mental conditions, very low trust, and extremely high expectations. Patients frequently have stated or unstated expectations about their surgical results, such as neophallic dimensions or vulvar appearance. As in any surgical endeavor, setting realistic expectations through patient education is critical. Some people may have an unspoken or unrecognized expectation that many of their problems will be solved after having what they may see as their definitive treatment for gender dysphoria.

To properly serve our patients, we must ask them about their transition history, their goals and desires so that we can offer the appropriate and realistic options. Especially when it comes to genital surgery, there are various options and considerations that need to be explored prior to making the definitive surgical plan. Without appropriate evaluation and discussion of all options, patients may find themselves remorseful and in need of secondary, more complicated surgeries.

Patients must make multiple consequential choices as they seek surgical care. For instance, trans-masculine patient seeking genital surgery must make multiple choices about their care: do they wish to remove the vagina; do they desire to stand to void, what scars they are willing to accept, and what their goals are regarding sexual functioning. Choosing between metoidioplasty and phalloplasty, or making the multiple decisions necessary for phalloplasty, requires extensive patient education about surgical risks and trade-offs. Trans-feminine patients may choose orchiectomy alone, vaginoplasty or vulvoplasty [2] (no vaginal canal construction). Patients come in to consultation with different levels of understanding about surgical options, and guiding patient choice requires asking about individual priorities.

Patient satisfaction may also be dependent on other unknown factors. We have encountered patients who chose metoidioplasty because they wanted a less-invasive and lower-risk surgery than phalloplasty but regretted this decision because what they really desired was the ability for penetrative intercourse. Likewise, we have seen patients who were unhappy with their metoidioplasty, because they chose that option when phalloplasty was not available. Similarly, trans-feminine patients who choose vulvoplasty to avoid preoperative hair removal or are deterred by necessary vaginal dilation requirements may later have a heightened desire for a vaginal canal that may worsen their gender dysphoria. Patients may choose not to share such thoughts with us, or they may not consciously be aware of them. This makes extensive education all the more important to achieve optimal informed consent and shared decision making.

Patient Education

As in any field, patients will present within a wide range of educational backgrounds, medical literacy, and intellectual capabilities. Furthermore, patients may have ample information from peers that may not be accurate or relevant to a particular surgeon's practice. Patient education should take into account the different challenges these factors bring, as well as the challenge anyone faces in understanding complex surgical options. We feel strongly that multiple modalities in education are important to account for patients with different educational levels, as well as the difficulty in retaining a high volume of new information from a single in-person consultation. Figures. 4.1 and 4.2 detail our center's patient flow and where they may interact with our multimodal patient education (Figs. 4.1 and 4.2).

For our patients seeking vaginoplasty/vulvoplasty, we mail an extensive written information packet prior to their initial office consult and then provide this written resource again when they arrive for their visit. This packet includes an Internet link to a video-recorded session of the surgeon giving a patient education talk about the surgery. This video is an option to educate patients with limited reading ability. Also, this chance to see and hear the surgeon speak ahead of a consultation does more than just deliver factual content; it allows the patient to develop a degree of familiarity or comfort with the surgeon prior to their face-to-face meeting, which can be intimidating.

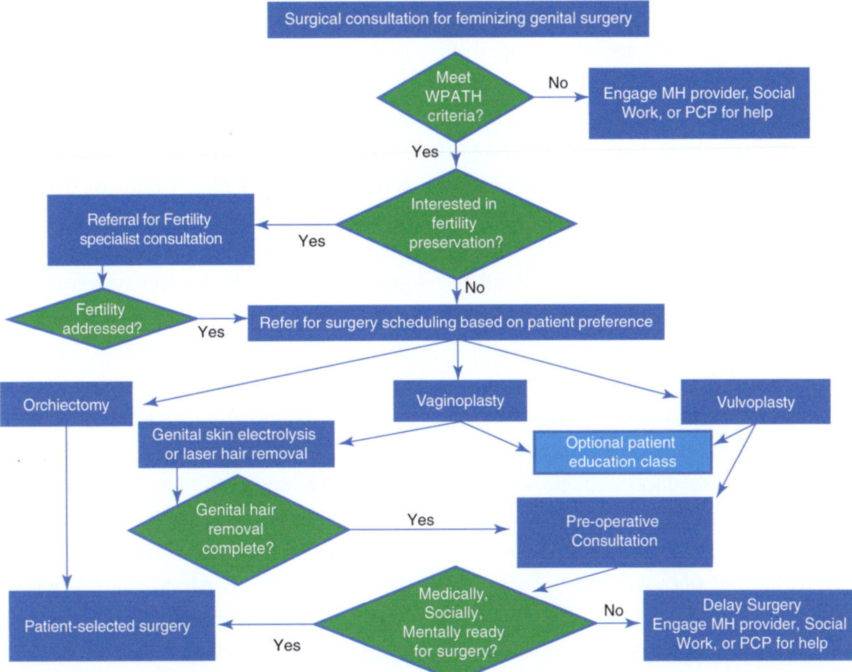

Fig. 4.1 Flowchart of patients referred for feminizing genital surgery

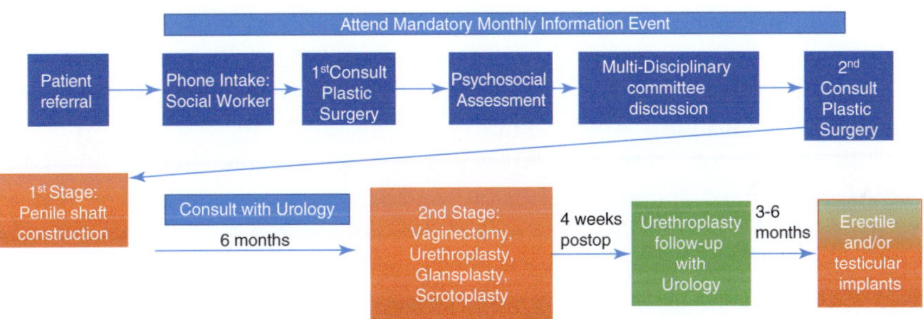

Fig. 4.2 Flowchart of patients referred for phalloplasty with urethroplasty

Prior to consultation, we encourage the patient to bring written questions, as well as their potential postsurgical caregiver, to the consultation. During the consultation, we show patients pictures of a range of surgical results, particularly of patients with different ages and body sizes, including good and less-than-ideal aesthetic results, as well as wound-healing difficulties. Each vaginoplasty/vulvoplasty and metoidioplasty consultation is 60 min long.

Patients seeking phalloplasty will be screened through an intake phone conversation to make sure they are aware of our requirements and also the versions and staging of offered procedures. This is particularly important for patients traveling from afar. The initial consultation is 60 min in length with the goal that the patient understands the offered services and surgical implications as it pertains to their anatomy and life circumstance. Mostly, patients return for a second consultation and an in-person consultation with our social worker.

One of the most important pieces of our patient education program is a monthly class specific to trans-feminine or trans-masculine genital surgery. These classes are taught by our program staff, partnering medical providers, and surgeons. Both patient and caregiver are encouraged to attend. Class registration is also extended to healthcare professionals including mental health or primary care providers who are wishing to deepen their knowledge on this topic as they care for patients seeking these surgeries. The focus of the class is to present information on optimal health and wellness (emotional and physical) for surgery, practical preparation for surgery, details of anatomy and surgery approach and technique, and what to expect during recovery and healing. Special attention is given to the role of caregiver to ensure both patient and caregiver are best prepared for what they can each expect. We often also have in attendance former patients who have been through surgery and recovery who can offer perspectives from their personal experience.

Patient Preparation for Surgery

Preparation is needed on multiple levels, including administrative, medical, psychological, and financial/social.

WPATH Letters of Support and Mental Health At the time of writing, World Professional Association for Transgender Health (WPATH) Standards of Care version 7 [3] is in use and requires patients undergoing genital surgery to have two letters in support of surgery from mental health professionals. Many patients and community members see this as an unnecessary barrier and "gatekeeping," and a step that cisgender patients undergoing surgery are rarely required to fulfill. It is the authors' belief that mental health evaluation and an ongoing relationship with a mental health provider is important for patients as they go through an inherently stressful process, and mental health support is something we should endeavor to offer all people undergoing life-changing surgery. Our program, as well as others, has looked to organ transplant programs and bariatric surgery programs as examples of surgical programs that consider mental health evaluation as a critical part of patient evaluation and preparation [4, 5].

Many patients seeking gender-affirming surgery that are young, independent, healthy, and have not experienced injury, illness, or prior surgery may be less prepared for or aware of what makes this process stressful. As such, it is important for patients to prepare for a temporary, but significant disruption to their life. For some people, asking for help and relying on caregivers can generate discomfort, while others may be socially or geographically isolated and have few resources for support available to them. We have experienced some patients minimizing the significance of these challenges in order to avoid delays in their care. Furthermore, many patients may not have experienced the physical pain or discomfort from surgery, the boredom associated with periods of strict bed rest, or the limitations in physical activity, all of which can be psychologically stressful. To further mitigate suspicions of gatekeeping, these perioperative stresses are pointed to as areas that can be well addressed in the context of a relationship with a mental health professional.

Finally, high patient expectations of aesthetic or functional results may predispose patients to be unhappy after surgery or to respond poorly to complications [6]. We have witnessed patients experience disappointment, frustration, anger, and depression when their expectations from surgery were unmet.

Medical Evaluation and Optimization Medical evaluation for gender-affirming surgery is no different than for other surgeries, with the caveat that reconstructive procedures using tissue transfer techniques inherently compromise blood supply. Optimization of the donor tissue prior to surgery is therefore of utmost importance. Anything affecting the microvascular anatomy should be addressed, that is, drugs, nicotine, diabetes. We require all patients to be nicotine-free in advance of surgery, as nicotine use is associated with poor wound healing and increased risk of flap complication or graft loss [7]. We perform urine nicotine and metabolite testing at the presurgical checkup 4 weeks prior to surgery. Likewise, we require that patients with diabetes have good management as measured by hemoglobin A1c levels less than 6.5. These requirements of nicotine cessation and diabetic control will exclude some patients from surgery [8]; however, given the importance of a good surgical outcome we believe this is justified.

Opioid and Substance Use Surgeons may need to address preoperative illicit substance use by patients, especially in the current climate of a crisis of opioid abuse in the United States. Patients who use or abuse opioids preoperative have been shown to have greater risk of complications after surgery [9]. Use of stimulants, alcohol, benzodiazepines, and other substances may also have negative implications for anesthetic management [10]. We do not routinely test for such substance use but will address it if suspected. We attempt to follow a strategy of harm reduction and help patients manage/treat their addiction with a goal of minimizing their risk after surgery. Patients taking chronic opioids prior to surgery are referred to pain management preoperatively to prepare for their postoperative care, and multimodal anesthetic and pain management efforts may help reduce the risk of opioid use or postoperative addiction [11].

Obesity Some patients will present with a body habitus too heavy to permit safe or effective surgery. With obesity, the distance between the skin and deep structures such as blood vessels increases. This is particularly an issue in phalloplasty surgery where the urethra created inside the free tissue transfer has a limited length. In metoidioplasty, the clitoris and urethra are fixed to the pubic bone, and obesity may mean even the best technical results are not visible or apparent to the patient. In vaginoplasty, obesity can make the vaginal canal dissection extremely difficult.

Many surgeons have body mass index (BMI) guidelines or cutoffs in patient selection. While published data is limited, some authors have found high BMI associated with more frequent complications after surgery [12]. BMI is only a rough guide however, as individual body fat distribution is more important than BMI measurement alone. Some patients may need to lose weight in order to be eligible for surgery, and this is often an uncomfortable conversation for the surgeon and the patient. We will sometimes schedule a surgery and provide a surgery date for patient a year or more in advance to give motivation for weight loss, then have a follow-up consult 6 months prior to surgery to check on progress with the understanding that if there is not progress in weight loss, then we may reschedule surgery. We always want to find a way to say "yes" to patients seeking gender-affirming surgery, and we have to balance the risk of complications with the harm of declining to provide an important treatment.

Social Support and Personal Preparedness Surgery and recovery requires extensive patient planning and resources. Patients will be off from work for long periods of time; we typically tell people to expect to be off from work for 6–8 weeks for vaginoplasty and 6 weeks after metoidioplasty. Phalloplasty in our center is broken into several stages, each of which has its own specific requirements and recovery period. Any genital surgery requires the patients to limit their walking since it creates friction and stress along the fresh suture lines. The importance of this cannot be overstated. Even when insurance pays for surgery, and time off from work is supported, a prolonged period without working can be a major financial stressor for patients. Patients must also prepare ahead with advanced food and household shopping, pre-purchasing recommended medical supplies (i.e., sanitary pads or gauze). We recommend that everyone undergoing gender-affirming genital surgery have at least one designated support person who can help the patient with tasks such as grocery shopping, picking up prescriptions or medical supplies, etc. In some cases, a support person may be asked to help with routine postoperative care such as drain management or even wound care. When it comes to phalloplasty, the support person may be called upon to help with genital wound care or dressing changes. We strongly recommend at least one support person attend the educational class specific to the patient's surgery and that there are backup plans for additional caregivers should the designate person not be able to fulfill all caregiving roles.

Physical Therapy Physical therapists have a role in helping patients prepare for surgery and recovery generally [13], and we have found their role to be invaluable in patients undergoing vaginoplasty. After vaginoplasty, the neovaginal canal passes through a new opening in the pelvic floor, and patients will need to perform self-dilation to prevent vaginal stenosis. Dilation may be uncomfortable for patients, and most people do not have much awareness of pelvic floor muscle function. We refer all patients to pelvic floor physical therapy (PFPT) before and after vaginoplasty, especially for education about pelvic floor relaxation to aid in dilation. We have found 40% of patients have pelvic floor dysfunction prior to surgery, and pelvic floor physical therapy before surgery can significantly reduce the rate of dysfunction after surgery [14]. PFPT is especially valuable in helping patients with the mechanics of dilation and coaching on relaxing the pelvic floor. Patients typically see PFPT before surgery and 3 weeks after surgery, about 1 week after they are taught self-dilation by the surgical team. Further PFPT follow-up is as-needed. Patients who have radial forearm phalloplasty are referred to occupational therapy for hand therapy while inpatients after phalloplasty.

Clinic and Hospital System Preparedness

Medical systems have much work to do to provide gender-affirming care. Currently, most health systems and electronic medical record (EMR) systems are poorly equipped to handle the incongruence between a person's assigned sex at birth and their affirmed gender. Evaluating a health system's skill in providing affirming care means looking at every point where a patient contacts the system, including phone calls to schedule an appointment, paperwork mailed to the

patient, signage in the waiting room, and importantly, how they are treated from clinic check-in to hospital discharge. While changing a health system or clinic's EMR, etc. can be very challenging, proper education of staff who will interact with patients is critical. Providing a truly affirming care experience requires attention to not only the tools available to the workforce, such as the medical record, but also the necessary awareness among the workforce and learners engaged in patient care of what it takes to be affirming to transgender patients.

Conceptually, this education is simple: fundamental education about gender dysphoria; the difference between gender identity, gender expression, and sexual orientation; and familiarity with use of affirmed name and pronouns. Language is important, and teaching people practical details about respectful use of language around gender diversity is critically important.

One of the most obvious goals is to always call a patient by their affirmed name and pronoun. This starts with intake forms that do not simply specify "Male or Female" but allow patients to comfortably provide their affirmed as well as legal name, and the pronouns they use. Staff should always respect these affirmed names and pronouns. But if someone makes a mistake, recognize the mistake, correct it, and move on.

Ideally, everyone should receive education in gender-affirming care and sensitivity, including those who contact the patient by telephone as well as in person. All members of the workforce interacting with the patient and their visitors should be trained including office staff, food service workers, parking attendants, pharmacy staff, nurses, everyone in the emergency department, all perioperative staff, and of course medical/surgical providers. It is important to note that even when the tools may be present to advise healthcare workers with regard to a patient's affirmed name, pronoun, or gender identity, it is the assumptions or unconscious biases at play that can lead the healthcare team member to inadvertently offend the patient by using gendered language such as Mister or Miss or Sir or

Ma'am that may correspond to the visual/verbal cues the team member perceives and interprets about the patient. For example, a trans-feminine patient with a deeper voice or facial hair may not be addressed affirmatively as female with her corresponding pronouns because she was perceived or assumed to be masculine, even when the medical record accurately reflects her female identity. This increased self-awareness of the worker combined with the appropriate training and tools are needed to ensure an affirming environment of care. Ideally, the healthcare environment also incorporates gender identity and gender expression as part of their nondiscrimination policies protecting gender-diverse patients and/or gender-diverse members of the workforce.

Workforce education can not only provide practical tools and tips for addressing patients affirmatively, it can also be useful to help others understand the context of the daily lives experienced by transgender patients. Transgender communities experience high rates of discrimination, violence, and trauma that impact the experience of trust and safety in many areas of life, including healthcare [15]. The goal is to help patients build resilience, health, and well-being by providing an affirming and trauma-informed environment of care for any encounter a patient has throughout the healthcare system, not just while accessing gender-affirming surgical care.

Trauma-Informed Care

Trauma is a widespread, harmful, and costly public health problem, and exposure to violence and trauma has been well-documented in trans/gender nonconforming (TGNC) communities. According to the 2015 US Trans Survey [15], one-third of respondents noted they were likely to avoid preventive/routine care in order to avoid further discrimination and trauma. The effects of trauma, left unaddressed or unrecognized, can hinder access to and utilization of care. For example, patients may be distressed by, unwilling, or unable to remove clothing for a physical examination. They may display discomfort when discussing personal questions that may be embarrassing or distressing. Some people may resist physical touch and/or struggle in relationships where a power dynamic is present, such as the patient–doctor relationship. Furthermore, carrying out routine aspects of a patient medical visit may result in disclosure of a current or past trauma; knowing how to respond to the patient in these circumstances can be essential to building the trust needed to provide care.

The care environment can be most effective when, in addition to a gender-affirming approach, we employ a Trauma-Informed Care approach [16]. Briefly, trauma-informed care refers to a patient-centered effort to recognize the risk of trauma history in a vulnerable population, to anticipate and understand how a patient's possible exposure to trauma might shape the way they respond to or interpret events in a health system or a provider's words or actions, and to proactively adjust to these challenges. This can include creating a soothing physical environment, training all staff in the principles of trauma-informed approaches, creating a sense of safety with the patient by establishing a respectful relationship, adopting collaborative and person-centered approaches, and offering choices and options to maximize a patient's sense of control [17]. The "4 R's" illustrate this approach [16]. A provider or system is trauma-informed when it *Realizes* the widespread impact of trauma and its understanding of potential paths of recovery; *Recognizes* the signs and symptoms of trauma in clients, families, staff, and others involved with the system; *Responds* by fully integrating knowledge about trauma into policies, procedures, and practices; and seeks to actively *Resist* re-traumatization.

It is important to distinguish that the physical healthcare environment is not the setting in which the mental health treatment, such as psychotherapy, takes place but rather the physical care is provided through a trauma-informed framework. This includes a process of evaluating policies and procedures based on an understanding of trauma; assuming every interaction with a trauma survivor may or may not activate a trauma response; and providing a corrective emotional experience. For those seeking services (and of the workforce as well), it often comes down to personal interactions that reflect sensitivity, respect, caring, transparency, and an understanding of trauma. Workforce education that is truly gender-affirming will also incorporate these principles of Trauma-Informed Care.

Conclusion

Gender-affirming care requires extensive education of the patient and their support network, both to prepare for surgery and recovery and also to appropriately manage expectations. Providers and health systems should make special efforts to provide respectful care. A trauma-informed approach can help mitigate the problems providers and health systems may encounter in caring for a group of people at high risk for trauma's harmful effects.

Take-Home Points
- Extensive patient education is critical to patient preparation and for setting realistic patient expectations of surgical outcomes
- A long history of bias and discrimination against transgender people in healthcare delivery means extensive efforts are needed to prepare a health system to provide affirming care
- Trauma-informed care is an approach to recognize the effects of trauma and discrimination in this population in order to provide better care

References

1. Safer JD, Coleman E, Feldman J, Garofalo R, Hembree W, Radix A, Sevelius J. Barriers to healthcare for transgender individuals. Curr Opin Endocrinol Diabetes Obes. 2016;23:168–71.
2. Jiang D, Witten J, Berli J, Dugi D. Does depth matter? factors affecting choice of vulvoplasty over vaginoplasty as gender-affirming genital surgery for transgender women. J Sex Med. 2018;15:902–6. https://doi.org/10.1016/j.jsxm.2018.03.085.
3. Coleman E, Bockting W, Botzer M, et al. Standards of care for the health of transsexual, transgender, and gender-nonconforming people, version 7. Int J Transgenderism. 2012;13:165–232.
4. Kuntz K, Weinland SR, Butt Z. Psychosocial challenges in solid organ transplantation. J Clin Psychol Med Settings. 2015;22:122–35.
5. Sogg S, Lauretti J, West-Smith L. Recommendations for the presurgical psychosocial evaluation of bariatric surgery patients. Surg Obes Relat Dis. 2016;12:731–49.
6. Waljee J, McGlinn EP, Sears E, Chung KC. Patient expectations and patient-reported outcomes in surgery: a systematic review. Surgery. 2014;155:799–808.
7. Rinker B. The evils of nicotine: an evidence-based guide to smoking and plastic surgery. Ann Plast Surg. 2013;70:599.
8. Giori NJ, Ellerbe LS, Bowe T, Gupta S, Harris AH. Many diabetic total joint arthroplasty candidates are unable to achieve a preoperative Hemoglobin A1c goal of 7% or less. J Bone Joint Surg Am. 2014;96:500.
9. Cron DC, Englesbe MJ, Bolton CJ, Joseph MT, Carrier KL, Moser SE, Waljee JF, Hilliard PE, Kheterpal S, Brummett CM. Preoperative opioid use is independently associated with increased costs and worse outcomes after major abdominal surgery. Ann Surg. 2017;265:695–701.
10. Moran S, Isa J, Steinemann S. Perioperative management in the patient with substance abuse. Surg Clin N Am. 2015;95:417–28.
11. Demsey D, Carr NJ, Clarke H, Vipler S. Managing opioid addiction risk in plastic surgery during the perioperative period. Plast Reconstr Surg. 2017;140:613e–9e.
12. Massie JP, Morrison SD, Maasdam J, Satterwhite T. Predictors of patient satisfaction and postoperative complications in penile inversion vaginoplasty. Plast Reconstr Surg. 2018;141:911e.
13. McIsaac DI, Jen T, Mookerji N, Patel A, Lalu MM. Interventions to improve the outcomes of frail people having surgery: a systematic review. PLoS One. 2017;12:e0190071.
14. Jiang D, Gallagher S, Burchill L, Berli J, Dugi D. Implementation of a pelvic floor physical therapy program for transgender women undergoing gender-affirming vaginoplasty. Obstet Gynecol. 2019;133:1–10.
15. James SE, Herman JL, Rankin S, Keisling M, Mottet L, Anafi M. The report of the U.S. transgender survey. Washington, DC: National Center for Transgender Equality; 2016.
16. Substance Abuse and Mental Health Services Administration. SAMHSA's concept of trauma and guidance for a trauma-informed approach. Rockville, MD: US Department of Health & Human Services; 2014.
17. Raja S, Hasnain M, Hoersch M, Gove-Yin S, Rajagopalan C. Trauma informed care in medicine. Fam Community Health. 2015;38:216–26.

Part II

Surgical Anatomy:
Transgender Female Patients

Surgical Anatomy: Orchiectomy and Fertility Preservation Options

Michael Owyong and Ranjith Ramasamy

Introduction

Over the past decade, there has been an increase in the number of patients undergoing gender-affirming surgery [1]. Therefore, we are likely to see a concomitant rise in the number of patients being referred to urologists for orchiectomy. Simple bilateral orchiectomy provides an effective means of achieving castrate levels of testosterone, allowing transgender female patients to use a lower dose of estrogen and discontinue spironolactone. Guidelines from the World Professional Association for Transgender Health recommend candidates for orchiectomy be independently evaluated by two qualified mental health professionals, and be accompanied by referral letters containing an assessment of the patient's psychosocial status, as well as the history and duration of any hormonal therapy [2]. Informed consent for the procedure should include a discussion of the option for either staged (early) orchiectomy—through an inguinal or scrotal approach—or single-stage orchiectomy and vaginoplasty, along with the risks and benefits of each technique and approach. Lastly, surgical candidates of childbearing age and/or with reproductive potential should be informed about options for fertility preservation, including

M. Owyong · R. Ramasamy (✉)
University of Miami Miller School of Medicine, Miami, FL, USA
e-mail: ramasamy@miami.edu

sperm cryopreservation, testicular sperm extraction, and testicular tissue cryopreservation, along with their risks, benefits, and costs.

Surgical Anatomy

Inguinal Region

Gross Anatomy

The skin of the inguinal region is relatively hairless, inelastic, and thick. Two layers of superficial fascia lie deep to the skin. Camper's fascia is the superficial layer of the superficial fascia. Camper's fascia is a layer of areolar tissue with its contained fat that varies in thickness with the nutritional status of the patient. The superficial inferior epigastric vessels run in this layer and can be encountered during inguinal incisions. Scarpa's fascia is the deep layer of the superficial fascia. Scarpa's fascia may be difficult to discern in older and obese patients and can be mistaken for the external oblique aponeurosis. However, Scarpa's fascia does not have parallel collagenous fibers and traction causes it to move with the skin to which it is attached.

Scarpa's fascia is also loosely connected to the innominate fascia of Gallaudet, which is the fascia overlying the external oblique aponeurosis. The superficial inguinal pouch, first described by Denis Browne, is a potential space between Scarpa's fascia and the innominate fascia. The

© Springer Nature Switzerland AG 2021
D. Nikolavsky, S. A. Blakely (eds.), *Urological Care for the Transgender Patient*,
https://doi.org/10.1007/978-3-030-18533-6_5

pouch lies lateral to the external/superficial inguinal ring and provides a space in which a cryptorchid testis may be found [3].

Between the pubic tubercle and the pubic symphysis, Scarpa's fascia remains unattached, leaving an opening for the spermatic cord. This abdominoscrotal passage can be felt as a ring around the examining finger and should not be confused with the external/superficial inguinal ring, which lies higher and is rarely palpable in the absence of a hernia.

Beneath Scarpa's fascia (and the innominate fascia of Gallaudet) lies the external oblique aponeurosis, whose fibers run downward and medially. The aponeurosis is attached medially to the upper border of the pubic symphysis and to the pubic crest up to the pubic tubercle.

The inferior margin of the external oblique aponeurosis folds dorsally on itself to form the inguinal (Poupart's) ligament (see Fig. 5.1).

The external oblique aponeurosis forms both the anterior wall and floor of the inguinal canal, which transmits the spermatic cord and the ilioinguinal nerve. Above the pubic tubercle, the fibers of the external oblique aponeurosis split to form the lateral edges/crura of the external inguinal ring. Transverse/intercrural fibers bridge the crura to form the superior edge of the external inguinal ring (see Fig. 5.2).

The transversalis fascia forms the posterior wall of the inguinal canal. The spermatic cord pierces the transversalis fascia lateral to the inferior epigastric vessels at the internal/deep inguinal ring. The internal inguinal ring lies midway between the anterior superior iliac spine and the pubic tubercle, above the inguinal ligament, and lateral to the external inguinal ring (see Fig. 5.3).

Both the internal oblique aponeurosis and transversus fascia pass over the inguinal canal to form its roof before fusing as the conjoint tendon and forming the posterior wall of the inguinal canal at the level of the external inguinal ring. Contraction of the internal oblique and transversalis muscles closes the roof of the inguinal canal against the floor, preventing herniation of intra-abdominal contents (see Fig. 5.4).

Arterial Supply and Venous Drainage

The superficial inferior epigastric artery and vein arise from the anterior surface of the femoral artery and vein below the level of the inguinal ligament. The superficial inferior epigastric vessels run within Camper's fascia across the line of an inguinal incision to the level of the umbilicus.

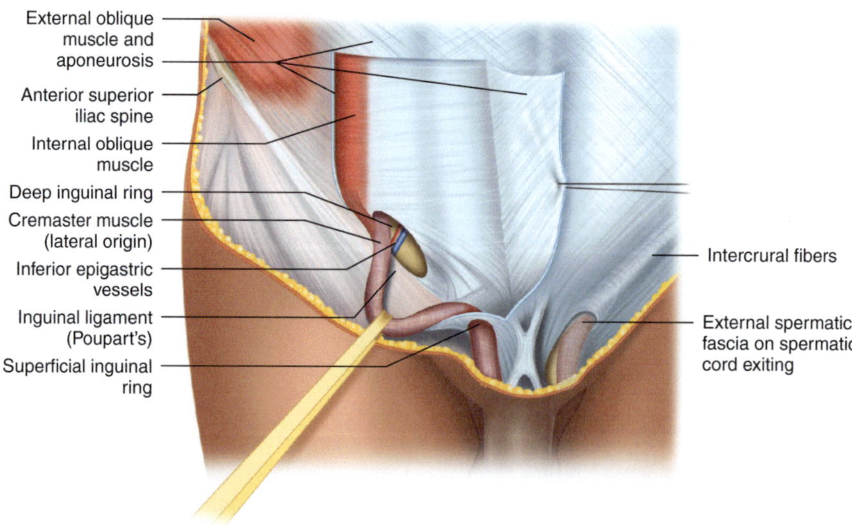

Fig. 5.1 Shelving edge of external oblique aponeurosis and its relationship to surrounding structures

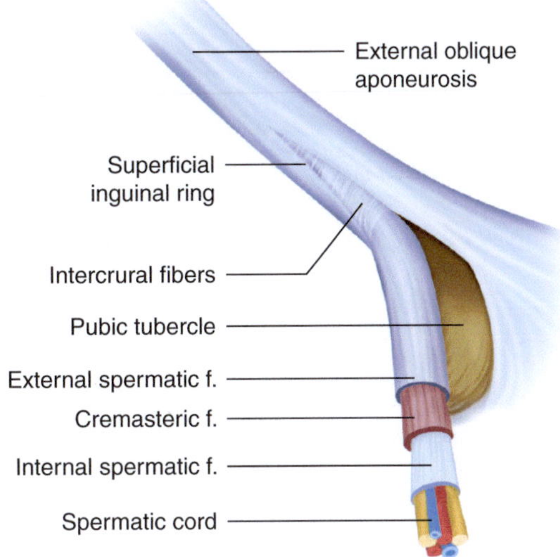

Fig. 5.2 View of the spermatic cord as it exits the external inguinal ring

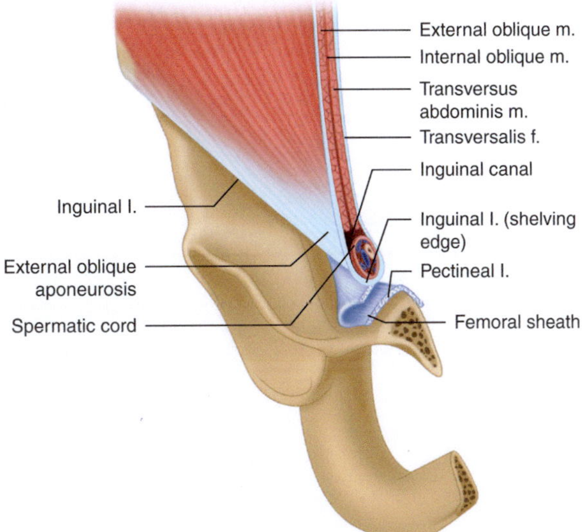

Fig. 5.3 View of the spermatic cord at the level of the internal inguinal ring

Scrotum

Gross Anatomy

The skin of the scrotum is pigmented and hair-bearing with abundant sebaceous and sweat glands, but has an absence of fat. Underlying the scrotal skin is the dartos smooth muscle, which is continuous with Colles fascia of the perineum, Scarpa's fascia of the abdomen, and dartos fascia of the penis. Depending on the tone of the under-lying dartos smooth muscle, the scrotal skin may be folded with transverse rugae or it may appear loose and shiny. The median raphe runs longitu-dinally in the midline from the urethral meatus to the anus. Deep to the raphe, the scrotum is divided by a septum into two compartments, each containing a testis (see Fig. 5.5).

The spermatic fasciae are layers of the abdominal wall that extend to form parts of the scrotal wall. The external oblique aponeurosis extends to form the external spermatic fascia. The internal oblique aponeurosis extends to form

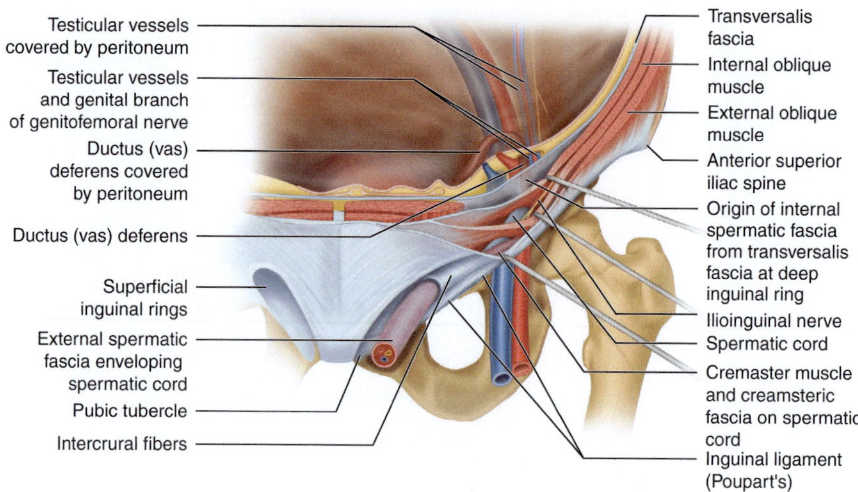

Fig. 5.4 Musculature of abdominal wall and their relationship to inguinal canal

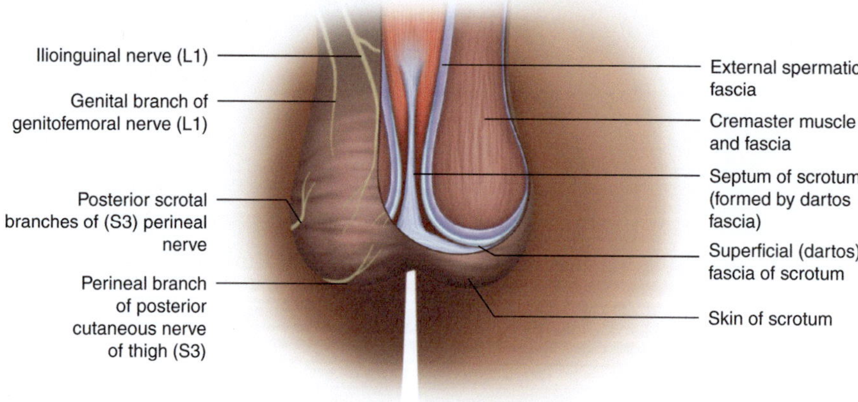

Fig. 5.5 Gross view of the nerves and layers of the scrotum

the cremaster muscle and fascia. And the transversalis fascia extends to become the internal spermatic fascia.

Deep to the internal spermatic fascia is the tunica vaginalis, which is derived from the vaginal process of the peritoneum. The parietal and visceral layers of the tunica vaginalis surround the testis. The tunica vaginalis is continuous with the testis posterolaterally, where it is attached to the scrotal wall. The gubernaculum fixes the testis at its inferior pole.

Arterial Supply

The anterior wall of the scrotum is supplied by the external pudendal arteries, which run parallel to the rugae and do not cross the median raphe. Branches of the perineal artery supply the posterior aspect of the scrotum. Arterial supply to the spermatic fascia is from the cremasteric, testicular, and deferential branches.

Venous Drainage

The anterior wall of the scrotum is drained by the external pudendal veins, which run parallel to the rugae and do not cross the median raphe. The perineal vein drains the posterior aspect of the scrotum.

Lymphatic Drainage

Lymphatic drainage from the scrotum travels to the ipsilateral superficial inguinal nodes. The lymphatic channels do not cross the median raphe.

Nerve Supply

The anterior wall of the scrotum is innervated by branches of the ilioinguinal and genitofemoral nerves, which run parallel to the rugae and do not cross the median raphe. The posterior aspect of the scrotum receives innervation from the scrotal branch of the perineal nerve and from the perineal branch of the posterior femoral cutaneous nerve.

Spermatic Cord

Gross Anatomy

The external spermatic fascia forms the outer tubular sheath surrounding the spermatic cord. If the external spermatic fascia is incised to the point where its sheath widens near the upper pole of the testis, the scrotal contents, even if enlarged, may be drawn into the wound. Deep to the external spermatic fascia are the cremasteric fascia and the internal spermatic fascia.

The major contents of the spermatic cord include the vas deferens, along with its corresponding artery, vein, and lymphatic, and the testicular artery and pampiniform plexus.

The vas deferens, also known as the ductus deferens, is a tubular structure with an outer diameter ranging between 1.5 and 2.7 mm [4]. Its embryologic origin is the mesonephric (Wolffian) duct. From the cauda epididymis to its termination at the ejaculatory duct, the vas deferens measures between 30 and 35 cm in length. The vas deferens is tortuous for the first 2–3 cm as it leaves the cauda epididymis and travels posteriorly along the spermatic cord before entering the pelvis lateral to the epigastric vessels. The outer adventitial connective tissue layer surrounding the vas deferens contains blood vessels and small nerves. Within this connective tissue layer, smooth muscle cells comprise the thick wall of the vas deferens.

Arterial Supply and Venous Drainage

The superior vesical artery gives off the deferential artery, which supplies the vas deferens. The venous drainage of the scrotal vas deferens is via the deferential vein, which drains into the pampiniform plexus.

Lymphatic Supply

Lymphatic drainage from the vas deferens travels to the external and internal iliac nodes.

Orchiectomy Techniques and Approaches

In addition to two referral letters from qualified mental health professionals, candidates for orchiectomy should have a persistent, documented diagnosis of gender dysphoria and a 12-month trial period of gender-affirming hormone therapy prior to undergoing irreversible surgical intervention. Once the decision to proceed with orchiectomy is made, a preoperative surgical consultation should take place with a discussion of the different operative techniques available and their advantages, disadvantages, and possible complications. We discuss in the following each technique and approach in detail and provide tips and tricks for the prevention and management of common complications.

Staged (Early) Orchiectomy

There is a current lack of evidence regarding the superiority of staged (early) orchiectomy—through an inguinal or scrotal approach—over single-stage orchiectomy and vaginoplasty. Therefore, the choice of technique and approach is based on patient preference and surgeon experience. In general, early orchiectomy provides significant medical benefit with minimal morbidity and is an option for patients not yet ready for vaginoplasty. With early orchiectomy, surgical technique and approach is of utmost importance in order to preserve the quality of scrotal skin and collateral tissues in anticipation of future vaginoplasty [5].

Inguinal Approach [6]

The surgical anatomic landmarks for a patient in the supine position include the anterior superior iliac spine, pubic tubercle, inguinal ligament, penis, and scrotum (see Fig. 5.6).

A curvilinear incision is made beginning cephalad and lateral to the pubic tubercle, extending laterally along Langer's lines. Langer's lines parallel the dermal collagen fibers and are oriented along lines of stress. They also correspond to the segmental thoracic and lumbar nerves. The incision is carried through the subcutaneous tissue onto the external oblique aponeurosis with electrocautery. The subcutaneous tissue may be further dissected off of the external oblique aponeurosis to clearly identify the inguinal ligament and aid with closure.

The external oblique aponeurosis is sharply opened over the inguinal canal extending medially to the external inguinal ring and laterally to a

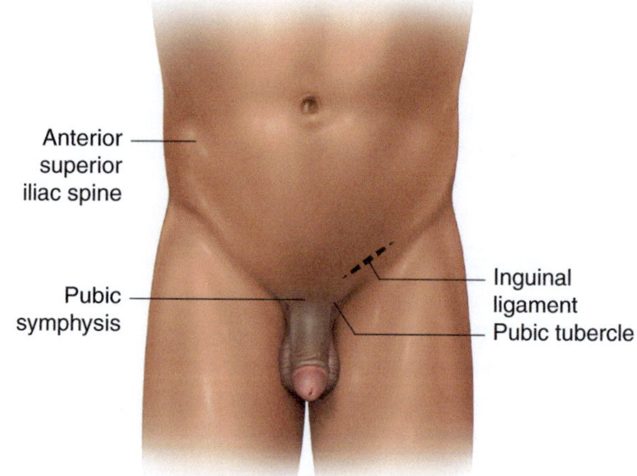

Fig. 5.6 Important anatomic landmarks during inguinal orchiectomy

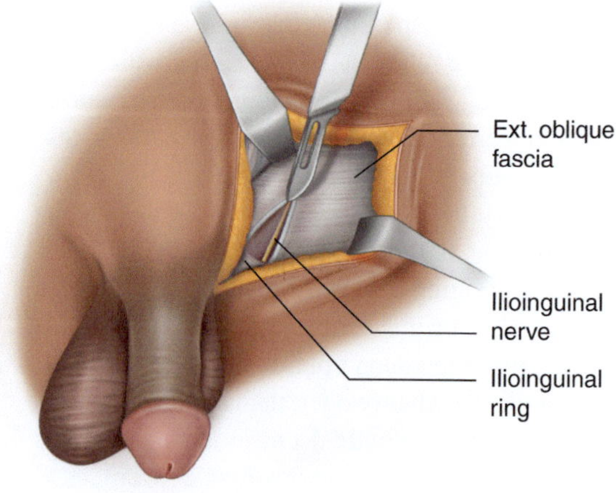

Fig. 5.7 Incision through the external oblique aponeurosis

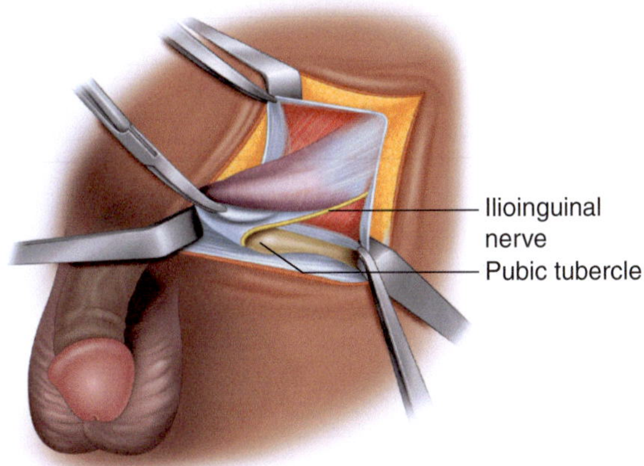

Fig. 5.8 Blunt dissection to circumferentially isolate spermatic cord

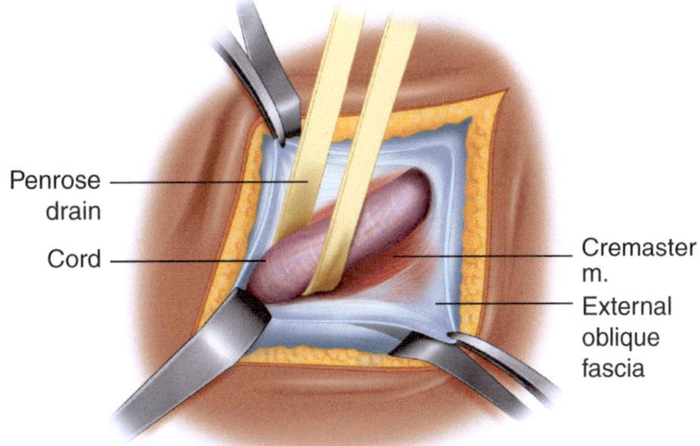

Fig. 5.9 Spermatic cord secured with a Penrose drain

point overlying the level of the internal inguinal ring. The ilioinguinal nerve lying on top of the spermatic cord is identified and dissected free from its investing external spermatic fascia and cremasteric musculature, and then retracted laterally out of harm's way (see Fig. 5.7).

Gentle blunt dissection at the level of the pubic tubercle with the aim of circumscribing the spermatic cord and cremasteric musculature is accomplished next (see Fig. 5.8).

The surgeon's finger should easily pass posterior to the cord along the floor of the inguinal canal. Care should be taken to avoid dissecting through the floor of the inguinal canal, as this increases the risk of developing a postoperative direct inguinal hernia. A Penrose drain can be used to secure the spermatic cord (see Fig. 5.9).

Delivery of the intact testicle within the tunica vaginalis can be facilitated by gently pushing the testicle from the base of the prepped hemiscrotum toward the incision. Gentle traction can be applied to the spermatic cord to aid this maneuver (see Fig. 5.10).

Further blunt dissection and/or electrocautery may be necessary to free the tunica vaginalis from its investing fascial layers. Subsequent to delivery of the testicle, the hemiscrotum will be invaginated at the level of the incision by the gubernaculum, which should be incised by electrocautery. The delivered testicle within the tunica vaginalis is then free and attached only by the spermatic cord (see Fig. 5.11).

The cord is dissected proximal to the internal inguinal ring. A handheld retractor can be used to elevate the internal oblique aponeurosis, reveal-

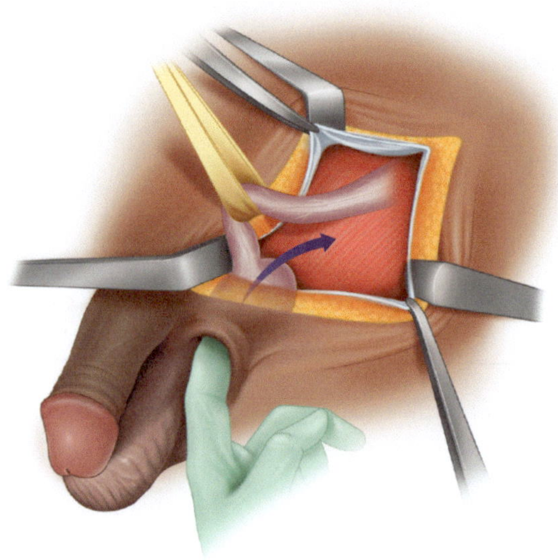

Fig. 5.10 Application of external force to gently deliver testis toward incision

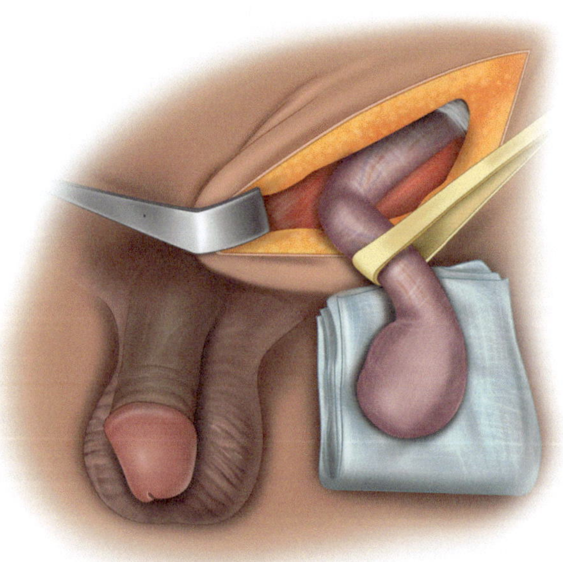

Fig. 5.11 Delivery of the intact testis

ing retroperitoneal fat. Electrocautery is used at this level to incise the cremasteric muscle fibers and skeletonize the cord, allowing clear visibility of the cord vasculature and vas deferens. The vas deferens is ligated and divided separately from the cord at this level with permanent suture. The cord proper is also doubly ligated and divided at this level with permanent suture. The surgical field is then irrigated and meticulous hemostasis is obtained.

The external oblique aponeurosis is approximated with running absorbable suture, taking care not to include the ilioinguinal nerve. If desired, long-acting local anesthetic for assistance with postoperative pain control can be applied at this time. The subcutaneous fascial tissue layers are approximated with running absorbable suture. The skin is then closed in a subcuticular fashion using running absorbable suture.

Scrotal Approach [7]

After shaving and sterile preparation of the scrotum, a single midline scrotal incision is made within the median raphe (see Fig. 5.12).

The incision is carried down to the septum and through the tunica vaginalis on either the right or left side. The testis is delivered into the wound and gentle traction is provided in order to expose the spermatic cord up to the level of the external inguinal ring. The vas deferens is then identified, ligated, and divided using a silk ligature. The cremasteric muscle is separated from the internal spermatic vessels and each is ligated separately using silk sutures (see Fig. 5.13).

After meticulous hemostasis is obtained, an identical operation is carried out on the contralateral side.

The dartos muscle is then approximated in an interrupted fashion using self-absorbing sutures. The wound is injected with local anesthetic and the skin edges are closed in a running subcuticular fashion with absorbable sutures, using two skin hooks at the apices to aid in closure (see Fig. 5.14).

At the end of the procedure, the wound is dressed with antibiotic ointment, dry fluffed gauze, and an athletic supporter.

Single-Stage Orchiectomy and Vaginoplasty

The general principles described earlier for performing a bilateral orchiectomy through a scrotal approach can be applied to perform a bilateral orchiectomy at the time of vaginoplasty and are described in detail in Chap. 6.

Prevention and Management of Complications

Surgical complications following orchiectomy are rare with an estimated incidence of less than 1% [1]. Reported complications include retroperitoneal hemorrhage, wound dehiscence, and hematoma/hematocele formation. We emphasize a few key points here to help avoid and manage these complications. First, meticulous control of the gonadal vessels is critical for preventing retraction into the retroperitoneum with subsequent hemorrhage. We also recommend a two- or three-layer closure of the subcutaneous tissue and skin layers to reduce the likelihood of wound disruption. Lastly, a scrotal support and "fluff" dressings

Fig. 5.12 Midline scrotal incision through median raphe

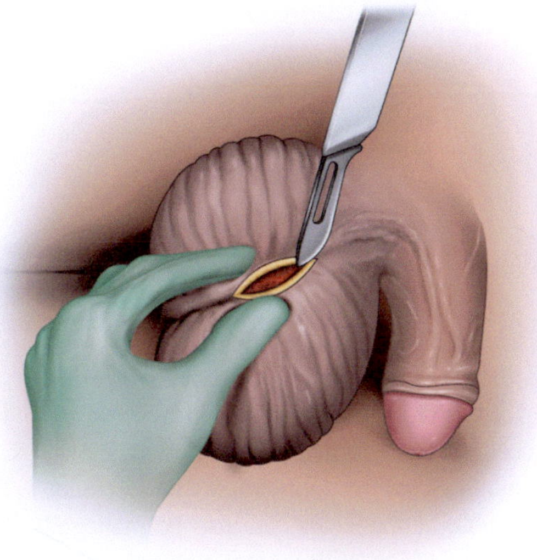

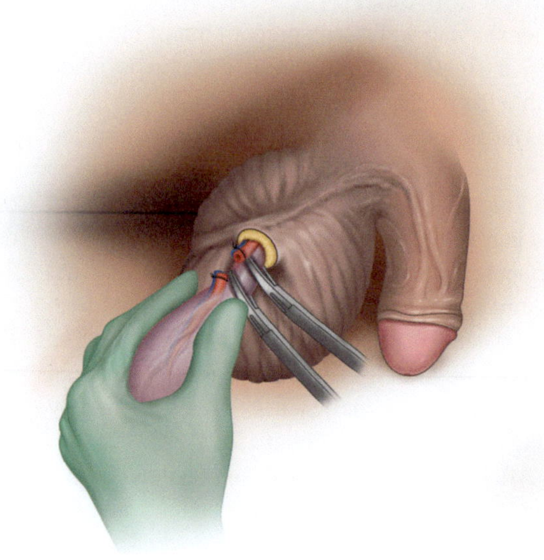

Fig. 5.13 Delivery of testis and ligation of spermatic cord

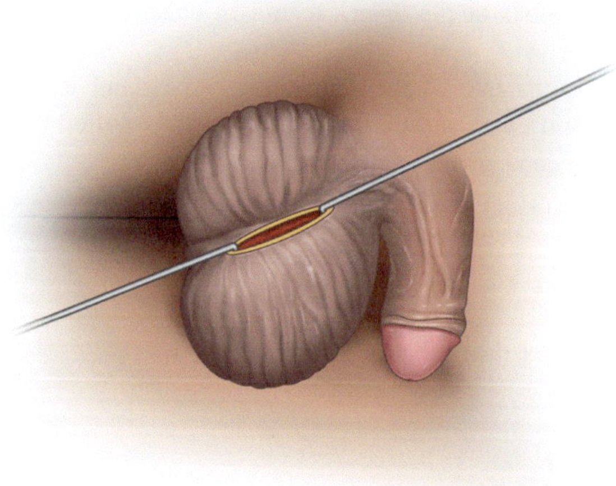

Fig. 5.14 Placement of apical skin hooks to facilitate closure

can minimize swelling and prevent formation of a hematoma/hematocele within the first 72 h.

It is important to note that cutaneous scrotal hematomas that arise in the postoperative period will resolve without intervention and can be managed conservatively with scrotal support, elevation, and intermittent application of ice packs. Small, stable hematoceles can also be managed in a similar fashion with scrotal support, elevation, and ice packs. However, large hematoceles require prompt drainage to prevent infection and prolonged pain.

Fertility Preservation Options

Patients undergoing feminizing surgery should be informed about options for fertility preservation, especially those patients who have not already reproduced. Many transgender adolescents elect to initiate gender-affirming hormones concurrently with gonadotropin-releasing hormone agonists to prevent the maturation of germ cells [8]. Guidelines from both the World Professional Association for Transgender Health and the Endocrine Society recommend a discussion of fertility preservation with transgender patients prior to the initiation of pubertal suppression and/or cross-sex hormone therapy [2, 9]. This is important as little is currently known regarding the effects of pubertal suppression with gonadotropin-releasing hormone agonists on future fertility potential. In addition, Lao and colleagues found a wide range of findings on review of testicular histology from orchiectomy specimens of male patients, who were on active estrogen supplementation therapy and underwent feminizing surgery [10]. As sperm production is androgen dependent, the use of estrogen supplementation therapy may affect spermatogenesis and maturation.

Despite publication of guidelines, the majority of patients undergoing feminizing surgery do not receive any counseling regarding future fertility prior to pubertal suppression and/or cross-sex hormone therapy. [8] De Sutter and colleagues conducted a survey of 121 transgender female patients and found that the majority of patients felt that fertility preservation options should be discussed and offered before starting hormonal treatment [11].

Options for fertility preservation include sperm cryopreservation, testicular sperm extraction, and testicular tissue cryopreservation.

Sperm Cryopreservation

Sperm cryopreservation is a viable method of fertility preservation for peripubertal and postpubertal patients undergoing feminizing surgery [12].

Semen samples are collected by masturbation after 2 or 3 days of abstinence. Cryoprotectants, such as glycerol and egg yolk, are added to the semen samples to prevent osmotic stress and maintain cell membrane integrity during freezing and thawing [13]. The samples then undergo storage in liquid nitrogen. McCracken and colleagues found that sperm concentration and total motile count in transgender women prior to hormone treatment were lower when compared to (cisgender)men that had recently fathered a child [14]. The etiology of these differences in semen parameters may be attributable to the use of tight undergarments. However, semen analysis can be performed prior to processing for cryopreservation and semen collection can be repeated every 2–3 days to ensure adequate sperm counts. Post-thaw sperm motility can also be assessed by setting aside one of the cryovials to be thawed. This method indicates how well sperm in the other remaining vials will survive when thawed later.

Due to the possibility of cryopreserved sperm to undergo cross-contamination with bacteria and/or viruses, several measures have been put into place [15]. Prior to sperm cryopreservation, donors and client depositors are routinely screened for sexually transmitted diseases, including HIV, hepatitis B, hepatitis C, syphilis, human T-lymphotropic virus, cytomegalovirus, chlamydia, and gonorrhea. Semen samples are then held in quarantine for at least 6 months and the donors/depositors are retested before the specimens can be released.

Transgender female patients are recommended to pursue sperm cryopreservation prior to the initiation of pubertal suppression and/or cross-sex hormone therapy. The presence of gender-affirming hormones at the time of semen collection has been found to be associated with abnormal semen parameters [16]. For patients using gender-affirming hormones, an average discontinuation time of 4.7 months is associated with recovery of normal semen parameters [16, 17].

Testicular Sperm Extraction

Testicular sperm extraction (TESE) becomes an option for sperm retrieval when factors such as patient age, anatomy, concerns about psychological impact, or azoospermia preclude the use of an ejaculated semen sample for subsequent cryopreservation. Lao and colleagues reported on a case of TESE at the time of feminizing surgery with successful sperm retrieval and cryopreservation [10].

Testicular Tissue Cryopreservation

Testicular tissue cryopreservation is a fertility preservation option in prepubertal boys and adolescents on pubertal suppression therapy. Because these patients have not yet entered puberty, they do not yet produce sperm and have no available mature gametes for cryopreservation. Current investigational protocols involving slow-freezing and vitrification have shown promise at successfully cryopreserving immature testicular tissue [18, 19]. However, since the option of prepubertal testicular tissue cryopreservation remains experimental, the Ethics Committee of the American Society for Reproductive Medicine recommends that decisions regarding gonadectomy for fertility preservation be delayed until adulthood [20].

Financial Considerations

Patients should be advised that these fertility preservation options are not available everywhere and can be very costly. Testicular sperm and tissue retrieval procedures may be covered by insurance or dedicated philanthropic funds for families who do not have adequate coverage. If possible, surgical procedures can be bundled with other necessary procedures to minimize the anesthetic exposure and cost. In addition, sperm cryopreservation and yearly storage costs are often not covered by insurance and can be prohibitive.

The financial cost of fertility preservation in pediatric patients can also be substantial. Since pediatric patients usually do not satisfy the definition of infertility (i.e., attempting to conceive for at least 12 months), families may end up paying out-of-pocket for fertility preservation services.

Conclusion

Simple bilateral orchiectomy in transgender female patients is an effective method of achieving castrate levels of testosterone. Two qualified mental health professionals should independently evaluate candidates for orchiectomy. The decision of either staged (early) orchiectomy—through an inguinal or scrotal approach—or single-stage orchiectomy and vaginoplasty should be based on patient preference and surgeon experience. Surgical candidates of childbearing age and/or with reproductive potential should be informed about options for fertility preservation, including sperm cryopreservation, testicular sperm extraction, and testicular tissue cryopreservation.

References

1. Lane M, Ives GC, Sluiter EC, Waljee JF, Yao T-H, Hu HM, et al. Trends in gender-affirming surgery in insured patients in the United States. Plast Reconstr Surg Glob Open. 2018;6(4):e1738.
2. Coleman E, Bockting W, Botzer M, Cohen-Kettenis P, DeCuypere G, Feldman J, et al. Standards of care for the health of transsexual, transgender, and gender-

Take-Home Points
- Simple bilateral orchiectomy in transgender female patients is an effective method of achieving castrate levels of testosterone.
- The choice of either staged (early) orchiectomy—through an inguinal or scrotal approach—or single-stage orchiectomy and vaginoplasty should be based on patient preference and surgeon experience.
- Surgical candidates of childbearing age and/or with reproductive potential should be informed about options for fertility preservation, including sperm cryopreservation, testicular sperm extraction, and testicular tissue cryopreservation.

nonconforming people, version 7. Int J Transgend. 2012;13(4):165–232.

3. Patel SR, Caldamone AA. Sir Denis Browne: contributions to pediatric urology. J Pediatr Urol. 2010;6(5):496–500.

4. Middleton WD, Dahiya N, Naughton CK, Teefey SA, Siegel CA. High-resolution sonography of the normal extrapelvic vas deferens. J Ultrasound Med. 2009;28(7):839–46.

5. Garcia M. PD25-06 Pre-vaginoplasty bilateral orchiectomy for transgender women: an efficient surgical technique that preserves collateral tissues and sensation. J Urol. 2017;197(4):e503–e4.

6. Elmajian DA, Venable DD. Radical orchiectomy. In: Smith JA, Howards SS, Preminger GM, Dmochowski RR, editors. Hinman's Atlas of Urologic Surgery. Amsterdam: Elsevier Health Sciences; 2016.

7. Tanrikut C, Goldstein M. Simple orchiectomy. In: Smith JA, Howards SS, Preminger GM, Dmochowski RR, editors. Hinman's Atlas of Urologic Surgery. Amsterdam: Elsevier Health Sciences; 2016.

8. Schelble A, Fisher A, Jungheim E, Lewis C, Omurtag K. Fertility preservation (FP) referral and follow-up in male-to-female (MTF) and female-to-male (FTM) transgender patients. Fertil Steril. 2017;108(3):e115–e6.

9. Hembree WC, Cohen-Kettenis P, Delemarre-Van De Waal HA, Gooren LJ, Meyer WJ III, Spack NP, et al. Endocrine treatment of transsexual persons: an Endocrine Society clinical practice guideline. J Clin Endocrinol Metabol. 2009;94(9):3132–54.

10. Lao M, Honig S. Evaluation of testis sperm extraction (TESE) and testis histology in the gender confirming surgery patient. Fertil Steril. 2016;106(3):e132–e3.

11. De Sutter P, Kira K, Verschoor A, Hotimsky A. The desire to have children and the preservation of fertility in transsexual women: a survey. Int J Transgend. 2002;6(3):97–03.

12. Keene DJ, Sajjad Y, Makin G, Cervellione RM. Sperm banking in the United Kingdom is feasible in patients 13 years old or older with cancer. J Urol. 2012;188(2):594–7.

13. Ball BA, Vo A. Osmotic tolerance of equine spermatozoa and the effects of soluble cryoprotectants on equine sperm motility, viability, and mitochondrial membrane potential. J Androl. 2001;22(6):1061–9.

14. McCracken M, Nangia A, Roby K, McLaren H, Gray M, Marsh C. Total motile sperm in transgender women seeking hormone therapy: a case-control study. Fertil Steril. 2018;110(4):e22.

15. Clarke GN. Sperm cryopreservation: is there a significant risk of cross-contamination? Human Reproduc. 1999;14(12):2941–3.

16. Adeleye A, Reid G, Mok-Lin E, Smith J. Fertility preservation for transgender females after gender affirming treatment is effective. Fertil Steril. 2017;108(3):e391.

17. Barnard E, Menke M, Witchel S, Dhar C, Montano G, Goodall J, et al. Fertility preservation outcomes in feminizing transgender patients: experience at a single institution. Fertil Steril. 2018;110(4):e282.

18. Keros V, Hultenby K, Borgstrom B, Fridstrom M, Jahnukainen K, Hovatta O. Methods of cryopreservation of testicular tissue with viable spermatogonia in pre-pubertal boys undergoing gonadotoxic cancer treatment. Hum Reprod. 2007;22(5):1384–95.

19. Poels J, Van Langendonckt A, Many MC, Wese FX, Wyns C. Vitrification preserves proliferation capacity in human spermatogonia. Hum Reprod. 2013;28(3):578–89.

20. Access to fertility services by transgender persons: an Ethics Committee opinion. Fertility and Sterility. 2015;104(5):1111–5.

Surgical Anatomy: Vaginoplasty

6

James J. Drinane and Richard A. Santucci

Abbreviations

FTM	female-to-male
GDD	Gender development disorder
GID	Gender Identity Disorder
IMA	inferior mesenteric artery
MTF	male-to-female
SMA	superior mesenteric artery
WPATH	World Professional Association for Transgender Health

Introduction

Vaginoplasty is a rewarding surgery owing to its predictable results and relative ease of performance. Vaginoplasty is the most commonly performed genital affirmation surgery. Successful vaginoplasty requires a detailed understanding of pelvic anatomy, and specific understanding of the patient's surgical goals. When executed well, most transgender women are very happy with their new anatomy and its function.

J. J. Drinane
Albany Medical College, Albany, NY, USA
e-mail: drinanj@amc.edu

R. A. Santucci (✉)
Brownstein-Crane Surgical Services,
Austin, TX, USA
e-mail: richard@brownsteincrane.com

History of the Procedure

Gender surgery has been ongoing for millennia, beginning with eunuchs (castrated males generally designated to perform specific social functions) and reported as far back as biblical times. There are reports of self-performed gender confirmation procedures as early as the seventeenth century, even to relieve gender dysphoria (found in personal diaries [1]). In South Asia, there is an ancient Hijra tradition, or "third sex," where boys voluntarily undergo demasculinization surgery usually consisting of penectomy, orchiectomy, and scrotectomy. When performed before puberty, the operation had the added effect of preventing the development of other secondary sexual characteristics.

The first gender-affirming surgery in the medical literature was reported by Dr. Magnus Hirschfeld who oversaw the surgical management of Lili Elbe in 1931 [2]. The first description of vaginoplasty itself was by Dr. Felix Abraham that same year. Abraham described a two-staged procedure [3]. When asked about the surgery he performed, he remarked "[it is] a kind of emergency surgery, necessary to save patients from worse self-inflicted procedures." With time, greater acceptance by society and the medical community has generated interest and developments in the global care of transgender patients with vastly improved outcomes in both form and function [3].

© Springer Nature Switzerland AG 2021
D. Nikolavsky, S. A. Blakely (eds.), *Urological Care for the Transgender Patient*,
https://doi.org/10.1007/978-3-030-18533-6_6

The most common means of performing vaginoplasty is a penile inversion technique, which has been modified in recent times. Penile inversion was first performed by Dr. Georges Burou, a French gynecologist, in the 1950s [1].

In 1965, Johns Hopkins University established the first multidisciplinary center for transgender care [4]. Here, experts in the medical, psychiatric, and surgical care of transgender patients were brought together in a team consisting of specialists in plastic surgery, gynecology, urology, endocrinology, psychiatry, and psychology. From the work of this group it was established that surgery for gender identity disorder was satisfying to patients who underwent the surgery.

Modern vaginoplasty techniques used in gender affirmation surgery have evolved from congenital vaginal reconstruction, adult reconstruction after pelvic resections for oncologic indications, and modifications of vaginoplasty as described for transgender women.

Demographics

Approximately, 0.61% of the global population (44 million individuals worldwide) can be diagnosed with gender dysphoria. However, some of these individuals do not desire surgery, or may not be candidates for it. It is estimated that approximately 1 in 37,000 natal males and 1 in 107,000 natal females have gender dysphoria. The true prevalence is likely greater [4].

In general, transgender male patients are more likely to seek treatment than transgender female patients. Compared with transgender women, transgender men are 4 times more likely to seek surgical treatment. The average age at transition is approximately 31 for transgender women, and these patients are more likely to be non-Caucasian and live in a rural setting, based on recent demographic studies [29].

It is unclear why there is a 4:1 discrepancy amongst transgender patients seeking surgery. Recent estimates indicate that about 1 in 12,000 transgender men and 1 in 30,400 transgender women undergo genital surgery for gender dysphoria each year [5]. With increased advocacy, acceptance, and access to care, it is likely that the numbers of transgender individual seeking care will rise in the future.

Preoperative Planning and Assessment

WPATH Guidelines

The World Professional Association for Transgender Health (WPATH) was formed in 1979 by Harry Benjamin to promote the understanding and treatment of gender dysphoria [6]. WPATH consists of professionals from many different disciplines such as medicine, psychology, law, social work, counseling, psychotherapy, family studies, sociology, anthropology, speech therapy, and sexology who are involved in the care of transgender individuals. WPATH publishes *Standards of Care for the Health of Transsexual, Transgender, and Gender Nonconforming People*, which contains guidelines on who is an operative candidate for both bottom and top surgery. It is in its seventh version [7].

The WPATH standards of care were established to increase and improve access to care for gender dysphoria given the scarcity of multidisciplinary gender clinics worldwide.

Currently, for those considering chest gender-affirming surgery ("top surgery"), WPATH [7] recommends that they have a letter from their treating mental health provider stating that they can cope with the psychological demands of the surgery, have been living as their desired gender for at least 12 months prior to surgery, and have reached the age of majority.

For patients seeking genital affirmation surgery, WPATH recommends: two letters from two different mental health providers, age of majority, and living as their desired gender for 12 months prior to surgery. One letter must come from an MD or PhD mental health professional, and must confirm long-standing, stable gender dysphoria, and the absence of any untreated mental illnesses that may interfere with decision making. A third letter is generally solicited from the patient's hormone provider, as WPATH recommends 12 months of continuous hormonal therapy prior to genital surgery [7]. In some cases, hormonal therapy is not possible or desired, and is not an absolute requirement.

It is recommended that the letters document the following:

1. The client's general identifying characteristics.
2. Results of the client's psychosocial assessment, including any diagnoses.
3. The duration of the mental health professional's relationship with the client, including the type of evaluation and therapy or counseling to date.
4. An explanation that the criteria for surgery have been met and a brief description of the clinical rationale for supporting the patient's request for surgery.
5. A statement about the fact that informed consent has been obtained from the patient.
6. A statement that the mental health professional is available for coordination of care and welcomes a phone call to establish this.

Our Practice Preferences

It is our practice to follow the WPATH guidelines as stated earlier [8]. We require our patients undergoing breast augmentation and bottom surgery to have a minimum of 12 months of continuous hormonal therapy prior to surgery, if hormone therapy is a part of their transition. The hormone provider letter should document the following: patient's legal and preferred name, date of birth, date patient relationship started and frequency of contact, date of therapy initiation and frequency of treatment and duration of therapy, and any contraindications to hormonal therapy.

Because transgender surgery is both potentially life threatening and essentially irreversible, we additionally require the mental health letters to document the following: patient's legal and preferred name, date of birth, date patient relationship started and frequency of contact, date of therapy initiation and frequency of treatment and

duration of therapy, a statement that the patient has been diagnosed with gender dysphoria, that the patient desires to live and be accepted as a member of the opposite sex, usually accompanied by the wish to make his/her body as congruent as possible with the preferred sex through surgery and hormonal treatments, the transgender identity has been present persistently for a least 2 years and the gender dysphoria is not a symptom of another mental health condition. The letter must also establish that gender dysphoria causes clinically significant distress or impairment in areas of social, occupational, or other important areas of functioning and that the patient has been living as the opposite sex for at least 12 months prior to surgery.

Considerations for Minors

With growing awareness that surgery allows for the physical expression of gender to be achieved, and increasing knowledge of the high risk of suicide and depression faced by patients who cannot get gender affirmation surgery, there have emerged patients under the age of 18 who desire surgical treatment of gender dysphoria. Some centers have begun treating these patients with puberty-suppressing medications such as GnRH analogs, aimed at relieving dysphoria/depression and preventing psychological harm by suppressing secondary sexual maturity at adolescence. Potentially, this relieves gender dysphoria and results in superior psychological and physical outcomes.

In general, WPATH does not recommend that minors undergo irreversible interventions such as genital surgery prior to reaching the age of majority [7]. However, these are not absolute contraindications to surgery, and future guidelines may suggest a safe and correct pathway to surgery for selected individuals under the age of 18.

Preoperative Patient-Related Factors

At the preoperative consultation, the goal is to determine if the patient can safely undergo surgery and cope with the psychiatric demands that their new anatomy will produce. Thus, it is imperative that they first obtain the mental health clearance as stated earlier. It is incumbent upon the surgeon to verify the diagnosis of gender dysphoria before surgery. According to J. J. Hage [6], "the surgeon remains responsible for any diagnosis on the basis of which he performs surgical interventions."

Patients also need to have been compliant with hormonal therapy, if chosen. It is also wise to assess any nicotine/tobacco use at this visit. Smoking or any nicotine use will impair wound healing and increase flap failure rates, and smokers should quit immediately and permanently. Similarly, obesity increases the risk of wound-healing complications [9–11]. Tobacco use should be halted a minimum of 6 weeks prior to surgery to reduce the risk of complications. If the patient's BMI is greater than 30, they are at increased risk of complications [11]. Many surgeons have an arbitrary BMI cutoff of 36, and patients are not offered genital reconstruction until this goal is met.

For transgender women seeking vaginoplasty, the physical exam should focus on past scars, body habitus, and note if a foreskin is present. It is particularly important to determine if there is an inguinal hernia and prior surgical scars on the penis or in the groin as these may affect the vascular supply and the ultimate length of the penile flap. The presence of hair on the penile shaft should be noted, as generally depilation of penile shaft hair is recommended preoperatively.

It is worth noting that the preoperative consultation can identify relative risk factors associated with higher rates of complications and these are not absolute contraindications to surgery. Lawrence, et al. reviewed 232 cases of transgender women and found that none regretted surgery outright and only 6% were occasionally regretful [12]. It is also important to set expectations for what surgery can realistically achieve. In our practice, we discuss societal, emotional, and sexual expectations postoperatively. Care for comorbid medical conditions are optimized preoperatively (excellent blood pressure control in hypertensive patients, excellent blood sugar control in diabetics) and "clearance" by treating specialists, if present, are mandatory.

Surgical Anatomy

Review of the Female Genital Anatomy

The goal of gender affirmation surgery is to create external genitalia that are congruent with the patient's desired gender. For transgender women, this involves the transformation of the penis, scrotum, and perineum into labia, clitoris, and vagina (Fig. 6.1).

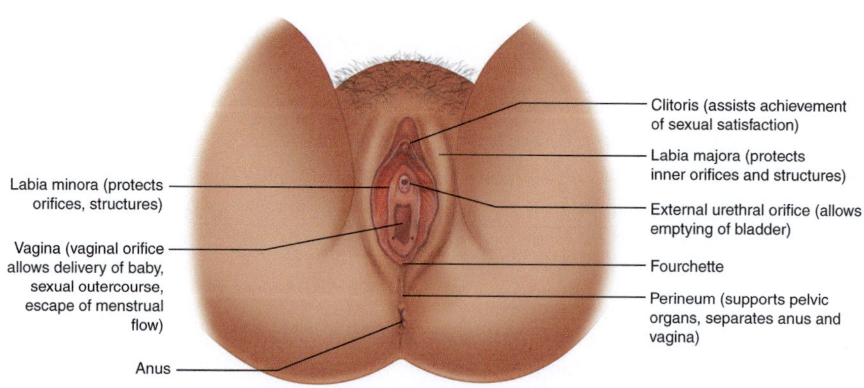

Fig. 6.1 Natal/Cis vagina with labeled structures

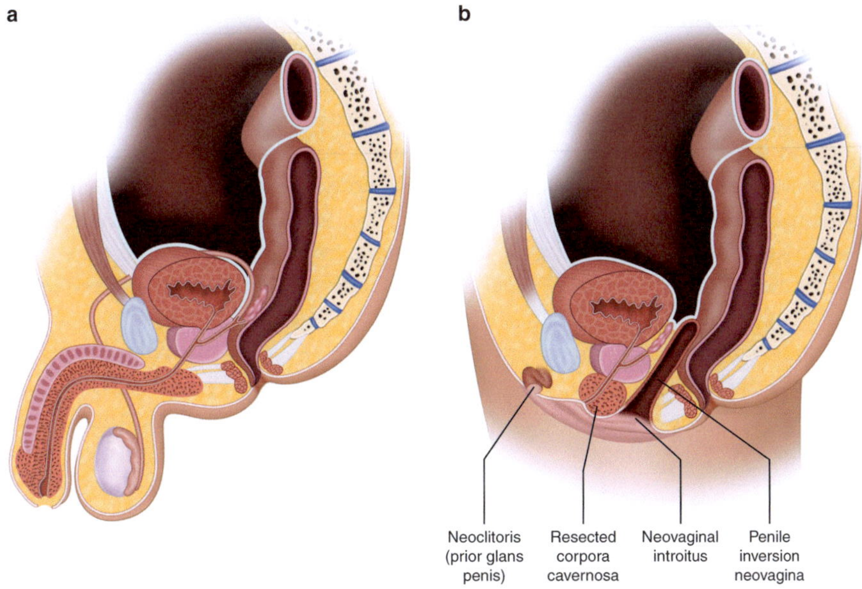

Fig. 6.2 Sagittal representation of natal male structures and the postoperative equivalent structures after vaginoplasty. (**a**) Natal male genital structures. (**b**) Typical anatomy of postoperative MTF patient after vaginoplasty

The creation of the neovagina in transgender women involves surgically creating a cavity between the rectum and the prostate internally. Externally, the labia minora, labia majora, introitus, and clitoris with its prepuce/clitoral hood are created. Finally, the urethra must be repositioned and shortened. To give the neovagina a normal appearance, the introitus, neovagina, labia minora, and clitoris and its hood should be hairless. A sagittal representation of the preoperative and postoperative anatomy is demonstrated in Fig. 6.2.

Aesthetic Parameters of Transgender Female Genitalia

The ideal vaginoplasty will create an aesthetically pleasing vagina. To do this, one must convert the natal male structures into a female appearance. This requires removal of the scrotum, formation of a sensate neoclitoris with prepuce, and feminine-appearing labia majora/minora [13].

Feminine-appearing labia majora will be smooth, graded in thickness from top to bottom and contiguous. They will coapt in the midline in some patients, usually those with higher amounts of subcuticular adipose tissue. Significant heterogeneity in labia majora size is present after vaginoplasty, just as in the natal female. The vestibule must also appear moist. The clitoris and its hood should be in the superior aspect and midline of the neolabia minora construct, with the neourethra approximately two-thirds the distance from the clitoris to the introitus. To prevent the clitoris from being placed too high, the authors recommend placing the neoclitoris at the line joining the adductor longus tendon similar to the landmark for puncture when performing a transobturator tap sling.

Creating a neovaginal cavity of sufficient depth and width to allow for penetrative sexual intercourse is important to many patients (although some patients may choose a simpler "zero depth" vaginoplasty in which a vaginal cavity is not surgically created). The cavity should measure approximately 14 cm deep by 6 cm in diameter to reduce the need for revision of the neovagina [30]. Larger and smaller introitus sizes may be possible/necessary depending on body habitus, just as in the natal female.

The ideal dimensions of the neovaginal cavity created are controversial. There is no "standard size" to create. However, based on FSTI scores of patients undergoing revision of the neovagina for inadequate depth it was found that a depth less than 6 cm was associated with an increased need for revision surgery [30]. It is worth noting that even if a neovagina of a sufficient depth is created, the cavity may shrink and become stenotic with time if regular intercourse is not had or dilations are discontinued [30].

Anatomy of Colon

The colon rarely may be used as an interposition flap to create the neovaginal cavity in transgender women. Due to this, a brief review of the clinically relevant anatomy of the colon is required.

The colon begins in the right lower quadrant at the cecum. The colon ascends along the right abdominal border as a secondarily retroperitoneal structure and proceeds toward the midline in the right upper quadrant. This portion of the colon is referred to as the ascending colon. The portion of colon traversing from right to left across the midline is the transverse colon. In some individuals this may be quite dependent and sag down to a much lower level than expected. In the left upper quadrant, the colon travels inferiorly toward the pelvis as the descending colon. Finally, as the colon takes a sharp turn into the pelvis it becomes the sigmoid colon, so named because of the sharp s-shape this portion of the colon assumes. The sigmoid colon joins the rectum. The rectum can be identified surgically by the coalescence of the tenia coli uniting to form an entire outer muscular layer and the lack of appendices epipolicae.

It is important to consider the segmental anatomy of the colon, because it has a well-defined and robust blood supply that permits its use as a pedicled visceral flap or "interposition graft." It is supplied by large named arteries off the inferior mesenteric (IMA) and superior mesenteric arteries (SMA). There is significant redundancy in the vasculature of the colonic angiosomes. The Marginal Artery of Drummond is an artery that is present approximately 80% of the time that directly connects the SMA and IMA angiosomes. Another SMA and IMA connection that may exist is the Arc of Riolan, which is also known as the meandering mesenteric artery.

If these are present, they allow one to perform aggressive mobilization and ligation of some vasculature of the colon when performing segmental colectomy or a pedicled colonic flap, as in vaginoplasty. However, great care must be taken to note the watershed areas if planning a large colonic flap to ensure that no ischemic colitis results. This is done clinically by observing for bleeding at the edges and color changes of the flap. Some have advocated using intravenous indocyanine green and the SPY system (Novadak Spy, Stryker, Kalamazoo, MI, USA) machine to ensure the remnants are viable. The segmental arterial supply and corresponding venous drainage of the colon is shown in Table 6.1. Clinically, the sigmoid colon may be mobilized on its mesentery creating a pedicled flap that may be used to elongate the vaginal cavity when sutured in place end-to-end, by keeping the proximal end sutured closed and the distal end in continuity with the neovagina. The advantages and disadvantages will be discussed later in more detail.

Table 6.1 Segmental blood supply of the colon

Segment	Arterial supply	Derivative artery	Venous drainage
Cecum	Anterior and posterior cecal	SMA	Anterior and posterior cecal
Ascending colon	Iliocolic, right colic	SMA	Iliocolic, right colic
Transverse colon	Right, middle and left colic	SMA&IMA	Right, middle and left colic
Descending colon	Left colic	IMA	Left colic
Sigmoid colon	Sigmoidal branches	IMA	Sigmoidal branches
Superior rectum	Superior hemorrhoidal	IMA	Superior hemorrhoidal

Anatomy of Perineum and Rectum

The perineum is defined as the region between the vulva or scrotum and the anus. Contained within this region are structures that are relevant to those performing vaginoplasty. Anteriorly, it is bounded by the pubic symphysis, posteriorly by the coccyx, laterally the inferior pubic and ischial rami with the roof formed by the pelvic floor, and the skin of the perineum forming the floor. The surface boundaries are the superior end of the intergluteal cleft posteriorly, laterally the medial thighs, and superiorly the penile base in males and the mons pubis in females.

It is separated into two triangles, the anterior urogenital and the posterior anal triangles by the line running between the bilateral ischial tuberosities (Fig. 6.3).

The urogenital triangle contains the external genitalia and the distal extent of the urinary tract. This area contains a complex layered anatomy distinct from the anal triangle. From superficial to deep, the layers are: skin, subcutaneous tissue, superficial perineal fascia, deep perineal fascia, perineal membrane, and finally the muscular pelvic floor (Fig. 6.4). The superficial perineal fascia has two layers: (1) Superficial layer, which is continuous with Camper's fascia; and (2) Colles fascia, which is continuous with Scarpa's fascia of the abdomen. The deep perineal fascia covers the perineal muscles and protruding structures of the pelvis (penis and clitoris). The perineal membrane is a tough fascia that provides an origin for the pelvic muscles of the external genitalia.

Between the layers of perineal fascia lie the perineal pouches [16]. These consist of the super-

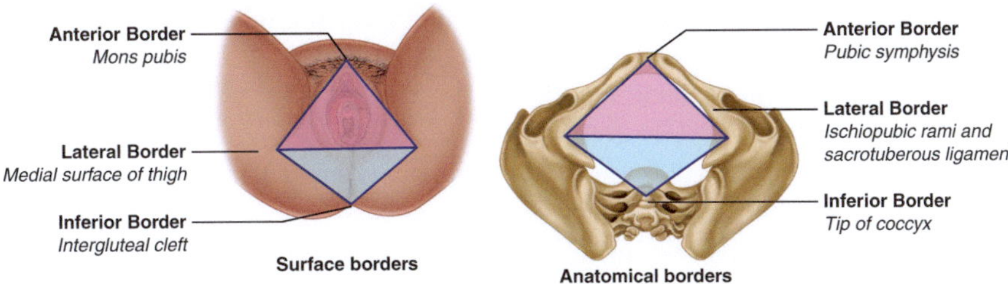

Fig. 6.3 The perineal triangles, contents, and borders

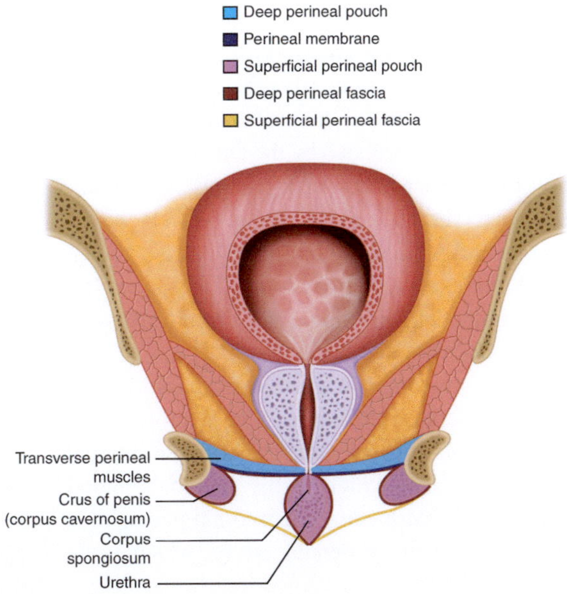

Fig. 6.4 The perineal fascial layers and perineal pouches

ficial and deep perineal pouches similarly to the perineal fascia. The deep perineal pouch is a potential space located between the deep fascia of the pelvic floor and the perineal membrane. It contains part of the urethra, external urethral sphincter, and the vagina in the female. In males, it also contains the bulbourethral glands and the deep transverse perineal muscles. The superficial perineal pouch is another potential space between the perineal membrane and the superficial perineal membrane. It contains the erectile tissues that form the penis and clitoris, and three muscles – the ischiocavernosus, bulbospongiosus, and superficial transverse perineal muscles. The greater vestibular glands (Bartholin's glands) are also located in the superficial perineal pouch. The pouch is bounded posteriorly to the perineal body.

The perineal body is an important structure that spans the anal and urogenital triangles and must be preserved. It is an irregular fibromuscular mass that is at the center of the perineum. It is made up of an amalgam of skeletal muscle, smooth muscle, elastin, and dense collagen fibers. It serves a point of attachment for the pelvic floor muscles and the perineum. The pelvic floor portion of levator ani, the bulbospongiosus, superficial and deep transverse perineal muscles, and both the external urethral and anal sphincters have insertions into it.

The anal triangle contains the external anal sphincter, ischiorectal fossae, and the anal aperture. It is bounded anteriorly by the posterior limit of the urogenital triangle, the theoretical line joining the two ischial tuberosities together. Posteriorly it is bounded by the coccyx, and laterally by the sacrotuberous ligaments. The dominant innervation to the perineum travels within its bilateral ischiorectal fossae, otherwise known as Alcock's canal. The ischiorectal fossae are fat-filled potential spaces that allow the rectum to expand during defecation.

The perineum is innervated primarily by the pudendal nerve. This nerve is derived from S2-S4 ventral rami. This nerve travels with the internal pudendal artery, which is the dominant blood supply to the perineum. The internal pudendal is derived from the pudendal artery, which is an internal branch of the internal iliac in the majority of individuals. The pudendal nerve and internal pudendal artery travel within Alcock's Canal.

Alcock's Canal is a space formed by the obturator fascia on the deep surface of the ischial tuberosities. It is found within the ischiorectal fossa and contains the internal pudendal artery and the pudendal nerve.

The pudendal nerve gives rise to the terminal innervation of the glans, scrotum, and the erogenous zones of the genitals and perineum. It must be preserved.

Similarly, the internal pudendal artery differentiates into the dominant pedicle for the penoscrotal skin. The penoscrotal skin is supplied by the dorsal penile arteries and the scrotal arteries for the penis and scrotum, respectively. These must be handled with care to prevent flap loss and wound-healing complications. The dominant venous drainage of this area is the deep dorsal vein of the penis, which drains in turn to the prostatic plexus.

Vaginoplasty Techniques

Today, there exist three well-described methods of creating a neovagina and external genitalia for transgender women. These are inversion vaginoplasty (usually with an additional scrotal skin graft), peritoneal vaginoplasty, and visceral interposition vaginoplasty. Each is described in detail below.

Current recommendations for management of hormones before surgery are in flux and are discussed in detail in Chap. 3. Typically, progesterone administration is halted 2 weeks prior to surgery to reduce the risk of venous thromboembolism (VTE). Many surgeons also halt estradiol, although we now allow up to 4 mg/day oral estradiol up until the day of surgery. We hold oral estradiol for 48 h after surgery and then restart at the patient's normal dose when they are ambulating.

Regardless of technique chosen, bowel prep is administered. Prior to induction of general anesthesia sequential compression devices are applied, and chemoprophylaxis against VTE is given per institutional policy. The patient is positioned in lithotomy using the surgeon's choice of positioning aid. The patient's temperature is regulated using a forced-air upper body warming blanket. Finally, after prepping and draping in a sterile fashion, the indwelling urinary catheter is inserted by the surgeon to ensure sterility since it is in the field. If robotic-assisted or laparoscopic harvest of bowel or colon is undertaken, the patient may be positioned differently.

With greater acceptance of gender dysphoria today, there are elderly or medically comorbid patients seeking surgical care as part of their treatment. In this group, it is recommended to investigate the potential for iliofemoral occlusive disease prior to embarking on surgery, with an angiogram or computed tomographic angiogram because of the small caliber of the vasculature supplying the pelvic skin. The skin of the flaps created in each technique is dependent on the terminal branches of the external pudendal deep and superficial branches (skin of external genitalia, perineum, medial thighs) and internal pudendal arteries (branches to bulb, penile urethra, and deep and dorsal penile branches). The external pudendal artery is derived from the common femoral artery as it branches just distal to the inguinal ligament. The internal pudendal artery arises from the internal iliac artery. Patients may choose a so-called zero depth vaginoplasty if they do not anticipate ever wanting vaginal penetration, or have comorbidities that may make this less involved surgery a safer option for them.

Standard Inversion Technique

Prior to scheduling surgery, the authors recommend the patient complete hair removal either by laser or electrolysis so that the penile shaft is hairless. This may reduce intravaginal hair growth postoperatively. We do not recommend scrotal hair removal as this tissue will be thinned to a split thickness skin graft and hair growth does not occur. Additional hair removal is at the patient's prerogative but is not necessary for successful surgery. Depilation may take up to 1 year

to complete, and this should be factored in when scheduling surgery. Hair removal should not be done within 2 weeks of surgery because it can damage some of the subdermal plexuses required to keep your penile skin flaps alive, and increases the risk of infection.

Penile disassembly and inversion vaginoplasty is the most common means of vaginoplasty used today.

When performing reconstructive surgery such as this, it is important to keep in mind what structures are being formed into which new structures, so that the patient can be marked appropriately, and the surgery conducted in an efficient manner. The labia majora are formed from the lateral periscrotal skin after orchiectomy, after removal of most of the scrotal cap for use as skin graft to augment the vaginal canal (Fig. 6.5). The clitoris is generated from the reduced glans. The labia minora are created from lateral neovaginal tissue, and the neoclitoris is brought through the center of the urethral flap to ensure a moist appearance of the vestibule, and allow for some lubrication with arousal. The penile urethra is shortened, spatulated, and everted allowing for creation of the inner labia minora, urethral meatus, and vestibular lining [14].

We and others use split thickness skin grafts harvested from the otherwise-discarded scrotum to augment the vaginal depth. It is sewn on to the inverted penile skin flap over a silicone mold (Fig. 6.6). Rarely, in cases of very large penis size or occasional uncircumcised patients with ample penile skin, this may not be required. Additional skin grafts are seldom required, but if so, they may be obtained from an elliptical skin incision via a pfannenstiel or lateral flank incision [15].

After positioning and draping the patient, the scrotum is marked out and injected with lidocaine or bupivacaine containing epinephrine to control bleeding and provide preemptive local anesthesia. The perineal body is identified and marked, indicating the location of the vaginal introitus. Some surgeons use a perineal flap to further augment the inverted penile skin vaginal lining, although we do not as we get excellent vaginal depth without it and it may introduce hair

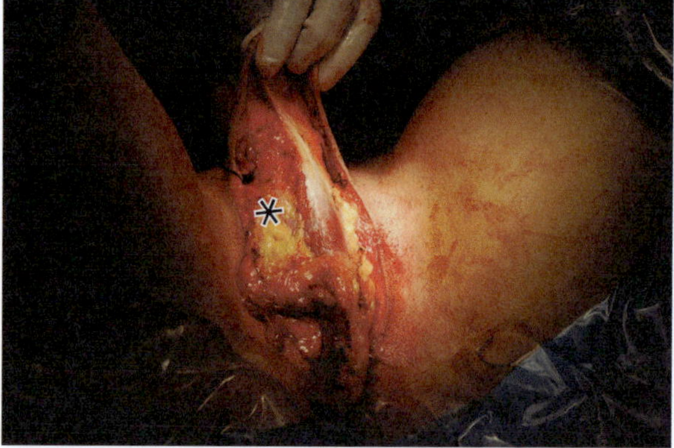

Fig. 6.5 Scrotum removed, sparing underlying fat for use in labia majora reconstruction. * Denotes subscrotal fat

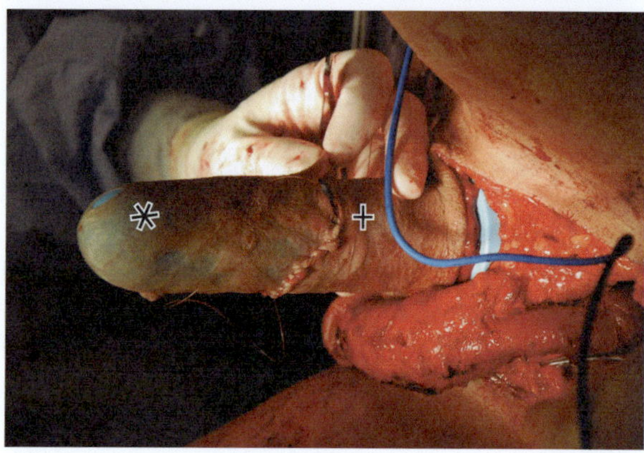

Fig. 6.6 Involuted penile skin flap is sewn to thinned scrotum to create neovagina. * Denotes scrotal skin graft; + Denotes penile skin flap

bearing skin into the introitus (Fig. 6.7). This is marked out if it is to be used. Typically, only a limited perineal flap will be used to create a tensionless posterior vaginal wall. The anterior limit is marked by measuring from the perineal body to the penoscrotal junction along the perineal midline raphe. The markings are joined in a "v-shaped" manner staying within the confines of the scrotal boundary creating smooth, graded, and continuous-appearing labia majora. The posterior limit of the flap is marked convexly parallel to the anus. By utilizing a "v-shaped" design, the risk of introital contracture is reduced. This flap is elevated in the extrasphincteric plane and centered anterior to the anus. Great care must be taken to avoid injury to the external sphincter and rectum. This flap is meant to be thin with its base elevated to create a broad subcutaneous pedicle without giving the posterior commissure a rectangular appearance.

Penile skin is then circumferentially dissected from the corona, preserving the dartos fascia maximally on the penile skin flap. The degloved penis is then delivered from the tubular skin flap.

After removal of scrotal skin, access to the testicles and spermatic cords is obtained via the midline incision, allowing for orchiectomy (Fig. 6.5). This is accomplished by resection of the spermatic cords at the external inguinal ring so they are not prominently visible or palpable.

After, orchiectomy, the vaginal cavity is created. A space is created between the rectum and the prostate. To do this, cautery is used to make a midline incision through the perineal fascia into the deep perineal pouch, taking care to avoid injury to its contents. The levator ani are identified and may need to be incised laterally using cautery to allow lateral expansion of the neovaginal cavity. Dissection continues until the peritoneal reflection is identified by following Denonvilliers fascia to its terminus (Fig. 6.8). While dissecting, it is imperative to avoid iatrogenic injury to the rectum. Dissection is complete once the cavity is at least 14×6 cm in dimension.

After the vaginal cavity has been created, the bulbospongiosus and ischiocavernosus muscles are resected (Fig. 6.9). By resecting these, the introitus is enlarged and the erectile structures of the penis are easily identified for later resection.

After identification of the erectile structures of the penis, the penis is disassembled. The glans is separated from the penis by dissecting deep to Buck's Fascia and identifying and maximally preserving the neurovascular pedicle to it. The urethra is separated from the glans at this point. The glans is then dissected proximally to the pubic symphysis, while maintaining its

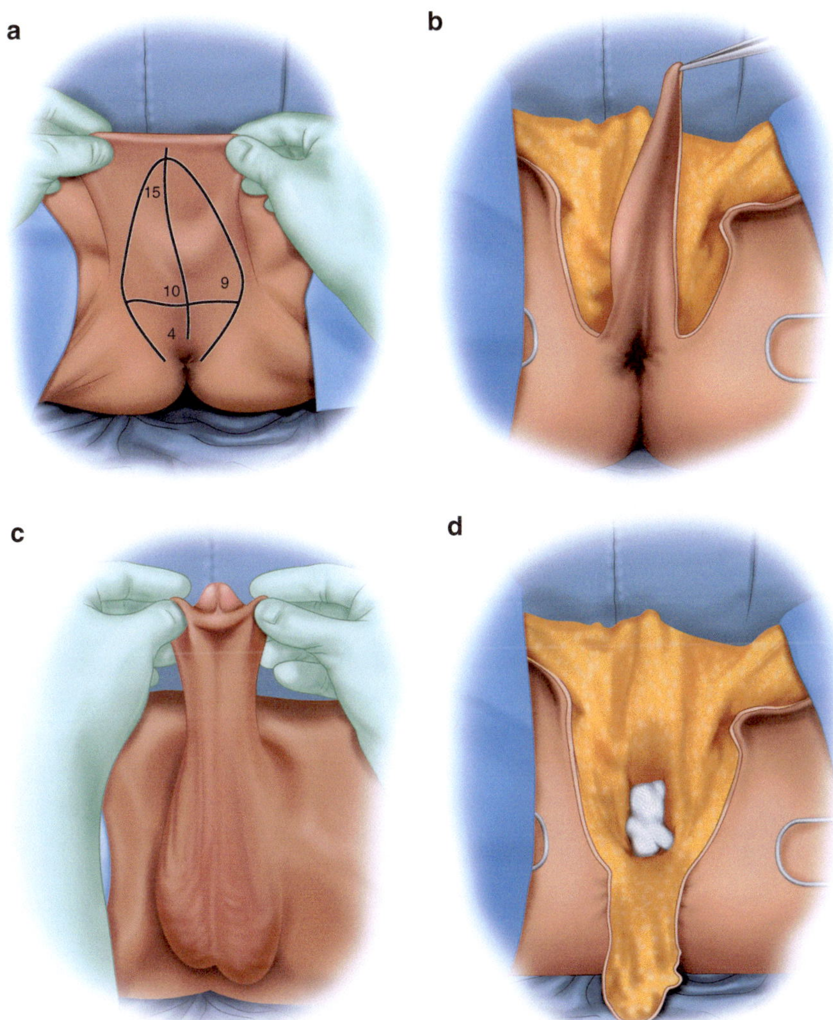

Fig. 6.7 (**a–e**) Creation of perineal skin flap to augment vaginal depth. (**a**) Scrotum held on stretch demonstrating markings of quadrangularly shaped skin flap design and measurements of 9–10 cm lateral from the perineal body, 4 cm posterior to perineal body and 10 cm anterior to perineal body with a total length of ~15 cm. (**b**) An example of an elevated perineal skin flap. (**c**) The penis is held on stretch to estimate size of the penile skin flap so that the surgeon may determine if the neovaginal cavity will require augmentation with either a flap or graft to enable sufficient depth. (**d**) An example of a completely dissected neovaginal space, perineal skin flap, and penile flaps with packing in the neovaginal cavity. (**e**) A sagittal representation of the neovaginal cavity created in relation to the pelvic structures

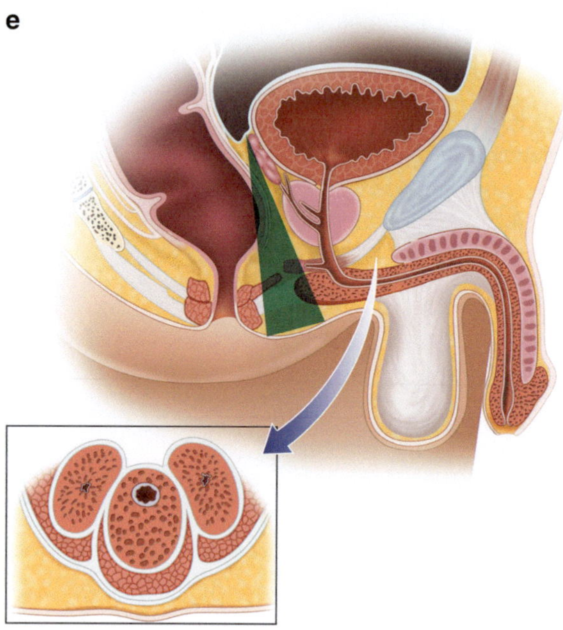

Fig. 6.7 (continued)

neurovascular pedicle. The penile urethra is circumferentially dissected and separated from the erectile tissue prior to resection.

At this point, the erectile tissue is resected at the pubis, leaving a short remnant to establish a base for the neoclitoris by suturing the remnants together [16]. Dissection of the glans neurovascular pedicle to the pubic symphysis exposes the bases of the corpora cavernosa, enabling their resection (Fig. 6.10). The corpora spongiousum is separated from the bulbar urethra, and then resected and oversewn here (Fig. 6.10). Resection of erectile tissue is necessary to prevent engorgement during arousal and limit penetration of the vagina. Prior to resection of the corpora, they should be suture ligated at their bases to prevent bleeding.

The neoclitoris is then fashioned from the dorsal glans (Fig. 6.10). At this point, the dorsal glans has been raised as a pedicled flap perfused by the dorsal penile artery and innervated by its dorsal penile nerve. This enables erogenous sensation. The glans is then shaped and sutured to the corporal base created previously. The neurovascular pedicle is sutured to the fascia of the anterior abdominal wall loosely affixed in place.

Now, the skin flaps are ready to be positioned. The penile flap/scrotal skin complex is advanced into the vaginal cavity after suturing the penile and scrotoperineal flaps together, creating a tubularized construct. They are then inverted and advanced into the neovagina. Fibrin sealant may be used to assist with flap inset. Drains are placed depending on surgeon preference, although we do not routinely place drains.

Next, the labia minora and clitoral hood must be constructed. This begins by making in incision in the penile skin flap and bringing the opened urethra/clitoris complex through it (Fig. 6.11). The neoclitoris is introduced to the flap at its superior extent leaving some redundancy above its inset to create a clitoral hood. The neoclitoris is brought through a small slit in the flap. Next, the neourethral meatus is placed in a position congruent with that of a natal female, usually, about two-thirds the distance from the introitus to the clitoris. See Fig. 6.12 for a visual representation of the completed vaginal cavity prior to insetting the labia majora and minora.

Lastly, the remaining scrotal skin is used to create the labia majora. This is done by tailoring it to the free edges of the wound and suturing it

Neovaginal cavity

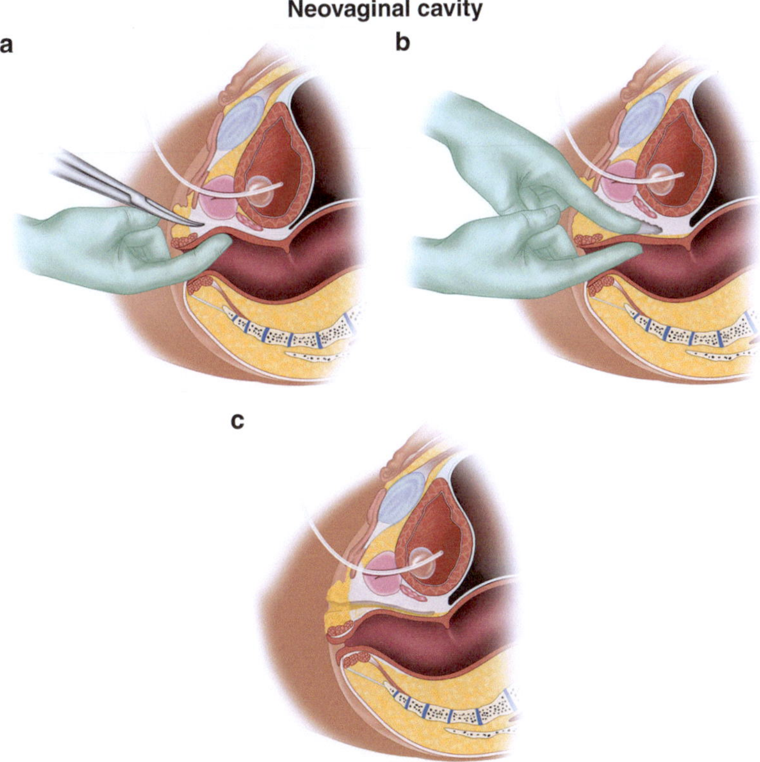

Fig. 6.8 (**a–c**) Penile Inversion Vaginoplasty sagittal anatomy of vaginal cavity dissection. (**a**) Dissection begins by incising the pelvic floor at the base of the penile bulb. (**b**) Dissection continues posterior to the penile bulb and posterior to the prostate. Care must be taken to stay anterior to Denovillier's fascia preventing rectal perforation. (**c**) Completed dissection of vaginal cavity in sagittal view: Dissection continues cephalad until the superior extent of the bladder is encountered. At this point a finger will be able to palpate the dome of the bladder. This provides a depth of 9–15 cm depending on patient anatomy. Care must be taken not to perforate the rectum during this dissection

Fig. 6.9 Bulbospongiosus muscle is dissected off the urethra and removed. * Denotes corpora spongiosum and urethra

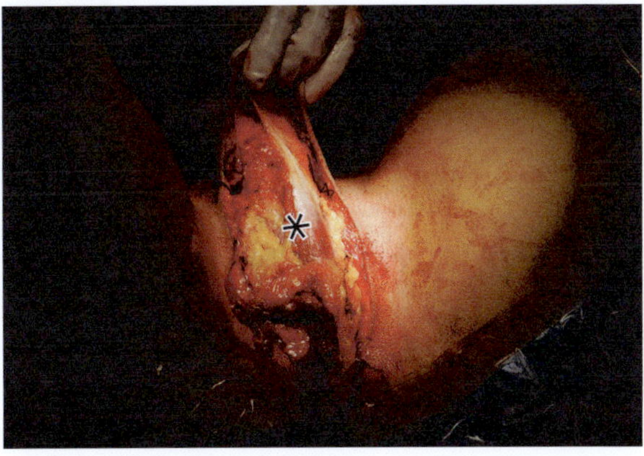

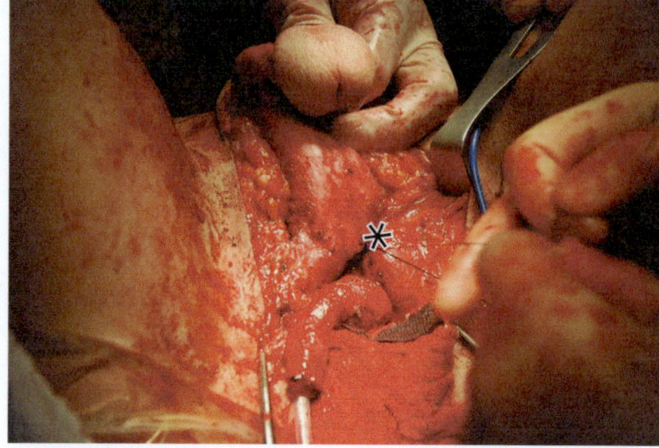

Fig. 6.10 Proximal corpora cavernosa is suture ligated to prevent bleeding prior to partial penectomy and clitoroplasty. * Denotes ligated corpora cavernosa

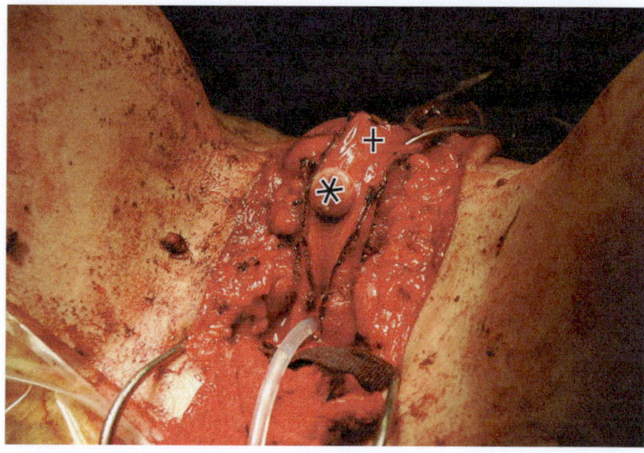

Fig. 6.11 Bulbar urethra is divided to seat neoclitoris. * Denotes neoclitoris; + denotes divided bulbar urethra

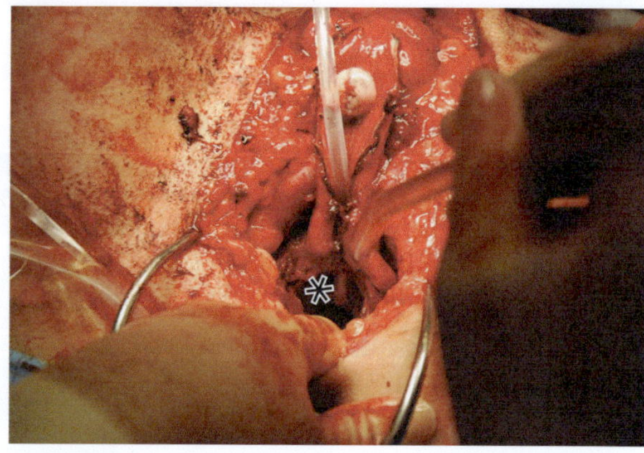

Fig. 6.12 Deep vaginal cavity is created between rectum and prostate. Cavity measures 14 cm deep × 6 cm wide. * Denotes neovaginal cavity

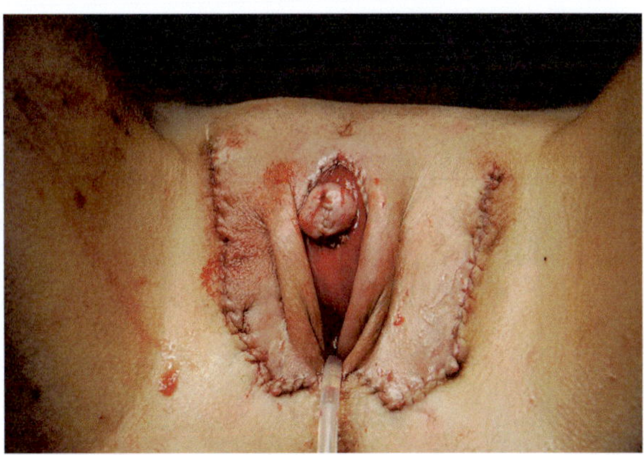

Fig. 6.13 Final result showing pink mucosal introitus, labia minora, and labia majora

closed in layers using the surgeon's choice of absorbable sutures (Fig. 6.13).

Finally, vaginal packing is placed in the vaginal cavity to serve as a bolster to improve the adherence and take of the flaps to the underlying tissue. This remains until post-op day 5–7, as does the urinary catheter.

If, postoperatively, the patient is not pleased with how the labia majora coapt, or if the clitoris is not adequately covered by labia majora, a second-stage labiaplasty can be performed later, which is beyond the scope of this chapter.

It is worth noting, there are variations of this operation reported and in use today. The most common modification uses a portion of the urethra in the introitus to lengthen the penile flap and lubricate the cavity [17]. Less commonly, the glans has been used to create a neocervix when desired [18].

Postoperatively, at our center, the patient is admitted to the hospital for 48 h. Early ambulation is assisted. When the vaginal packing is removed on post-op day 5–7, the urinary catheter is also removed.

After removing the packing, scheduled vaginal dilation is begun. Most surgeons have their patients dilate the vaginal cavity three or four times a day for the first 6 weeks. The frequency of dilation is gradually reduced over the next 3 months. Ultimately, the patient will need to self-dilate their neovagina only two to three times a week. The authors also recommend intermittent intravaginal douching to remove intravaginal debris, starting 1 month postoperatively and continuing two to three times a week as needed.

Visceral Interposition (Fig. 6.14)

Typically, visceral interposition vaginoplasty is reserved for cases of congenital vaginal agenesis, grossly insufficient penile length, and some revision vaginoplasty cases. Either small bowel or sigmoid colon may be used, although sigmoid is most common.

It is used rarely in primary gender affirmation surgery because it requires an intra-abdominal operation to harvest the viscera, and carries with it increased risks associated with laparotomy and potential colon anastomosis leak. Prior to sigmoid interposition vaginoplasty, the patient must have a colonoscopy to exclude malignancy. Many patients complain of foul-smelling mucous discharge afterward. Furthermore, an annual speculum exam of the sigmoid vagina is required to assess for possible malignancy.

Intestinal vaginoplasty does have some benefits that make it an option for revision cases. It provides a vascularized, tubular structure that provides its own mucous allowing for an easier

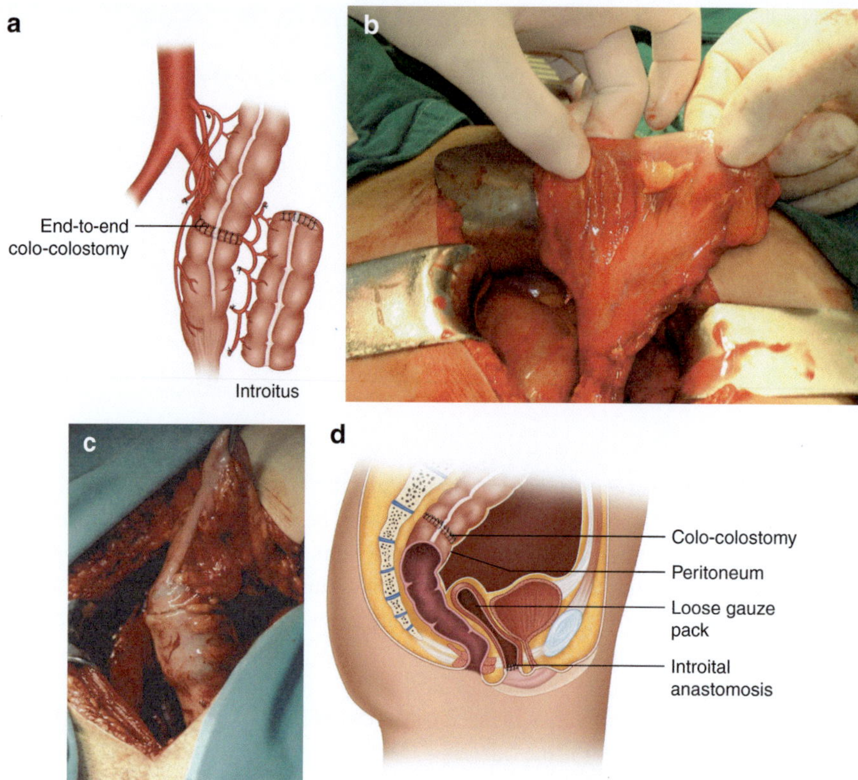

Fig. 6.14 (**a**) Blood supply to the sigmoid colon and rectum. Harvesting of the rectosigmoid segment for vaginal construction. (**b**) A very short segment of rectosigmoid colon with highly mobile mesentery is harvested. (**c**) Colorectal anastomoses as performed using staple devices. (**d**) Two semicircular incisions are made (inset). Vascularized lateral flaps are created and completely mobilized to anastomose with sigmoid segment as deep as possible. (**b**, **c**: from Djordjevic et al. [31])j Dsm_2494 3487..(DjordD

inset into a previously operated field from prior vaginoplasty. It also reduces the possibility of needing continuous dilations.

It is recommended that two teams perform intestinal vaginoplasty. Most commonly, a total laparoscopic approach or a hand-assisted laparoscopic approach (HALS) is used to obtain the colon. If HALS is used, it is recommended that a Pfannensteil incision be used for the hand port to minimize the risk of incisional hernia and scarring.

A segment of 12–15 cm of bowel is required. The segment is transferred in an isoperistalic direction and sutured end-to-end into the vaginal cavity, and the fecal stream united intra-abdominally by the general surgery team. The colon is mobilized in a manner similar to that of a low anterior resection (Fig. 6.15). The mesentery of the donated colon may be sutured to the pelvic brim to prevent torsion. If possible, it is recommended to place omentum between the suture lines. Then the external genitalia are created as described previously.

Postoperatively, the cavity is packed for 48–72 h. The urinary catheter remains for the same amount of time. Postoperative antibiotics are stopped after 24 h post-op. VTE chemoprophylaxis is stopped once the patient is ambulatory. The patient is taught how to dilate her introitus.

Peritoneal Vaginoplasty

Recently, some centers have begun to augment the inverted penile flap canal utilizing pelvic peritoneum to line the deep neovaginal cavity. This was originally proposed for neovaginal con-

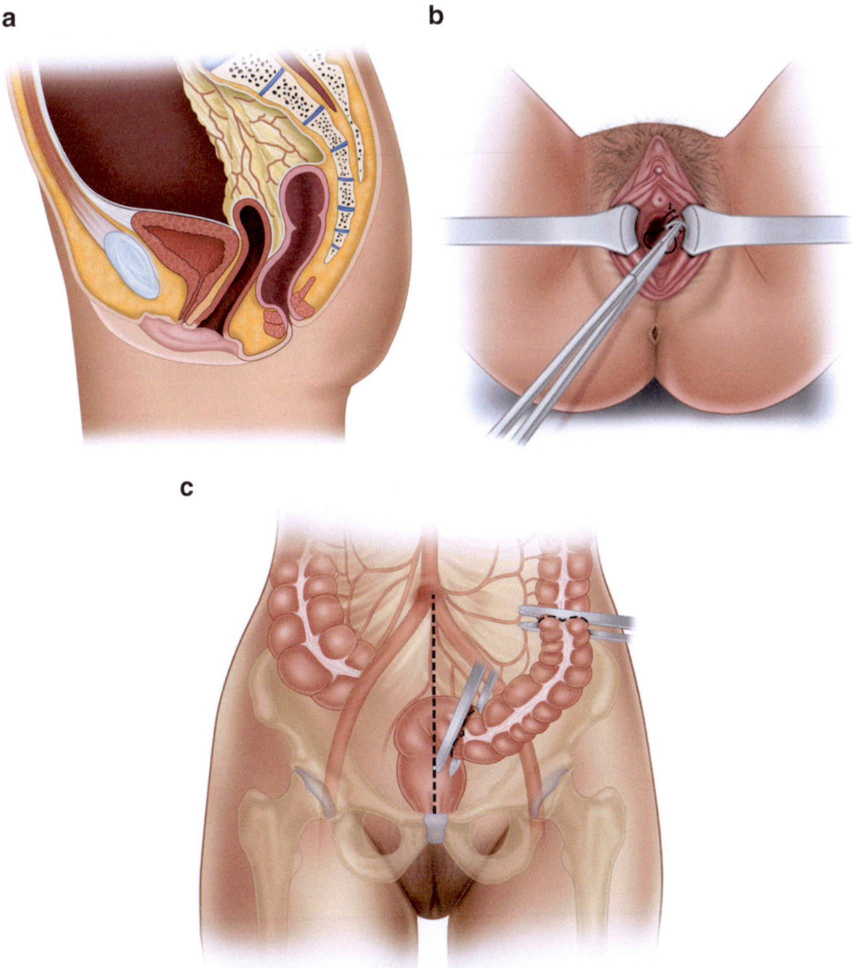

Fig. 6.15 (**a–c**) Visceral interposition vaginoplasty. (**a**) A schematic representation of pelvic anatomy in a sagittal view after inset of a visceral interposition neovaginal flap. (**b**) The surgeon's view when insetting the distal end of the visceral neovaginal flap to the cutaneous neovaginal flap. (**c**) A diagrammatic representation of pedicled colon flap harvest using linear staplers

struction in patients with vaginal agenesis as a result of Mayer-Rokitansky-Kurster-Hauser Syndrome (Fig. 6.16). This was first reported in 1969 by Davydov [19].

Augmentation of the neovaginal cavity with pelvic peritoneum in transgender women may have advantages, especially in cases of insufficient penile skin perhaps in patients who had puberty blockade. However, it adds time, expense, and complexity to the operation, which may not be necessary, as standard inverted penile flap vaginoplasty with scrotal skin graft augmentation achieves excellent vaginal depth in the

majority of patients. Figure 6.17 demonstrates the relation of surrounding structures to the dissection depth for a cis-male pelvis to serve as a guide to the surgeon.

The operation commences similarly to the standard penile inversion and disassembly technique, with some differences (Fig. 6.18). The surgeon creates the neovaginal cavity between the bladder and rectum as previously described. Pincers are used to grasp the peritoneum and a small incision is used to drain the rectovesicular pouch. After this, the incision is enlarged and with retraction (upward, anteriorly, and posteri-

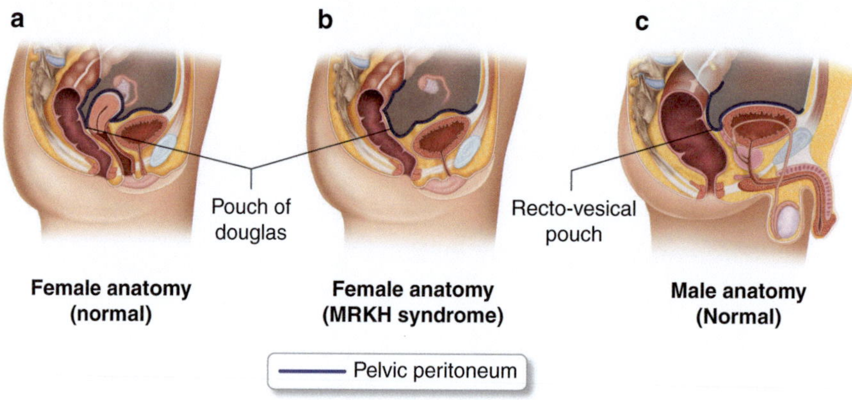

Fig. 6.16 (**a–c**) Sagittal representation of the anatomy present in (a) cis-female, (b) cis-female with MRKH Syndrome, and (**c**) cis-male

Fig. 6.17 Sagittal representation of the depth of neovaginal cavity dissection in relation to surrounding cis-male pelvic structures to guide the surgeon intraoperatively

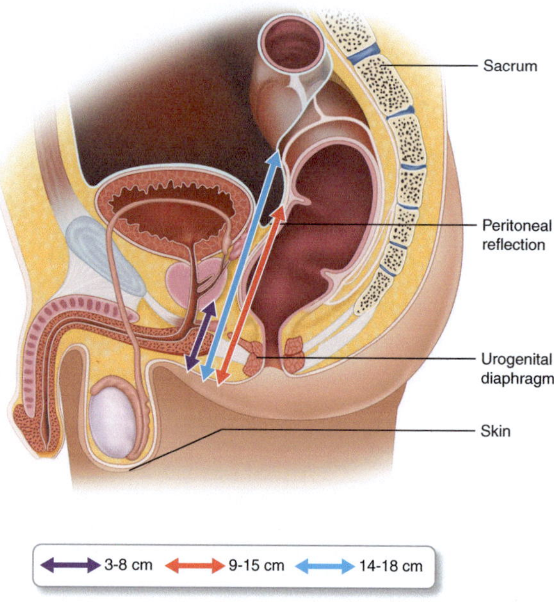

orly), the posterior pelvic peritoneum is pulled down to the vaginal cavity and sutured to the introitus using interrupted sutures of 0 chromic. The caudal end of the cavity is then sutured closed after verifying that there is adequate depth of the vagina for penetration. This typically is 10–12 cm in length. Care must be taken to tack the anterior rectum to the peritoneum to prevent an enterocele from developing. Finally, as before, a vaginal dilator, mold, or packing is placed in the vagina to enable the space to stay patent.

It may take up to 6 months for the entire neovagina to re-epithelialize with nonkeratinized stratified squamous epithelium of the peritoneum.

After Discharge Care Pathway

Upon discharge, patients are educated about the expected milestones. They are instructed to engage in light activity, lifting not more than 15

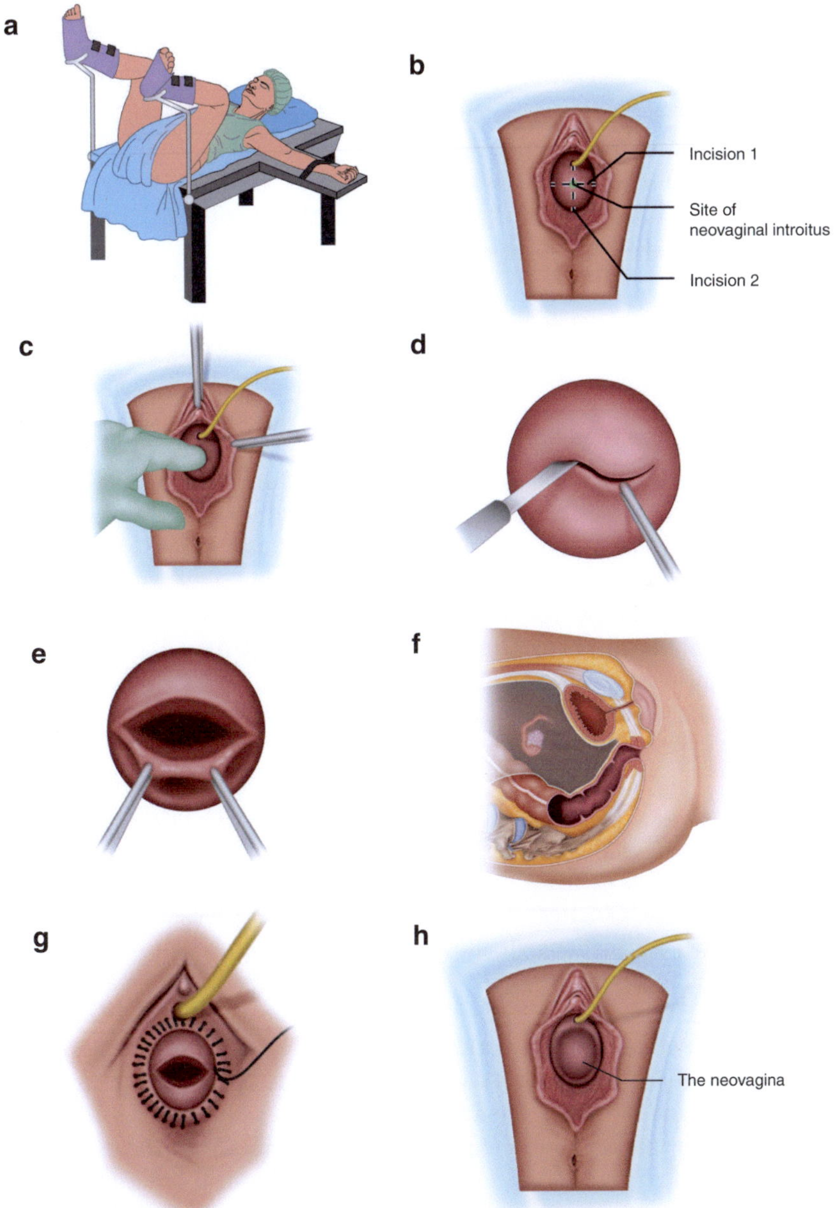

Fig. 6.18 (**a–h**) Operative details for peritoneal vaginoplasty. (**a**) Standard operative positioning for vaginoplasty using stirrups. (**b**) A schematic representation of the planned incisions for creation of a peritoneum augmented vaginal introitus. (**c**) The area of dissection is identified by palpating the posterior pelvic peritoneum prior to beginning dissection. (**d**) The posterior pelvic peritoneum is incised beginning the dissection of the flap. (**e**) The initial elevation of the posterior peritoneal flap. (**f**) Sagittal representation of the anatomy present in a cis-female. (**g**) Peritoneal flap is sutured to the cutaneous portion of the neovagina using 0 chromic sutures. (**h**) Peritoneal flap is inset into neovagina

pounds and maintaining pelvic rest for at least 6 weeks after surgery. If patients are traveling for surgery, it is recommended that they stay near their operating surgeon for at least 2 weeks before traveling home.

At discharge, they are encouraged to wear loose clothing. It is recommended they avoid tight elastic straps in the groin to ease the post-op edema. The authors recommend patients place an absorbent pad in their underwear. Ambulation and leg elevation are encouraged, and time spent sitting is limited in an attempt to reduce swelling of the perineum.

After 6 weeks, they can return gradually to their activities without restriction. They can engage in sexual intercourse at this time as well.

Outcomes

Patient Satisfaction

Appropriately selected patients are extremely satisfied after undergoing vaginoplasty. For many, this represents the culmination of their journey to have the world see them as they see themselves by having gender-affirming genital surgery. There are several preoperative factors that can help the surgeon avoid operating on patients likely to experience dissatisfaction with vaginoplasty. These include: personal and social stability, age over 30 at the time of surgery, and a well-defined support system.

Sexual Function

Vaginoplasty provides an excellent tool for patients desiring gender affirmation as it allows for urologic and sexual function in over 90% of patients undergoing the operation. Recently, German researchers surveyed their patients who had primary inversion vaginoplasty performed between 2004 and 2010 and found that over 90% of them were able to achieve regular orgasms [20].

Revision Rates

Little data currently exist on surgical revision rates. In the past, vaginoplasty was a two-stage procedure with a planned labiaplasty. However, as surgical techniques evolved, vaginoplasty has evolved in most centers into a single-stage operation. The most common reason for revision is introital stenosis, which is reported to be 4.1% in penile inversion vaginoplasty and 1.2% of vis-

ceral vaginoplasties according to a recent systematic review performed by Horbach et al. in [21]. The management of this must be tailored to each individual patient.

Patient Regrets

According to Lawrence et al. [27], regret after gender affirmation surgery is rare. They reported in their review of over 200 patients that 0 patients outright regretted having the feminizing surgery. They did find however, that approximately 6% of their patients experienced occasional regret. They found that dissatisfaction was due to poor surgical results, not due to other factors associated with poor satisfaction as stated above.

Complications

Immediate Perioperative Complications

Fortunately, vaginoplasty is a safe and effective procedure with an acceptably low complication rate [22–28]. Injury to the bladder, urethra, and rectum are rare, but can occur. If injury to one of these vital surrounding structures occurs, intraoperative diagnosis and treatment is best. If there is a rectal injury it should be closed in layers.

Other early complications include: abscess, surgical site infection, flap loss, failure of skin graft take, insufficient vaginal cavity depth, urinary stream abnormalities, and dehiscence. Dehiscence, usually of the inferior vaginal introitus where the penile flap edge is at most risk for tissue ischemia, is most common.

Vaginal Stenosis

The introitus or vaginal canal can become strictured and stenotic. If the patient is able to tolerate it, this can be managed with serial dilations. If the vaginal introitus only is narrowed, y-v plasty: usually bringing in perineal skin to enlarge the opening may be curative. Revision vaginoplasty, usually with placement of skin grafts into incision made in the vagina, may be required. In some severe/recalcitrant cases, it may be necessary to create a new neovaginal lining with either viscera or pelvic peritoneum.

Rectovaginal Fistula

Occasionally, rectovaginal fistulas do occur after vaginoplasty, despite careful technique. They may occur early or late. Most often, these patients will have had a rectal injury that was repaired and failed, or an undiagnosed rectal injury. If this occurs, they will require fecal diversion, resection of the fistula, and revision of the vaginoplasty.

Conclusions

Vaginoplasty is a safe, effective and satisfying operation for MTF patients. It provides the transfemale with a functioning vagina that is cosmetically pleasing. The neovagina allows for erogenous sensation to be preserved and full sexual function postoperatively. The complication profile is sufficiently low to warrant widespread adoption of vaginoplasty into the standard armamentarium of surgeons performing bottom surgery.

Take-Home Points
- Vaginoplasty is the most common bottom surgery performed.
- It is recommended to follow WPATH guidelines for genital surgery and obtain letters from treating mental health providers (two per WPATH) and one from hormone provider verifying they are ready for surgery and have completed 12 months of continuous hormonal therapy.
- Penile Inversion Vaginoplasty is the most common method for creation of neovagina.

- Alternative vaginoplasty techniques include visceral interposition, and peritoneal vaginoplasty.
- Complication rates are low with most complications related to wound-healing issues that are managed conservatively with local wound care.
- Patients report excellent functional and cosmetic outcomes after surgery, including the ability to achieve climax.
- Revision rates are low with neovaginal stenosis being the most common reason for revision surgery.

References

1. Edgerton MT, Knorr NJ, Callison JR. The surgical treatment of transsexual patients limitations and indications. Plast Reconstr Surg. 1970;45(1):38–50.
2. Ettner R, Monstrey S, Coleman E, editors. Surgery: male-to-female patients. In: Principles of transgender medicine and surgery. New York: Routledge; 2016.
3. Hirschfeld M. Die intersexuelle konstitution. Jahrbuch fur Sexuelle Zwishenstufen. 1923;23:3–27.
4. Schechter LS. The surgeon's relationship with the physician prescribing hormones and the mental health professional: review for version 7 of the World Professional Association for Transgender Health's Standards of Care. Int J Transgend. 2009;11(4):222–5.
5. Monstrey S, Hoebeke P, Dhont M, De GC, Rubens R, Moerman M, Hamdi M, Van KL, Blondeel P. Surgical therapy in transsexual patients: a multi-disciplinary approach. Acta Chir Belg. 2001;101(5):200–9.
6. Hage JJ. Medical requirements and consequences of sex reassignment surgery. Med Sci Law. 1995;35(1):17–24.
7. Coleman E, Bockting W, Botzer M, Cohen-Kettenis P, DeCuypere G, Feldman J, Fraser L, Green J, Knudson G, Meyer WJ, Monstrey S. Standards of care for the health of transsexual, transgender, and gender-nonconforming people, version 7. Int J Transgend. 2012;13(4):165–232.
8. Brownstein & Crane Surgical Services (US). Process and fees: Letter requirements [internet]. San Fransico (CA); [cited 2018 Sep 30]. Available from: http://brownsteincrane.com/process/.
9. Krueger JK, Rohrich RJ. Clearing the smoke: the scientific rationale for tobacco abstention with plastic surgery. Plast Reconstr Surg. 2001;108(4):1063–73.
10. Chen CC, Collins SA, Rodgers AK, Paraiso MF, Walters MD, Barber MD. Perioperative complications in obese women vs normal-weight women

who undergo vaginal surgery. Am J Obstet Gynecol. 2007;197(1):98–e1.

11. Olsen MA, Higham-Kessler J, Yokoe DS, Butler AM, Vostok J, Stevenson KB, Khan Y, Fraser VJ. Developing a risk stratification model for surgical site infection after abdominal hysterectomy. Infect Control Hosp Epidemiol. 2009;30(11):1077–83.

12. Lawrence AA. Factors associated with satisfaction or regret following male-to-female sex reassignment surgery. Arch Sex Behav. 2003;32(4):299–315.

13. Seitz IA, Wu C, Retzlaff K, Zachary L. Measurements and aesthetics of the mons pubis in normal weight females. Plast Reconstr Surg. 2010;126(1):46e–8e.

14. Schechter LS. Surgical management of the transgender patient. Elsevier Health Sciences; 2016.

15. Hage JJ, Karim RB. Abdominoplastic secondary full-thickness skin graft vaginoplasty for male-to-female transsexuals. Plast Reconstr Surg. 1998;101(6):1512–5.

16. Saylor L, Bernard S, Vinaja X, Loukas M, Schober J. Anatomy of genital reaffirmation surgery (male-to-female): vaginoplasty using penile skin graft with scrotal flaps. Clin Anat. 2018;31(2):140–4.

17. Perovic SV, Stanojevic DS, Djordjevic ML. Vaginoplasty in male transsexuals using penile skin and a urethral flap. BJU Int. 2000;86(7):843–50.

18. Malloy TR, Noone RB, Morgan AJ. Experience with the 1-stage surgical approach for constructing female genitalia in male transsexuals. J Urol. 1976;116(3):335–7.

19. Davydov SN. Colpopoeisis from the peritoneum of the uterorectal space. Akush Ginekol. 1969;45(12):55.

20. Hess J, Henkel A, Bohr J, Rehme C, Panic A, Panic L, Rossi Neto R, Hadaschik B, Hess Y. Sexuality after male-to-female gender affirmation surgery. Biomed Res Int. 2018;2018:9037979.

21. Horbach SE, Bouman MB, Smit JM, Özer M, Buncamper ME, Mullender MG. Outcome of vaginoplasty in male to female transgenders: a systematic review of surgical techniques. J Sex Med. 2015;12(6):1499–512.

22. Monstrey S, Hoebeke P, Dhont M, De GC, Rubens R, Moerman M, Hamdi M, Van KL, Blondeel P. Surgical therapy in transsexual patients: a multi-disciplinary approach. Acta Chir Belg. 2001;101(5):200–9.

23. Bowman C, Goldberg JM. Care of the patient undergoing sex reassignment surgery. Int J Transgend. 2006;9(3–4):135–65.

24. De Cuypere G, TSjoen G, Beerten R, Selvaggi G, De Sutter P, Hoebeke P, Monstrey S, Vansteenwegen A, Rubens R. Sexual and physical health after sex reassignment surgery. Arch Sex Behav. 2005;34(6):679–90.

25. Lawrence AA. Factors associated with satisfaction or regret following male-to-female sex reassignment surgery. Arch Sex Behav. 2003;32(4):299–315.

26. Lobato MI, Koff WJ, Manenti C, da Fonseca SD, Salvador J, Fortes MD, Petry AR, Silveira E, Henriques AA. Follow-up of sex reassignment surgery in transsexuals: a Brazilian cohort. Arch Sex Behav. 2006;35(6):711–5.

27. Smith YL, Van Goozen SH, Kuiper AJ, Cohen-Kettenis PT. Sex reassignment: outcomes and predictors of treatment for adolescent and adult transsexuals. Psychol Med. 2005;35(1):89–99.

28. Crissman HP, Berger MB, Graham LF, Dalton VK. Transgender demographics: a household probability sample of US adults, 2014. Am J Public Health. 2017;107(2):213–5.

29. Reed HM, Yanes RE, Delto JC, Omarzai Y, Imperatore K. Non-grafted vaginal depth augmentation for transgender atresia, our experience and survey of related procedures. Aesthet Plast Surg. 2015;39(5):733–44.

30. Buncamper ME, Van der Sluis WB, De Vries M, Witte BI, Bouman MB, Mullender MG. Penile inversion vaginoplasty with or without additional full-thickness skin graft: to graft or not to graft? Plast Reconstr Surg. 2017;139(3):649e–56e.

31. Djordjevic ML, Stanojevic DS, Bizic MR. Rectosigmoid vaginoplasty: clinical experience and outcomes in 86 cases. J Sexual Med. 2011;8(12):3487–94.

Complications of Vaginoplasty

7

Amanda C. Chi, Melissa M. Poh,
and Polina Reyblat

Introduction

Greater acceptance and integration of transgender persons into our society as well as expansion of benefits for care associated with gender transition have led to the increased interest in gender affirmation surgery from both the transgender and surgical communities. There has been a nearly threefold increase in volume of gender-affirming surgery in recent years [1]. The rise in number of gender-affirming genital surgery will also result in more patients with a history of genital surgery seeking care, making it imperative for urologic surgeons to be able to recognize and manage various issues and complications that can arise post gender-affirming surgery.

Transfeminine genital surgery is a complex and multistep reconstructive surgery that generally consists of bilateral orchiectomy, penile disassembly, creation of neovaginal cavity between the rectum and the urogenital structures (prostate and bladder), labiaplasty, clitoroplasty, vaginoplasty, and urethral reconstruction. The overall goal of the surgery is to create a perineogenital complex that is both functional and feminine in appearance. A vaginal vault is created for the patient who desires a neovagina, which will require dilation to maintain patency. "Shallow-depth" or "zero-depth" vaginoplasty where a neovaginal canal is not created can also be offered. There are three main approaches for vaginoplasty: (1) genital skin flap; (2) intestinal vaginoplasty; (3) non-genital flaps. Genital skin flap based method, specifically the penile inversion approach, is currently most commonly used as primary surgery. Intestinal vaginoplasty has established itself as a procedure used predominantly for patients with paucity of available penile or scrotal skin or as a salvage operation. These approaches can be supplemented with robotic-assisted peritoneal flap dissection to augment the neovaginal canal – a method that is gaining popularity [2]. This chapter focuses on complications associated with penile skin inversion vaginoplasty.

A. C. Chi
Urology Department, Kaiser Permanente West Los Angeles Medical Center, Los Angeles, CA, USA
e-mail: Amanda.C.Chi@kp.org

M. M. Poh
Department of Plastic Surgery, Kaiser Permanente West Los Angeles Medical Center, Los Angeles, CA, USA
e-mail: Melissa.M.Poh@kp.org

P. Reyblat (✉)
Urology Department, Kaiser Permanente Los Angeles Medical Center, Los Angeles, CA, USA
e-mail: Polina.X.Reyblat@kp.org

Brief Overview of Complications and Outcomes

As with any complex surgery, adhering to reconstructive surgical principles and attention to detail can minimize postoperative complications. Complications can range from minor, which are

© Springer Nature Switzerland AG 2021
D. Nikolavsky, S. A. Blakely (eds.), *Urological Care for the Transgender Patient*,
https://doi.org/10.1007/978-3-030-18533-6_7

easily treatable, to major, which require additional surgical interventions and ongoing medical care. Urological *intraoperative complications* include rectal injury, bladder/urethral injury, and persistent bleeding in the rectoprostatic space encountered during the dissection of the vaginal vault. *Early in the postoperative period*, commonly encountered complications are rectovaginal fistula, urethrovaginal fistula, urinary retention, urinary tract infections, periurethral bleeding, neovaginal prolapse, tissue necrosis, graft loss, granulation tissue formation as well as wound dehiscence, abscess and hematoma formation. *In the months to years following vaginoplasty*, a urologist may encounter urethral malposition leading to deviated stream, meatal stenosis, granulation tissue formation, vaginal stenosis/loss of depth, bulge at introitus, neovaginal hair, recurrent urinary tract infections, as well as a variety of voiding dysfunction and pelvic pain complaints. Patients also may present with dissatisfaction of clitoral sensation as well as cosmetic appearance of the perineogenital complex. The overall incidence of complications after vaginoplasty ranges from 15% [3] to 70% [4] with reoperation rate of 21.7% [5] to 48% [4]. Minor issues, such as small amounts of granulation tissue or small wound dehiscences, are ubiquitous and expected. Satisfaction with vaginoplasty is reported to be high across multiple studies. Manrique et al. showed a satisfaction rate with penile inversion vaginoplasty of 88% (71–99%) with overall results, 86% (66–98%) with functional outcomes, and 86% (71–96%) with aesthetic outcomes. Ability to reach orgasm was 75% (57–89%) [3]. Hess et al. reported patient reported satisfaction post vaginoplasty from retrospectively collected surveys [6]. In this cohort of post vaginoplasty patients with median 5 years follow-up, 90.2% reported that their expectations for life as a woman were fulfilled and 85.4% saw themselves as women; 85.4% were satisfied or very satisfied with their outward appearance as a woman; 74% were satisfied or very satisfied with their functional outcome. The same group looked into sexual function outcomes and reported that of those who engaged in sexual intercourse, 55.8% rated

their orgasms to be more intense than before and 20.8% felt no difference [7]. Most patients were satisfied with the sensitivity of their neoclitoris (73.9%). Patients who experienced excessive bleeding, poor cosmetic outcome, and prolonged pain tended to have lower satisfaction [4]. The high incidence of complications related to transfeminine vaginoplasty highlights the importance of thorough informed consent with these patients preoperatively. This chapter aims to review most common complications encountered by a urologist and address the evaluation and management of these complications.

Intraoperative Complications

Rectal Injury

Rectal injury is the most dreaded intraoperative complication during vaginoplasty. It occurs during the dissection of the neovaginal canal along Denonvilliers' fascia, which lies between the rectum and the prostate. The formation of the neovaginal canal is best performed by applying principles described by Hugh Hampton Young in 1904, in his approach to perineal prostatectomy [8]. "Denonvilliers' fascia is observed beneath the extensor anal sphincter. The rectourethral muscle is resected to approach the apex of the prostate gland. Prostatic fascia covering the prostatic base is opened with blunt, and sharp dissection laterally and superiorly, and intrafascial area is entered." Of note, his approach relies on a hypertrophied prostate gland, as it was originally developed as a treatment of benign prostatic enlargement and later adopted for the treatment of carcinoma of the prostate. While this approach is anatomically reliable and reproducible, dissection around a small prostate proves to be more challenging. Because patients undergoing vaginoplasty have been on feminizing hormones for at least 12 months (WPATH SOC guidelines) and may be of a younger age, they tend to have smaller prostates that can make dissection difficult. Intraoperative rectal injury has been reported to be 1–5% [9, 10]. Intraoperative recognition of a rectal injury is of paramount importance since the development of a rectovaginal fistula after a recognized and repaired rectal injury is less likely [11]. Preoperative bowel preparation is helpful to empty the rectum and reduce the infection burden if a repair is needed at the time of surgery. A small and sharply made rectal injury can be repaired primarily in multiple layers. Bulbospongiosus muscle can be rotated and used as an additional layer to bolster the repair. The assistance of colorectal surgeons in the assessment and repair of the rectal injury can be helpful to evaluate the need for a more extensive repair or possible diversion. Furthermore, they can also help assess the integrity of the repair with endoscopic techniques if warranted. In our practice, if a patient has a rectal injury, we postpone removal of vaginal packing until 2 weeks after the initial surgery. To decrease the likelihood of infection, vaginal packing is replaced with a new packing under sedation approximately 1 week postoperatively. The integrity of the repair is also assessed endoscopically by the colorectal surgeon at this time. This vaginal packing is then removed 1 week later (2 weeks post vaginoplasty) and routine dilation protocol ensues.

Bladder or Urethral Injury

Bladder or urethra can be entered when neovaginal canal dissection plane is taken too anteriorly. Urethral injury occurs in 0–4.0% of cases [12]. Primary repair should be completed at the time of injury. As with other intraoperative injuries to the urinary tract, a watertight repair in one or two layers using absorbable sutures should be performed. A urethral catheter should be maintained for urinary diversion. After small repairs, a urethral catheter should be maintained in place for approximately 6 days postoperatively. In more extensive repairs, a longer period of catheter drainage may be required, typically for 14 days postoperatively. Voiding cystourethrogram can be completed prior to catheter removal to confirm urethral/bladder integrity if deemed necessary by the surgeon.

Pelvic Floor Muscle Dissection Associated Complications

Wide dissection of the pelvic floor muscles is important in order to develop adequate width of the introitus. Failure to divide the anterior levator ani muscles may lead to difficulty in dilation and a narrow introitus. This dissection is best performed with slow and meticulous cautery. Bleeding from branches of the internal pudendal artery typically occurs, requiring suture ligation of these vessels in addition to electrocautery. In our experience, hemostasis is best controlled with 2-0 Vicryl on UR-6 needles, which allow placement of sutures at these steep angles. Hemostasis of the neovaginal space is critical prior to placement of the penile skin flap/scrotal skin graft complex into the canal. While the packing placed into neovagina will aid with tight apposition between the skin graft and surrounding tissue bed in the neovaginal space, formation of a hematoma in the neovaginal canal can prevent take of the skin flap and graft. In the long term, graft loss can lead to the development of granulation tissue and possible vaginal stenosis.

Early Postoperative Complications

Periurethral Bleeding and Hematoma Formation

Postoperative surgical bleeding occurs in 3–12% of patients [13, 14], where blood transfusion is required in 1–7% of patients [4, 5, 12]. The most likely source of bleeding is corpus spongiosum tissue. Bleeding at urethral edge at the meatus can often be managed at bedside with either a hemostatic agent dressing or suture. In our practice, we evert the mucosa of the urethral meatus and close the corpus spongiosum for hemostasis with a running 5-0 Maxon suture prior to maturing the urethral meatus. Prevention of hematoma formation inside the neovaginal canal is critical for graft take and avoidance of neovaginal prolapse. Drains are placed under the mons region and the labia majora to help detect persistent

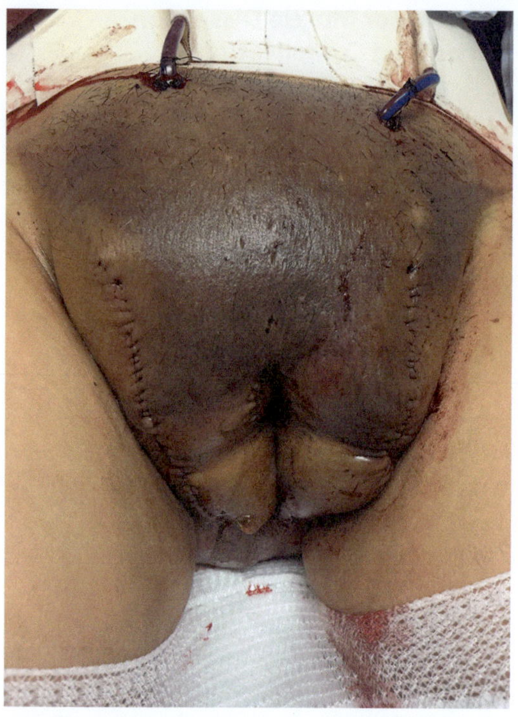

Fig. 7.1 Large hematoma, post penile inversion vaginoplasty

bleeding and evacuate usual postoperative fluid. In situations of an expanding hematoma, additional drainage or operative evaluation of the surgical field and reestablishment of hemostasis may be necessary. Meticulous hemostasis during each step of the case, well-fitted vaginal packing maintained in place with labial sutures, and pressure dressing at the conclusion of the case will minimize this undesirable complication (Fig. 7.1).

Urinary Retention

Urinary retention after vaginoplasty is usually transient and self-limited. Studies have reported a rate of urinary retention of 9–13% [4, 9]. For patients who are unable to adequately empty their bladder at the time of the voiding trial, a urethral catheter should be replaced. In our practice, patients will undergo a second voiding trial

on their first postoperative visit, which is typically 5–7 days after the initial attempt. The majority of our patients regain their ability to volitionally void by the time of the second voiding trial. An effort should be made to decrease narcotic pain medication use, treat constipation, and encourage ambulation. Additionally, since these patients still have their prostate glands, initiating a course of alpha-blockers for patients can be helpful. In rare cases when urinary retention persists, patients can learn to self-catheterize every 4–6 h. Clean intermittent catheterization allows patients to attempt volitional voiding before passing the catheter each time. As residual urine measured from each catheterization decreases, patients can self-transition to voiding entirely on their own.

Urinary Tract Infections

Postoperative urinary tract infections (UTIs) range from 4.4% to 7% [4, 9] according to most reports. One study reports postoperative UTI rates as high as 32% [15]. Due to presence of indwelling urethral catheters, patients are at higher risk for bacterial colonization and symptomatic infection. Prior to antibiotic treatment, providers should confirm presence of UTI symptoms such as dysuria, frequency, urgency, and/or fevers. Urine culture should be obtained prior to starting empiric therapy and treatment should be tailored based on culture results. Asymptomatic bacteriuria should not be considered as UTIs and should not be treated.

Neovaginal Prolapse

Prolapse of neovaginal skin is a rare complication reported in 0% [16] to 3% [17] of cases of penile inversion vaginoplasty. Prolapse in cases using intestinal segment appear to be as high as 8% [18]. Majority of prolapse presents in the first 6 months after surgery. Bucci et al. proposed placement of fixation stitches, where one absorbable suture is placed at the apex of the penoscrotal cylinder and fixed to Denonvilliers' fascia and two additional sutures are placed at the posterior/midpoint of the flap and fixed to the pre-rectal fascia [19]. In our practice, the cylindrical penoscrotal skin flap/graft is saturated with fibrin sealant (TISSEEL, Baxter) prior to placement into the neovaginal canal. After placement of skin flap, the neovagina is tightly packed to ensure surface apposition. At the conclusion of the case, the labia majora are sutured together to maintain vaginal packing in place. To date, there are no reports on long-term outcomes or results of patients who underwent sacrocolpopexy for neovaginal prolapse. Few reports, using either open [20, 21] or laparoscopic [22] transabdominal sacrocolpopexy approaches showed successful outcomes.

Graft Loss

Graft loss is a rare complication seen in less than 4% of the cases [5, 13]. Smoking and cardiovascular comorbidities seem to correlate with increased risk. Hematoma development in the neovaginal canal can prevent skin graft take. Hence, meticulous hemostasis within the neovaginal canal and well-fitted vaginal packing/bolster are paramount. In our series, loss of penile skin graft occurred in one patient due to postoperative bleeding leading to operative exploration, and in another patient who had a BMI over 40 (Fig. 7.2). From our experience, we observed that over time, the neovaginal canal will re-epithelialize even after a significant initial skin loss. In addition, adherence to the dilation protocol will maintain patency of the neovagina. If dilation is stopped, vaginal stenosis or shortening of the canal will likely occur.

Granulation Tissue

Granulation tissue inside the neovagina is one of the most common complications of the penile inversion vaginoplasty. While some authors

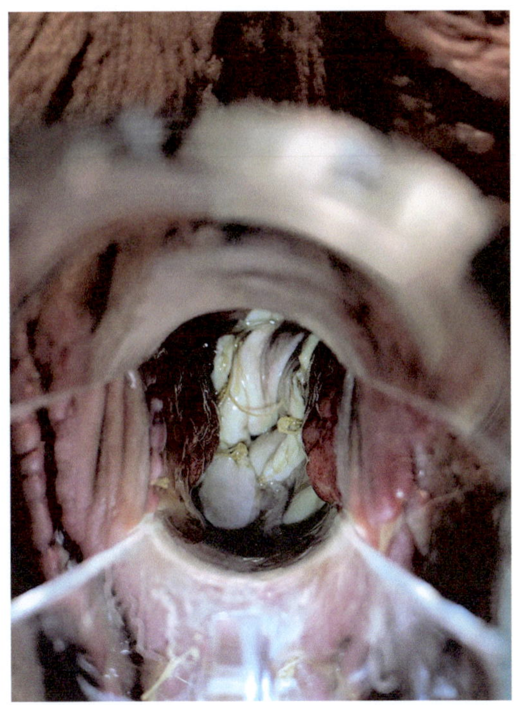

Fig. 7.2 Loss of graft, patient with BMI >40

report incidence between 7% and 26% [4, 10], most contemporary surgeons tend to agree that some degree of granulation tissue will occur in the majority of patients. Granulation tissue can occur in any area where there is an open wound, typically from tissue necrosis. It is often seen in the neovaginal canal but can also be present on the vulva, particularly the posterior fourchette (Fig. 7.3a). Patients may report blood-tinged discharge on the dilator or spotting. Other patients, particularly those with a large volume of granulation tissue, may report pain. The mainstay of treatment is application of silver nitrate to the area over several weeks to months, depending on the amount of granulation tissue. In rare occasions of patient intolerance to in-office treatment, or high burden of granulation tissue, an exam under anesthesia performed to allow more extensive treatment with silver nitrate is required. Patients with extensive amount of granulation tissue can experience wound contracture and progressive narrowing or shortening of neovagina.

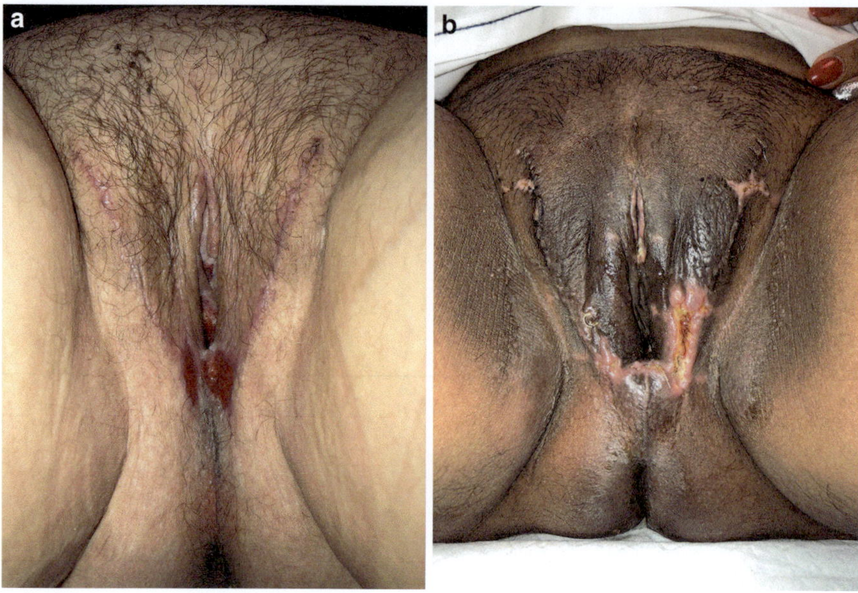

Fig. 7.3 (**a**) Granulation tissue at posterior fourchette. (**b**) Wound dehiscence

Some providers advocate the use of MediHoney (commercially available for purchase) to be placed at the tip of the dilator during dilation. There are no studies to date demonstrating clinical benefit of those applications. It is critical that patients do not stop vaginal dilation during the healing period.

Wound Dehiscence

Wound dehiscence is a common early postoperative complication and is related to tension on the incisions, particularly at the posterior fourchette (Fig. 7.3b). To minimize the dehiscence, the penile skin flap should be elevated off of the mons at the level of the fascia to allow for more advancement of the tissue. Younger or thinner patients usually require more dissection off the fascia to mitigate the lack of laxity inherent in older or heavier patients. Local wound care and patience usually leads to complete healing. Depending on the location, the dehiscence can lead to granulation tissue, which can be treated as previously described. Again, patients should continue dilation per protocol.

Delayed Complications

Vaginal Stenosis

Vaginal stenosis is a devastating complication since it nullifies one of the main surgical goals: creating a functional neovaginal canal. It can be categorized as introital or canal stenosis. Introital stenosis can also lead to loss of depth of the canal due to difficulty with complete dilation. Symptomatic narrowing of the introitus was reported in 12% (range 4.2–15%) of the cases [13] and usually can be managed by stricturoplasty, commonly with combination of advancement flaps. In some instances, additional skin grafts may be required to enlarge the circumference of the introitus. Neovaginal canal stenosis is reported as 7% (1–12%) [12, 13]. Many patients are geographically distant from the centers where their surgeries were performed thus preventing consistent follow-up, so these studies may be limited. Many patients in the past may also lack resources or interest in pursuing further intervention. Stenosis of the neovagina can be caused by one or a combination of factors: poor adherence to dilation protocol; difficulty/pain with dilation;

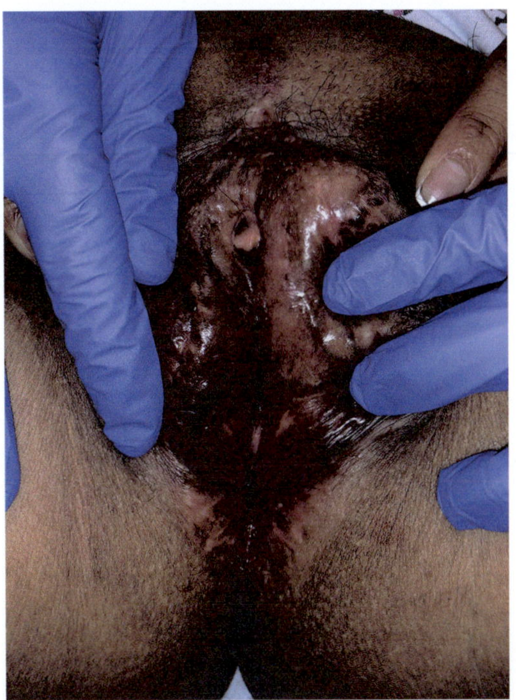

Fig. 7.4 Stenosis of vaginal canal

progressive scar contracture associated with lack of graft take and/or granulation tissue development (Fig. 7.4).

Challenges with dilation can be brought on by a variety of reasons: pain, underlying pelvic floor dysfunction, lack of privacy or supportive environment to perform dilations or change in personal goals and intentional abandon of the vaginal canal. Pain and pelvic floor dysfunction could be due to insufficient dissection of the levator ani complex at the time of the neovaginal canal formation. In addition, preexisting pelvic floor dysfunction can contribute to difficulty in relaxing pelvic floor muscles during dilation. In recent retrospective review by Dugi et al., 42% of patients undergoing vaginoplasty had preexisting pelvic floor dysfunction that were identified preoperatively [23]. Timely intervention with pelvic floor therapy demonstrated improvement in pelvic floor function leading to successful dilation [23]. In patients who experience pain with dilation due to granulation tissue, therapy should focus on treatment of granulation tissue while maintaining consistent dilation schedule.

Neovaginal canal stenosis requires surgical intervention for reestablishment of the full-length canal. Pedicled intestinal segment and peritoneal flap vaginoplasty [2] have become the two most commonly employed options that avoid external scars and use of skin grafts elsewhere on the body. It is well-established that repeat dissection in the rectoprostatic space, particularly from a perineal approach, carries an increased risk of rectal and bladder injury when compared to primary vaginoplasty [11]. Secondary intestinal vaginoplasty has higher rates of revision surgeries (79% (23) vs. 21.7% [5]), as well as carries additional risks and potential complications associated with an intra-abdominal surgery and a bowel anastomosis, such as bowel obstruction, anastomotic leak, diversion colitis, and mucocele due to a closed blind loop of intestine if stenosis occurs. In some cases, the intestinal neovagina had to be removed due to infection leading to necrosis of the colonic segment and recurrent stenosis related to ischemia [24]. Peritoneal flap vaginoplasty has emerged as a safe option for these challenging cases. This approach utilizes a combined transabdominal and perineal approach similar to the one described by Davydov in 1969 [25] as a treatment for vaginal agenesis. Similar to intestinal vaginoplasty, peritoneal flap vaginoplasty may also play a significant role as a primary surgery, particularly for patients with limited source of genital skin flap [2].

Rectoneovaginal Fistula

Development of a rectoneovaginal fistula is one of the most undesirable complications of vaginoplasty. It can occur after an unrecognized rectal injury or after a failed repair of a recognized rectal injury. In a retrospective review of records of 1082 transgender women by Sluis et al. [11], 8 of 997 (0.8%) patients who underwent primary vaginoplasty developed rectoneovaginal fistulae. Rate of fistula formation was higher, at 6.25%, in secondary vaginoplasties. Out of 21 patients who had rectal injuries that were repaired intraoperatively, 4 (19%) still developed rectoneovaginal fistula shortly after the operation. Others are thought to be due to unrecognized rectal injury at the time of dissection [11]. Patients were initially managed with low residue diet. Unfortunately, only one fistula resolved spontaneously while on low residue diet. The remaining patients underwent surgical repair of the fistula employing various interposition grafts or flaps.

Diagnosis of the rectoneovaginal fistula requires clinical suspicion and congruent physical exam findings (Fig. 7.5a). Patients typically will describe stool or gas emanating from the neovaginal canal. Presence of fecal matter in the neovaginal vault should prompt neovaginal speculum exam and rectal exam in order to confirm the presence of fistula. Imaging studies such as gastrografin enema, endoscopy, CT, or MRI, can support the diagnosis, but are rarely necessary. Similar to treatment of any rectovaginal fistula, fecal diversion with temporary colostomy is typically necessary to optimize chance of resolution. Failure of resolution of fistula with conservative measures requires excision of the fistula and repair of rectal and neovaginal defect with interpositioning local tissue. Patients should be counseled on the potential of neovaginal canal stenosis if neovaginal dilation is interrupted for a pro-

longed period of time. In the past, patients were instructed to cease dilation to allow the neovaginal canal to close, thus treating the fistula but leading to loss of the neovaginal canal. We have repaired a rectoneovaginal fistula through a transvaginal approach and using gracilis flap interposition (Fig. 7.5b). The repair was completed 3 months after the patient underwent diverting colostomy, corresponding to 6 months after her initial vaginoplasty. At 1 month after repair, we reestablished an every-other-day dilation schedule performed by the surgeon for 2 weeks and then allowed the patient to resume dilation on her own at 3 months post repair. In this manner, the patient's width and depth of her neovaginal canal was preserved.

Urethroneovaginal Fistula

Reported incidence for urethroneovaginal fistula ranges from 0.8% to 3.9% [17, 26, 27]. This likely occurs due to unrecognized urethral injury or breakdown of a repaired urethral injury. In patients with a distal urethroneovaginal fistula, one can consider excising the distal bridge of tis-

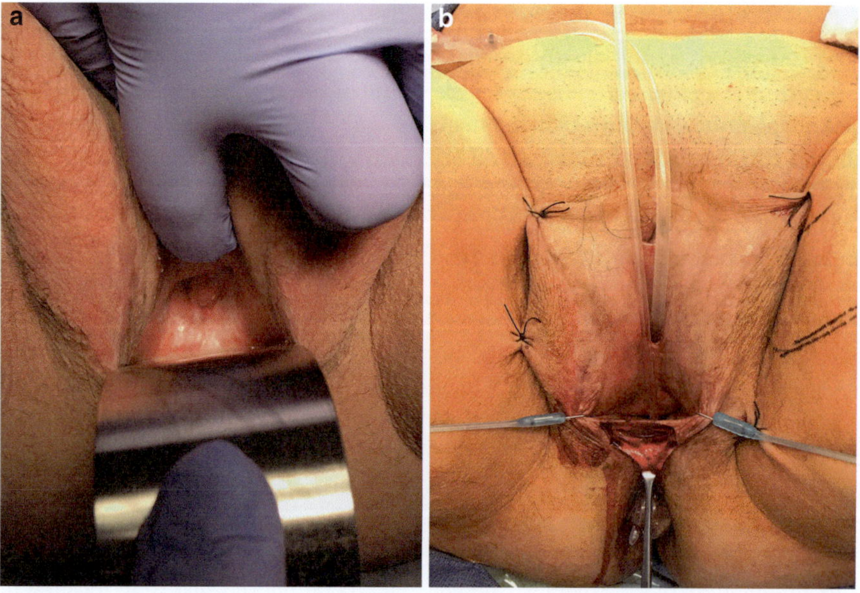

Fig. 7.5 (a) Rectovaginal fistula. (b) Repair of the rectoganical fistula, transvaginal approach

sue, resulting in a more recessed urethral meatus. In the case of a more proximal fistula, the fistula can be repaired transvaginally to close the neovaginal defect and urethral defect with local interpositioning flaps.

Urethral Stricture and Urethral Malposition

The most likely location of a urethral stricture post vaginoplasty is at the urethral meatus. The reported incidence of meatal stenosis varies widely, with most authors noting 1–6% [16, 17, 26] and one group noting 40% [27]. The rates of meatal stenosis in vaginoplasty techniques that transect the urethra at the meatus versus those that preserve the posterior urethral plate to span between the neoclitoris and urethral meatus have not been parsed out. Complaints of new onset obstructive urinary symptoms such as weak stream or feeling of incomplete emptying should raise suspicion for urethral stricture disease, particularly in those patients who did not have these symptoms prior to vaginoplasty. Patients with urethral strictures can also present with urinary retention and frequent urinary tract infections. Meatal stenosis can usually be diagnosed on physical exam (Fig. 7.6). In patients who are not in urinary retention and maintain normal renal function, we prefer to avoid dilation of the stenotic segment and plan for definitive surgical reconstruction. Dilation will alter anatomy, making it more difficult for the surgeon to ensure that the entire stenosed segment has been excised. During urethroplasty, a small caliber catheter is placed via the stenotic meatus to help delineate urethra. A circumscribing incision is made and corpus spongiosum and urethra is dissected sharply away from surrounding tissue. Care is taken to develop the plane along the corpus spongiosum to maintain blood supply to the urethra and adjacent skin flap. The stenotic fragment is transected sharply and urethral edge is spatulated ventrally to ensure a large caliber urethral meatus. We place a running suture circumferentially to evert urethral mucosa and for hemostasis. A V

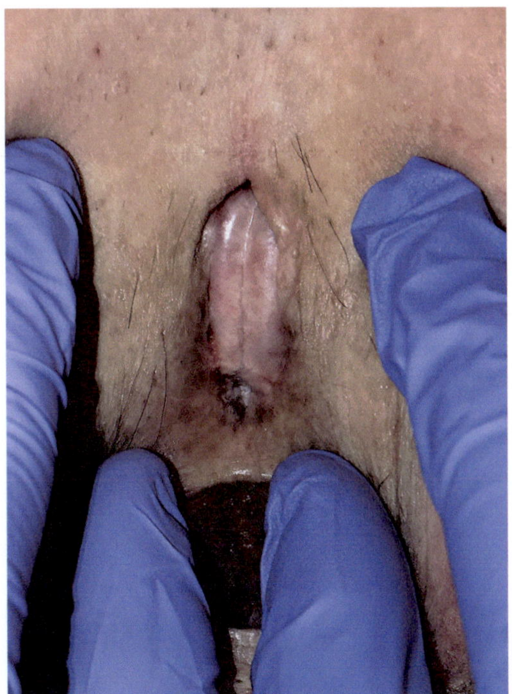

Fig. 7.6 Meatal stenosis

flap is created from the anterior neovaginal wall and advanced into the posteriorly spatulated portion of the urethra. Urethral meatus is then matured with interrupted 4-0 Vicryl sutures. A catheter remains in place for 5–7 days postoperatively.

The urethral meatus can also be anteriorly malpositioned, leading to deviation of the urine stream in a forward direction when the patient sits to void. This issue frequently presents as a complaint of urine spraying over the edge of the toilet seat, a need to bend the torso forward, or the use a deflective device (e.g., towel) to direct the urine stream downward. This anterior urethral angle can be corrected by an approach similar to the one described above. In some instances where the attachment of the corpus spongiosum to the crus of the corpora cavernosum was not dissected adequately at the time of the initial operation, more significant periurethral dissection is needed to free up the urethra. Once the urethra has been mobilized adequately to allow it to drop into a position suitable to generate a downward stream, the meatus can be matured as described above. The skin or tissue anterior to the new meatus position has to be closed to compensate for the change urethral position.

Urethral Bulb Bulge

A periurethral bulge that hangs into the distal anterior vaginal canal can present in patients when there is inadequate tapering of corpus spongiosum tissue at bulbous urethra at the time of the vaginoplasty. Patients describe it as a sensation of engorged erectile tissue around the urethra and vaginal opening, particularly during arousal, causing problems with intercourse, pain, discomfort or dysphoria (Fig. 7.7a). In addition to inadequately tapered corpus spongiosum, the bulge can also be due to incompletely resected bulbospongiosus muscle. Correction of the bulge can be achieved transvaginally, typically with an incision through the inverted penile skin flap that overlies the urethra (Fig. 7.7b). The skin flaps are raised and dissection is carried more deeply to expose any remaining bulbospongiosus muscle, which should be excised completely. If there is excessive corpus spongiosum, an indwelling catheter should be placed to delineate the course of the urethra and the ventral aspect of the spongiosum can be tapered to parallel the urethra. The edges of the trimmed corpus spongiosum can be closed with 4-0 Vicryl. In our practice, we maintain vaginal packing and urethral catheter for approximately 5 days in patients with large anterior neovaginal wall incisions to help with adherence of the overlying penile skin flap. If needed, this intervention can be combined with urethral repositioning, labiaplasty, clitoroplasty, or other cosmetic revisions of the perineogenital complex [28].

Lower Urinary Tract Function

Multiple steps of the vaginoplasty can lead to altered voiding dynamics such as dissection of the neovaginal canal, resection of bulbospongiosus muscles, tapering of the corpus spongiosum, and mobilization of the urethra. The impact of these procedures on voiding function has not been studied in-depth. Hoebeke et al. retrospec-

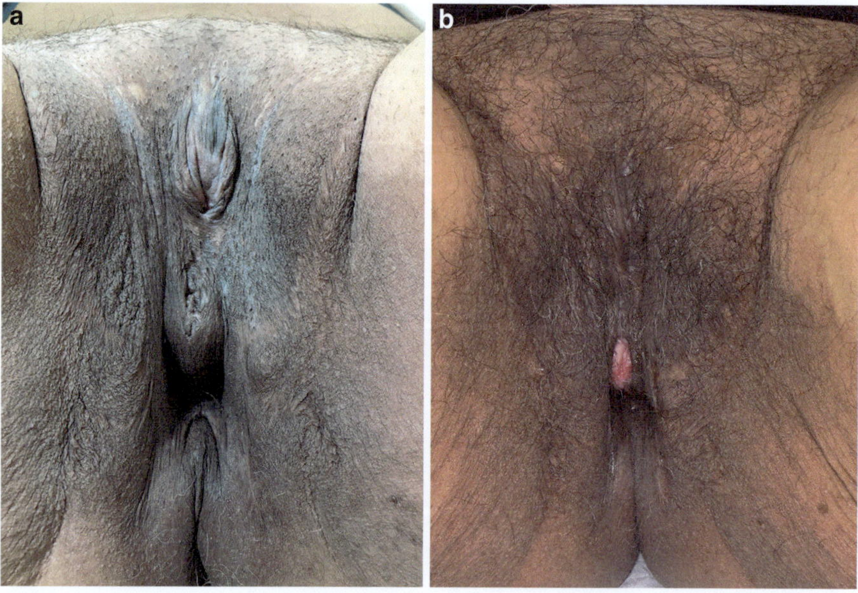

Fig. 7.7 (**a**) Urethral bulb bulge at introitus. (**b**) Urethral bulb bulge, post-revision

tively queried voiding patterns and lower urinary tract symptoms by administering questionnaires to patients after gender-affirming surgery [15]. This study gathered data on 31 transgender female patients. Six patients (19.3%) reported that their voiding function was worse than before the surgery and reported loss of urine via dribbling, urge or stress incontinence. Although patients are at risk for external urethral sphincter injury during neovaginal canal dissection, there are currently no reported data specific to stress urinary incontinence. It is possible that an intact internal urethral sphincter function helps dampen potential effects of a weakened or injured external urethral sphincter.

In Hoebeke's group, 10 patients (32%) reported urinary tract infections (UTI) with a mean episode rate of 1.7, although the definition of a UTI was not clearly outlined and presence of urinary symptoms or UTIs prior to surgery was not documented [15]. In another small retrospective review by Kuhn et al., there were no UTIs reported by 18 surveyed patients, but "diverted stream, overactive bladder and stress urinary incontinence were noticed to be a common problem" [29]. In larger cohorts (>100 patients), UTIs were seen in 4.4–7% of patients [4, 9]. In our practice, we administer American Urological Association Symptom Index (AUA-SI) preoperatively and postoperatively at 3, 6, 9, and 12 months. The results of the first 50 patients can be seen in Table 7.1. With this small cohort, we have yet to identify trends in change of lower urinary tract symptoms in our patients. In our early data, the two patients with high AUA-SI (19 and 15) were found to have meatal stenosis that have since been treated.

Changes in voiding symptoms warrant careful physical examination, which can be supplemented with noninvasive flowmetry and post-void residual measurement with bladder ultrasound. Using the AUA-SI and taking thorough preoperative survey of voiding function are helpful for identifying and documenting changes in voiding function. Prostate-related voiding symptoms should also be considered in post-vaginoplasty patients. Surgically correctable conditions such as urethral stricture or meatal malpositioning should be addressed prior to or concurrently with functional therapies for voiding symptoms.

Hair in the Neovaginal Canal

Careful and meticulous preoperative removal of hair employing permanent methods is the only measure to minimize hair formation in the neo-

Table 7.1 Mean AUA-SI scores prior to and at 3,6,9,and 12 months following vaginoplasty

	Incomplete emptying[a]	Frequency[a]	Intermittency[a]	Urgency	Weak stream[a]	Hesitancy[a]	Nocturia (void per night)	Total (0–35)[b]	Quality of life score (0–6)[c]
Pre-Op	0.31	1.21	0.23	0.42	0.19	0.077	1.2	3.6	1.0
1 months post-op	0.54	1.1	0.86	0.49	0.91	0.27	1.4	5.6	1.4
3 months post-op	0.59	1.2	0.69	0.88	0.66	0.28	1.2	5.5	1.7
6 months post-op	0.46	1.1	0.54	0.77	0.54	0.15	0.92	4.5	1.1
9 months post-op	0.83	1.8	1.3	1.2	1.0	0.42	1.6	8.1	1.7
12 months post-op	1.3	2.3	1.0	2.0	0.83	0.17	1.8	9.5	1.3

[a]*Score* from 0(never) to 5(always)

[b]*Extent of LUTS* 0–7: mild, 8–19: moderate, 20–35: severe

[c]*Quality of life*: 0: delighted, 1: pleased, 2: mostly pleased, 3: mixed,4: mostly dissatisfied, 5: unhappy, 6: terrible

vaginal canal. As the skin (penile shaft and scrotal skin) used for lining the canal is inherently hair-bearing, this process can be laborious, prolonged, expensive, and painful. In general, depending on a patient's hair density and tolerance, it can take 6–12 months to deem the scrotum, perineum, and penile shaft cleared of hair. Even with these stringent requirements, there will be dormant hair follicles that are not detected and eliminated over the course of treatment sessions. Use of depilatory creams has been described, but the results remain anecdotal. Alternatively, the process of scraping or burning the hair follicles from the scrotal skin graft or the penile skin flap at the time of vaginoplasty have been reported; however, these techniques risk injuring or thinning the dermal layer, which can lead to compromised blood flow or a thin graft that will lead to more contraction.

Hair growth in the vaginal canal after vaginoplasty may lead to increase in discharge, discomfort with dilation or intercourse, unpleasant odor, formation of nests of hair, concretions, and calculi (Fig. 7.8a, b). Hair can be removed during routine visits utilizing vaginal speculum and ring forceps. Unfortunately, this technique is only temporary. Post-vaginoplasty electrolysis at the introitus can be performed but to a limited degree.

Clitoral Exposure/Cosmesis

Requests for revision due to external genitalia cosmetic appearance are common and generally not considered as a complication. Rate of revision of the perineogenital complex ranges from 25% to 50% [10, 13, 30]. These revisions can include additional clitoral coverage by reconstruction of clitoral hood, formation of more defined labia minora, or reduction of labia majora (Fig. 7.9). Timing of revisions should be at least 3 months from the date of the original surgery to allow for tissues to settle and edema to resolve. In some cases, the posterior fourchette forms a ridge, making dilation and intercourse more difficult. This ridge can be revised by re-advancing the perineal flap. Clitoroplasty and labiaplasty can be completed as an outpatient surgery and can be combined with revision of urethral meatus or a urethral bulb bulge (Fig. 7.9b, c).

Conclusion

Penile inversion vaginoplasty provides a safe and effective technique in appropriately selected patients to achieve the goals of constructing a functional neovaginal and a feminine-appearing

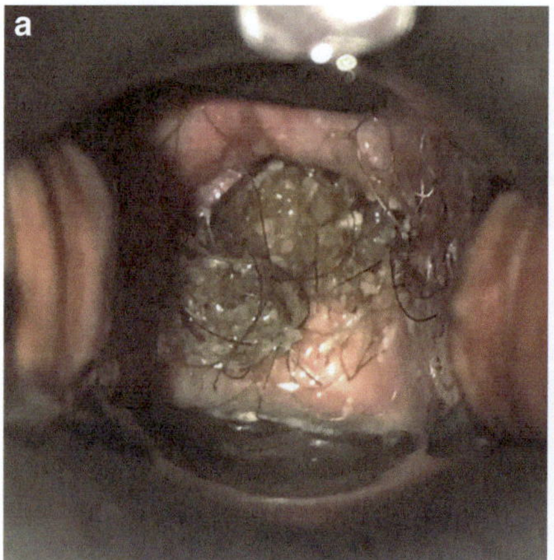
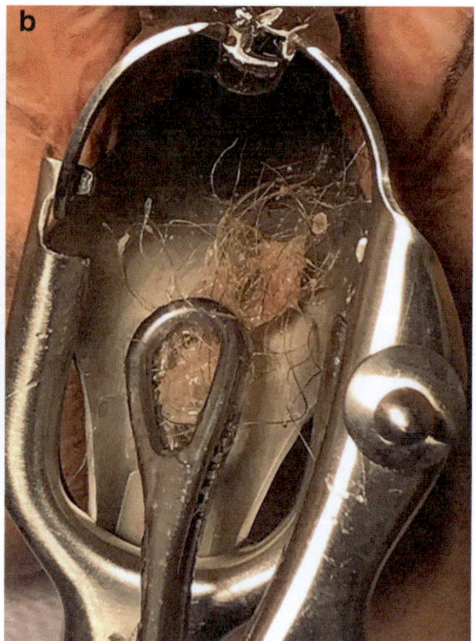

Fig. 7.8 (**a**) Hair in the neovaginal canal. (**b**) Hair in the neovaginal canal

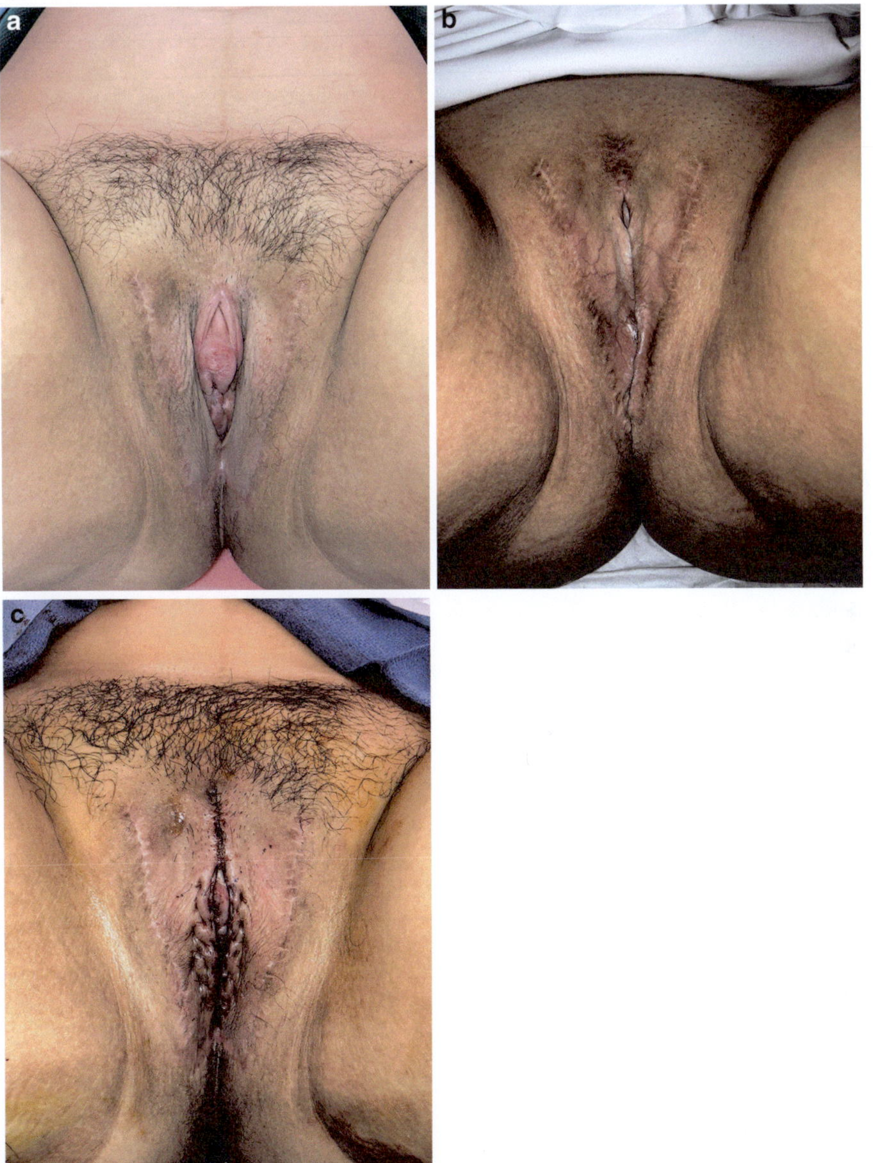

Fig. 7.9 (**a**) Three months after penile inversion vaginoplasty. Overexposed clitoris. Not well-defined labia minora. (**b**) Revision labiaplasty and clitoroplasty. (**c**) Six weeks after revision operation

perineogenital complex. Post-vaginoplasty patients can present with complications ranging from minor and nonoperative to those that may require multiple surgical interventions. Thorough preoperative discussions with the patient and even supporting friends and family are extremely important to ensure patients' understanding of the possible short-term and long-term complications related to this procedure. Broadening medical school and postgraduate curriculum to improve understanding of gender-affirming surgical procedures and related anatomy can strengthen the ability of healthcare providers to provide care for these patients.

Take-Home Points

- Wound-related events (granulation tissue, some wound breakdown) are ubiquitous, respond well to local care, and mostly self-limited.
- Recto-neovaginal fistula develops in most of unrecognized rectal injuries and a small proportion of recognized and repaired rectal injuries.
- Commitment and compliance with vaginal dilation is a cornerstone of long-term success and preservation of the neovaginal canal.
- About 25–50% of patients will require a second surgery to improve appearance of the perineogenital complex, achieve better voiding angle, reduce urethral bulb bulge.
- Urethral meatus strictures develop in a small subset of patients and require surgical correction.
- Collaborative approach of plastic surgeons and reconstructive urologists is critical in comprehensive evaluation and treatment of postsurgical events and complications.

References

1. Canner JK, Harfouch O, Kodadek LM, Pelaez D, , Coon D, Offodile AC, Haider AH, Lau BD. Temporal trends in gender-affirming surgery among transgender patients in the United States. JAMA Surg 2018;153(7):609–616.
2. Jacoby A, Maliha S, Granieri M, Dy G, Bluebond-Langner R, Zhao L. Robotic Davydov Peritoneal Flap Vaginoplasty for Augmentation of Vaginal Depth in Feminizing Vaginoplasty. J Urol. 2019;201(6):1171–6.
3. Manrique O, Adabi K, Martinez-Jorge J, Ciudad P, Nicoli F, Kiranantawat K. Complications and patient-reported outcomes in male-to-female vaginoplasty-where we are today: a systematic review and meta-analysis. Ann Plast Surg. 2018;80(6):684–91.
4. Massie J, Morrison S, Van Maasdam J, Satterwhite T. Predictors of patient satisfaction and postoperative complications in penile inversion vaginoplasty. Plast Reconstr Surg. 2018;141(6):911–21.
5. Dreher PC, Edwards D, Hager S, Dennis M, Belkoff A, Mora J, Tarry S, Rumer KL. Complications of the neovagina in male-to-female transgender surgery: a systematic review and meta-analysis with discussion of management. Clin Anat. 2018;31(2):191–9.
6. Hess J, Rossi Neto R, Panic L, Rübben H, Senf W. Satisfaction with male-to-female gender reassignment surgery—results of a retrospective analysis. Dtsch Arztebl Int. 2014;111(47):795–801.
7. Hess J, Henkel A, .Bohr J, Rehme C, Panic A, Panic L, Rossi Neto R, Hadaschik B, Hess Y. Sexuality after male-to-female gender affirmation surgery. Biomed Res Int [Internet]. 2018 2018, 9037979, 7 pages. https://doi.org/10.1155/2018/9037979.
8. Young H. The early diagnosis and radical cure of carcinoma of the prostate. J Urol. 1905;16:315–21.
9. Buncamper ME, van der Sluis WB, van der Pas RS, Özer M, Smit JM, Witte BI, Bouman MB, Mullender MG. Surgical outcome after penile inversion vaginoplasty: a retrospective study of 475 transgender women. Plast Reconstr Surg. 2016;138(5):999–1007.
10. Gaither TW, Awad MA, Osterberg EC, Murphy GP, Romero A, Bowers ML, Breyer BN. Postoperative complications following primary penile inversion vaginoplasty among 330 male-to-female transgender patients. J Urol. 2018;199(3):760–5.
11. Van der Sluis WB, Bouman MB, Buncamper ME, Pigot GL, Mullender MG, Meijerink WJ. Clinical characteristics and management of neovaginal fistulas after vaginoplasty in transgender women. Obstet Gynecol. 2016;127(6):1118–26.
12. Hadj-Moussa M, Ohl D, Kuzon W. Feminizing genital confirmation surgery. Sex Med Rev. 2018;6(3):457–68.
13. Horbach SE, Bouman MB, Smit JM, Ozer M, Buncamper ME, Mullender MG. Outcome of vaginoplasty in male-to-female transgenders: a systematic review of surgical techniques. J Sex Med. 2015;12(6):1499–512.
14. Papadopulos NA, Zavlin D, Lelle JD, Herschbach P, Henrich G, Kovacs L, Ehrenberger B, Machens HG, Schaff J. Combined vaginoplasty technique for male-to-female sex reassignment surgery: operative approach and outcomes. J Plast Reconstr Aesthet Surg. 2017;70(10):1483–92.
15. Hoebeke P, Selvaggi G, Ceulemans P, De Cuypere G, T'Sjoen G, Weyers S, Decaestecker K, Monstrey S. Impact of sex reassignment surgery on lower urinary tract function. Eur Urol. 2005;47(3):398–402.
16. Perovic S, Stanojevic D, Djordjevic M. Vaginoplasty in male transsexuals using penile skin and a urethral flap. BJU Int. 2000;86(7):843–50.
17. Krege S, Bex A, Lümmen G, Rübben H. Male-to-female transsexualism: a technique, results and long-term follow-up in 66 patients. BJU Int. 2001;88(4):396–402.
18. Djordjevic M, Stanojevic D, Bizic M. Rectosigmoid vaginoplasty: clinical experience and outcomes in 86 cases. J Sex Med. 2011;8(12):3487–94.

19. Bucci S, Mazzon G, Liguori G, Napoli R, Pavan N, Bormioli S, Ollandini G, De Concilio B, Trombetta C. Neovaginal prolapse in male-to-female transsexuals: an 18-year-long experience. Biomed Res Int [Internet]. 2014;2014:240761, 5 pages. https://doi.org/10.1155/2014/240761.

20. Loverro G, Bettocchi C, Battaglia M, et al. Repair of vaginal prolapse following penoscrotal flap vaginoplasty in a male-to-female transsexual. Gynecol Obstet Invest. 2002;53(4):234–6.

21. Frederick R, Leach G. Abdominal sacral colpopexy for repair of neovaginal prolapse in male-to-female transsexuals. Urology. 2004;64(3):580–1.

22. Condous G, Jones R, Lam AM. Male-to-female transsexualism: laparoscopic pelvic floor repair of prolapsed neovagina. Aust N Z J Obstet Gynaecol. 2006;46(3):254–6.

23. Jiang D, Gallagher S, Burchill L, Berli J, Dugi D 3rd. Implementation of a pelvic floor physical therapy program for transgender women undergoing gender-affirming vaginoplasty. Obstet Gynecol. 2019;133(5):1003–11.

24. van der Sluis WB, Bouman MB, de Boer NK, Buncamper ME, van Bodegraven AA, Neefjes-Borst EA, Kreukels BP, Meijerink WJ, Mullender MG. Long-term follow-up of transgender women after secondary intestinal vaginoplasty. J Sex Med. 2016;13(4):702–10.

25. Davydov S. Colpopoeisis from the peritoneum of the uterorectal space. Akush Ginekol (Mosk). 1969;45(12):55–7.

26. Reed H. Aesthetic and functional male to female genital and perineal surgery: feminizing vaginoplasty. Semin Plast Surg. 2011;25(2):163–74.

27. Rossi Neto R, Hintz F, Krege S, Rubben H, Vom Dorp F. Gender reassignment surgery – a 13 year review of surgical outcomes. Int Braz J Urol. 2012;38(1):97–107.

28. Karim R, Hage J, Bouman F, Dekker J. The importance of near total resection of the corpus spongiosum and total resection of the corpora cavernosa in the surgery of male to female transsexuals. Ann Plast Surg. 1991;26(6):554–6.

29. Kuhn A, Hiltebrand R, Birkhäuser M. Do transsexuals have micturition disorders? Eur J Obstet Gynecol Reprod Biol. 2007;131(2):226–30.

30. Raigosa M, Avvedimento S, Yoon T, Cruz-Gimeno J, Rodriguez G, Fontdevila J. Male-to-female genital reassignment surgery: a retrospective review of surgical technique and complications in 60 patients. J Sex Med. 2015;12(8):1837–45.

Part III

Surgical Anatomy: Transgender Male Patients

Surgical Anatomy - Hysterectomy for Transgender Men

Olivia H. Chang and Cecile A. Ferrando

Introduction

For transgender men, the most commonly performed genital surgery is a total hysterectomy – surgical removal of the uterus and cervix. In the National Transgender Discrimination Survey of nearly 28,000 transgender individuals, 14% of the transgender male respondents had undergone hysterectomy, while 57% of the respondents reported that they would like a hysterectomy someday [1]. While we have some data, it is difficult to estimate the true prevalence of and characteristics of transgender men who desire hysterectomy. The currently published prevalence rates do not accurately reflect the desire for surgery or describe the accessibility of hysterectomy for transgender males. There remain structural barriers for these patients, including poor access to care and lack of insurance coverage. There are also unfortunate patient–provider barriers, such as patient's fear of provider discrimination or lack of provider education on transgender health needs [2, 3]. In our experience, younger individuals are seeking hysterectomy. In a recently published study by our group, using a national surgical quality improvement database, we found that the mean age of transgender men undergoing hysterectomy was 24 ± 14 years old [4]. This finding has important implications with regard to how patients are counseled, especially as it pertains to their fertility options.

Not all transgender men undergo genital surgery as part of the gender affirmation process. For some, surgery can be medically necessary to treat gender dysphoria [5]; for others, hysterectomy may be indicated for treatment of pain, abnormal uterine bleeding and/or uterine fibroids [6, 7]. In addition, the decision to proceed with a hysterectomy may relieve transgender men of the need for continued cervical cancer screening or eliminate their risk of experiencing abnormal uterine bleeding that can sometimes be associated with testosterone therapy. Seeking gynecologic care for these issues can be distressing for transgender men as waiting at a women's health office with cisgender women can exacerbate gender dysphoria and speculum exams can be emotionally and physically traumatizing for patients [8]. Providers who offer hysterectomy to transgender men for gender affirmation or for other gynecologic indications must be sensitive to the unique needs of these patients.

O. H. Chang (✉) · C. A. Ferrando
Cleveland Clinic Foundation, Section of Female
Pelvic Medicine and Reconstructive Surgery,
Department of Obstetrics and Gynecology,
Cleveland, OH, USA
e-mail: chango@ccf.org; ferranc2@ccf.org

© Springer Nature Switzerland AG 2021
D. Nikolavsky, S. A. Blakely (eds.), *Urological Care for the Transgender Patient*,
https://doi.org/10.1007/978-3-030-18533-6_8

Pelvic Anatomy of the Transgender Man

The internal reproductive organs consist of the uterus, cervix, fallopian tubes, and ovaries. The external genitalia consist of the labia majora, labia minora, clitoris, and perineum [9, 10]. Due to exogenous hormone therapy, there are variations to the internal and external genitalia. Testosterone therapy can cause clitoromegaly, and thinning of the vaginal epithelium from the loss of the intermediate and superficial layers of the vagina [11].

Uterus

The uterus is a hollow muscular organ with three layers forming the uterine wall – endometrium, myometrium, and serosa. It is positioned in the pelvis, anterior to the sigmoid colon and posterior to the bladder. In a nulliparous woman, the uterus is roughly 8 cm in length, 5 cm in width, and 2.5 cm in thickness. Blood supply to the uterus is supplied by the uterine artery, which is a branch of the anterior division of the internal iliac artery. The uterine arteries branch at the level of the junction of the cervix and uterine body and travel superiorly to anastomose with the ovarian arteries.

Fallopian Tubes

The fallopian tubes extend from the uterine fundus toward the ovaries as a pair of the tubular structures known as the oviducts. The fallopian tubes are separated into four portions from medial to lateral, including the isthmus, ampulla, infundibulum, and the fimbriae. Fallopian tubes range in length from 1 to 14 cm. The vascular supply of the fallopian tubes comes from the uterine and ovarian vessels.

Ovaries

The ovaries, or the gonads, are a pair of off-white structures roughly the size of an almond. The ovaries are found lateral to the uterus. They remain in their anatomic location with support from the utero-ovarian ligament, infundibulo-pelvic ligament, and the mesovarium. The vascular supply of the ovaries includes the ascending branches of the uterine artery, and the ovarian arteries, which are direct branches of the aorta below the renal vessels.

Cervix

The most distal part, or the "neck," of the uterus is the cervix. The cervix itself is dense with collagenous connective tissue. Within the cervix there is an endocervical canal with columnar epithelium, and an ectocervix with stratified squamous epithelium. There is a transformation zone called the squamo-columnar junction – this is where cervical dysplasia most commonly is found. The vascular supply of the cervix comes from the descending branch of the uterine arteries.

Vagina

The vagina is a tubular structure that serves as a conduit from the cervical portion of the uterus to the introitus of the external genitalia. Its vascular supply includes the vaginal artery with other collateral blood supply. The vagina is supported proximally by cardinal and uterosacral ligaments. It is supported distally by the levator ani and bulbocavernosus muscles. At the most distal portion of the vagina is the hymen. It is a thin, partially perforated membrane at the entrance. There are variations in the size and shape of the hymen, as a result of individual variation and sexual activity.

External Genitalia

The vulva is the term used to describe the external genitalia that is visible and consists of the labia majora, labia minora, vestibule, clitoris, and perineum. These structures are vascularized by the pudendal vessels that come off of the anterior division of the internal iliac artery. The clitoris, derived from the genital tubercle, is the most ventral structure. It is covered by the clitoral hood. The vaginal introitus is flanked by the paired structures of the labia majora and labia minora. The labia majora are longitudinal cutaneous folds of adipose tissue. Within the vulva is the vestibule. It is embryologically derived from the urogenital sinus and contains mucous-secreting glands that provide moisture and lubrication to the introitus.

Ureters

The ureter exits the renal pelvis bilaterally. It travels along the psoas muscles, and crosses over the common iliac vessels as it enters the pelvis, and courses medial to the internal iliac arteries. As the ureters descend ventrally and medially toward the bladder, they travel below the uterine arteries as they insert into the cardinal ligament structure then enter the trigone of the bladder.

Important Considerations

The critical portions of a hysterectomy are the following: (1) identification of the location and course of the ureters bilaterally; (2) transection of the uterus from its blood supply; (3) creation of a colpotomy; and (4) retrieval of the surgical specimen (uterus) followed by the closure of the vaginal cuff. A thorough understanding of pelvic anatomy is crucial for those performing hysterectomy in order to avoid intraoperative injury and perioperative morbidity.

Hysterectomy for a Transgender Man

Box 8.1 World Professional Association for Transgender Health's Criteria for Hysterectomy and Ovariectomy for Transgender Men

1. Two referrals from mental health providers for genital surgery
2. Persistent, well-documented gender dysphoria
3. Capacity to make a fully informed decision and to consent for treatment
4. Age of majority in a given country
5. If significant medical or mental health concerns are present, they must be well controlled
6. Twelve continuous months of hormone therapy as appropriate to the patient's gender goals*

*unless the patient has a medical contraindication or is otherwise unable or unwilling to take hormones

World Professional Association for Transgender Health Criteria

Like all providers caring for transgender patients, surgeons performing hysterectomy for transgender men should use the World Professional Association for Transgender Health (WPATH) Standards of Care (SOC) as a guide for evaluation and management of patients. The SOC list specific criteria for hysterectomy and oophorectomy for transgender men seeking genital affirmation surgery (Box 8.1). These guidelines do not apply to transgender men whose indication for hysterectomy is medical or gynecologic.

Currently, WPATH recommends two mental health letters of referral for genital surgery, which includes hysterectomy. We suspect that as the SOC continue to be revised, this recommendation may change specifically for patients who desire a hysterectomy. A second letter for this surgery is thought to be burdensome to some patients. Per WPATH, patients must have the capacity to make an informed decision to consent for treatment and they must be medically optimized with mental health support. The purpose of the 12 continuous months of hormone therapy is to introduce a period of reversible estrogen suppression before the patient undergoes irreversible surgery [8].

Perioperative Considerations

When counseling patients for surgery, it is important to have an extensive presurgical discussion with the patient. We propose a presurgical checklist as seen in Box 8.2 to guide providers in counseling patients prior to a hysterectomy and any additional procedures. We believe that it is critical that any and all gender affirmation surgeries be offered by surgeons who are well versed in not only their specialty, but also transgender care. Even if a surgeon is technically capable of performing a hysterectomy, it is important that they understand transgender-specific care in order to ensure that patients are cared for appropriately and responsibly.

Box 8.2 Preoperative Checklist for Transgender Men Undergoing Genital Surgery

- Ensure that the patient meets the WPATH criteria for surgery
- Review the risks and benefits of the various modes of hysterectomy
- Review the patient's desired extent of gender affirmation surgery and the surgeon's and the hospital institution's capacity to perform these procedures*
- Discuss concurrent procedures
- Discuss the likely cosmetic and functional outcomes, and the possible need for further revisions
- Inform the patient of the complication rate for each procedure
- Provide fertility counseling and referral to a specialist as needed
- Pregnancy test on the day of surgery
- Management of testosterone preoperatively and VTE prophylaxis intraoperatively

*if there are no qualified personnel, patients should be referred to the appropriate consultants

---

Operating Room Environment

While the surgeon may be an expert in gender affirmation surgeries, the anesthesia and nursing team may be less familiar with the unique needs and challenges of the surgery and this should be considered on the day of surgery. A collaborative approach is needed to provide optimal care [12]. The team should be familiar with the patient's gender identity and preferred pronouns prior to the start of pre-anesthesia care. If there is any uncertainty, it is appropriate for staff members to ask about gender identity and preferred pronouns. This practice has been implemented in the community health setting for many years [13], and it is appropriate to apply it to perioperative practices. To reduce delays on the day of surgery, the Institute of Medicine recommends having this information documented in the electronic health records to improve efficiency on the day of surgery [14].

Pregnancy Testing

All transgender men who are of reproductive age should have a pregnancy test prior to surgery. Not all transgender men are on testosterone therapy and without exogenous cross-sex hormone therapy, ovulation is likely. In addition, ovulation suppression is not perfect on testosterone therapy, especially if patients are not always compliant with their treatment. As a result, all patients should undergo pregnancy screening with a urine human chorionic gonadotropin test (urine pregnancy test) with reflex serum testing pending results.

Management of Testosterone

Transgender men may be on testosterone therapy, which may be administered via the parenteral or transdermal routes [11, 15]. Testosterone therapy is associated with higher erythropoietin production and an elevated hematocrit (polycythemia) [11, 15, 16]. A large systematic review revealed clinically insignificant changes in cardiovascular measures such as blood pressure after initiation of testosterone therapy, as well as inconsistent changes in liver and renal function after therapy [16].

There is anecdotal concern about an increased risk of venous thromboembolism (VTE) perioperatively, given that many patients are polycythemic on testosterone. However, in a cohort of 50 transgender men on an average of 10 years of testosterone therapy, none of the men reported a history of VTE or cardiovascular events [17]. The same observations were made in an Austrian retrospective cohort study of 89 transgender men [18]. In a meta-analysis by Elamin et al. ($N = 651$ transgender men), few patients had a cardiovascular event or VTE while on testosterone therapy; in fact, the incidence of any adverse event associated with testosterone therapy was low in this analysis [19]. No studies have specifically reported on the incidence of VTE in transgender patients undergoing hysterectomy while on testosterone therapy.

While there are no guidelines regarding the management of testosterone therapy in the perioperative period, the above data can be used to make decisions about perioperative management. It is reasonable to allow patients to continue their testosterone therapy and to practice venous thromboembolism prophylaxis based on risk stratification, which is dependent on the patient's medical history, surgical approach, and perceived period of immobility. For patients undergoing vaginal or laparoscopic surgery without a history of VTE, early mobilization and mechanical prophylaxis such as compression stockings or sequential compression devices may be sufficient. In our practice, all patients are offered same day discharge to help with early mobilization to reduce the risk of postoperative VTE.

Fertility Counseling

Over half of the transgender men surveyed by Wierck et al. reported a desire to have children ($n = 27/50$, 54%). Auer et al. conducted a cross-sectional survey of 90 German transgender men and found that none of the men who were already undergoing testosterone therapy pursued any fertility-preserving options prior to initiation. However, in this study, 57.1% of the men would have postponed gender affirmation hormone treatment to preserve their fertility had they been given the option. More transgender men reported a desire for children before, compared to after, initiation of hormone therapy (53% compared to 25%, $p = 0.049$) [20]. In another study, 37.5% of surveyed men reported that they would consider germ cell preservation if presented with the option [21]. Data exist showing that even after initiation of testosterone therapy, it is possible for transgender men to have genetically related offspring [22], and so it remains an important part of the preoperative discussion regardless of whether or not patients have initiated testosterone therapy [23].

One method of germ cell preservation is oocyte retrieval followed by oocyte or embryo cryopreservation. While oocytes may be retrieved from ovarian tissue even if the patient has been exposed to testosterone therapy [22, 24], most patients undergo oocyte retrieval prior to initiating testosterone therapy [23, 25], as there is conflicting evidence on the effect of exogenous testosterone on ovarian morphology [26, 27]. Providers should make sure to describe the process to their patients before referring them for specialist consultation. Patients should know that the process of retrieval involves serial pelvic exams and transvaginal ultrasounds, which could be distressing and uncomfortable [28]. Furthermore, ovarian stimulation is required, which means that patients have to discontinue their testosterone therapy and initiate feminizing treatments such as gonadotropin therapy. This can also be very stressful for patients and it may worsen their gender dysphoria. These discussion points are an important part of preoperative counseling and should not be used to deter patients from pursuing fertility treatments but should be mentioned to make them aware of what the process entails.

One emerging method of fertility preservation is cryopreservation of ovarian tissue [29]. For ovarian tissue preservation, the cumulus–oocyte complex is recovered from the antral follicles and can undergo in vitro maturation, followed by cryopreservation. This is an emerging technology that has been used in women with cancer or ovarian insufficiency [30, 31]. One study by De Roo et al. looked at ovarian histology in transgender men following one or more years of exogenous testosterone treatment. In their cohort, they were able to show in vitro maturation potential of the cumulus–oocyte complex from ovaries that were removed at the time of hysterectomy in these men [22]. Nevertheless, the biggest limitation of this technology is that it is only offered at selected centers and it remains experimental [32].

As technology evolves, it is likely that there will be more sophisticated mechanisms for oocyte retrieval and cryopreservation for all patients, including transgender men. In the meantime, it is crucial that providers discuss fertility preservation options with patients before they undergo surgery [32–34].

Choosing the Route of Surgery

Between 2013 and 2016, per the national database of the American College of Surgeons' National Surgical Quality (NSQIP), the most common mode of hysterectomy for patients with a designated male gender was laparoscopic (57.2%), followed by laparoscopic-assisted vaginal hysterectomy (20%), abdominal hysterectomy (15.2%), and vaginal hysterectomy (7.7%) [4]. Most surgeons performing gender affirmation hysterectomies perform laparoscopic hysterectomies as it is minimally invasive and patients can be discharged the same day. We review the different types of approaches to perform a hysterectomy, although the optimal route of surgery is the one that the surgeon feels most competent performing.

Vaginal Approach

The American College of Obstetricians and Gynecologists recommend a vaginal approach to hysterectomy whenever possible [35]. In a Cochrane review comparing different surgical approaches to hysterectomy for benign disease, the authors concluded that vaginal hysterectomy was associated with faster return to normal activities and fewer complications [36].

There may be concerns that vaginal hysterectomy is more difficult to perform in transgender men compared to cisgender women as a result of a higher incidence of nulliparity in this group as well as less compliant and atrophic vaginal epithelium as a result of chronic testosterone use [7, 37]. Obedin-Maliver et al. compared 33 transgender men and 850 cisgender women who underwent vaginal hysterectomy. They found that there were no differences between the groups in anesthesia time, estimated blood loss, intraoperative complications, acute postoperative complications, and delayed postoperative complications [6]. The main limitation of this study is that the transgender cohort was very small, precluding generalizability; however, the paper does support the feasibility of a vaginal approach to a hysterectomy, particularly in the hands of skilled pelvic surgeons. We believe that a vaginal approach should always be taken whenever possible as it is the least invasive mode and is associated with favorable outcomes.

Minimally Invasive Abdominal Approach

Despite the benefits of vaginal surgery, the most commonly published approach for gender affirmation hysterectomy in transgender men is conventional laparoscopy. WPATH recommends a laparoscopic approach toward hysterectomy for gender affirmation [8].

Laparoscopic hysterectomies are performed using three to four 5-mm trocars placed through the abdominal wall. Larger trocars can also be used for specimen removal or for suturing the vaginal cuff if determined to be necessary by the surgeon. Small trocars are ideal as the incisions are discreet and allow patients to conceal their surgical scars.

Although data are sparse, hysterectomies performed laparoscopically in transgender men may be associated with a lower incidence of complications than those performed in cisgender women. O'Hanlan et al. performed a retrospective chart review of 493 patients who underwent total laparoscopic hysterectomy with oophorectomy. This cohort included 41 transgender men and 552 cisgender women. When compared to cisgender women, transgender men had significantly less blood loss and a shorter duration of surgery. This is likely because the transgender men cohort had smaller uteri overall (mean weight 118.02 g ± 115.6 g) compared to the cisgender women cohort (mean weight 167.14 ± 108.4), $p < 0.001$ [7].

When compared to abdominal hysterectomies, laparoscopic hysterectomies are associated with shorter duration of hospital stay, fewer wound infections, shorter mean return to activities and improved quality of life postoperatively [35, 36]. The two approaches to hysterectomy have similar adverse events with comparable rates of bowel injury, vascular injury, and bleeding. However, laparoscopic hysterectomies were 2.44 times more likely to be associated with a lower urinary tract injury though the overall incidence is very low [36]. A thorough understanding of pelvic anatomy and the trajectory of the ureters can decrease the risk of injury.

Some surgeons may offer robotic-assisted laparoscopic hysterectomy. Studies have not shown a clear advantage between robotic-assisted versus traditional laparoscopy when comparing length of hospital stay, total operating time, conversion to laparotomy or total blood loss [36, 38]. At this time, there is insufficient evidence to determine the most advantageous option of the two. The decision to perform traditional versus robotic-assisted laparoscopy should be dependent on the surgeon's skillset and the hospital facilities.

Open Abdominal Approach

Abdominal hysterectomies are performed through an abdominal incision that can be made vertically or transversely on the abdomen. Choice of incision depends on the size and dimensions of the uterine specimen and the surgeon's experience. This approach toward hysterectomy is typically reserved for patients with a large uterus or with a history of multiple abdominal surgeries who are at higher risk for intraoperative injury. We have already mentioned the benefits of minimally invasive surgery, including vaginal and laparoscopic. Open abdominal surgery should really only be performed when the risks associated with minimally invasive surgery outweigh its benefits.

Vaginal Exam and Vaginal Cuff Closure

In transgender men undergoing hysterectomy, there may be a higher incidence of vaginal laceration from uterine manipulation placement or specimen (uterine) retrieval due to atrophic changes in the vaginal epithelium. Providers should be mindful of this during surgery in order to minimize trauma. Often, vaginal lacerations will need primary closure repairs, so a vaginal exam is warranted at the conclusion of the hysterectomy. Severe vaginal atrophy as a result of testosterone therapy may also place patients at risk of poor healing and postoperative vaginal cuff dehiscence. To avoid this, we recommend a two-layered closure with delayed absorbable suture and a prolonged period of pelvic rest (up to 12 weeks) postoperatively.

Complications Associated with Hysterectomy

Complications of hysterectomy include those that are inherent to any abdominal or pelvic surgery. The possible surgical complications include: surgical site infection, need for blood transfusion, and injuries to the urinary tract (bladder and ureters), bowel, and blood vessels. In the previously mentioned NSQIP database study, transgender men were not more likely than cisgender women to experience a postoperative complication after a hysterectomy, even after controlling for major medical comorbidity, mode of surgery, and age [4]. The incidence of postoperative complications was reported to be 3.4% in the transgender men group compared to 3.3% in the control group, $p = 0.92$. An important finding of this study, however, was that vaginal and laparoscopic approaches to hysterectomy were associated with a lower risk of developing any postoperative complication when compared to the abdominal approach (adjOR 0.04, 95% CI 0.002–0.17; adjOR 0.09, 95% CI 0.04–0.18, respectively) [4]. These findings further support the aforementioned: minimally invasive options for hysterectomy, either laparoscopic or vaginal, should be offered to all transgender men given the lower risk of associated postoperative complications compared to the abdominal approach. In choosing the type of minimally invasive approach, there should be shared decision-making between the patient and surgeon, accounting for the patient's preferences and the surgeon's expertise.

Concurrent Procedures at the Time of Hysterectomy

The decision to pursue concurrent procedures at the time of hysterectomy should be made in advance, depending on the patient's desires and the surgeon's/institution's capabilities. We discuss a list of possible concurrent procedures at the time of hysterectomy (Box 8.3). A multidisciplinary approach to care should be taken to ensure that the patient is adequately counseled on the risks and benefits of all procedures.

Concurrent Vaginal Vault Suspension

A vaginal vault suspension, or colpopexy, is the attachment of the vaginal apex to ligaments within the pelvis, including the uterosacral and sacrospinous ligaments. Colpopexy is often performed for the treatment of pelvic organ prolapse, but it can also be performed at the time of hysterectomy to prevent pelvic organ prolapse from occurring in the future.

It has been estimated that 2.9% of women experience pelvic organ prolapse in their lifetime [39]. In a retrospective cohort of cisgender women presenting to a urogynecology clinic,

---

Box 8.3 Optional Concurrent Procedures at the Time of Hysterectomy

1. Vaginal vault suspension
2. Salpingectomy
3. Oophorectomy
4. Vaginectomy
5. Mastectomy and chest reconstruction

Harris et al. compared characteristics between parous and nulliparous women. They found that nulliparous women were less likely to present with pelvic organ prolapse compared to their parous counterparts [40]. Other studies have shown that parity, vaginal delivery, age, and body–mass index are significantly associated with the development of pelvic organ prolapse in cisgender women [41]. Not all, but many transgender men presenting for hysterectomy are nulliparous. While it is safe to say that the transgender man's likelihood of developing pelvic organ prolapse is dependent on the risk factors he possesses, we suspect that his risk is lower compared to that of a cisgender woman.

There is currently a paucity of prospective data on the use of concurrent vaginal vault suspension at the time of hysterectomy for any patient undergoing surgery, and there are no data specifically reporting on concurrent suspension in transgender men. While there are trials underway [42], at this time, there is insufficient evidence to recommend routine prophylactic vaginal vault suspension at the time of any hysterectomy. As mentioned, if we extrapolate data from the cisgender woman population, nulliparous transgender men are much less likely to experience pelvic organ prolapse in their lifetime. As such, until more data are available, the decision to perform a prophylactic suspension should be left to the surgeon and the patient after thorough preoperative counseling.

Concurrent Salpingectomy and Oophorectomy

In individuals who desire hysterectomy but wish to preserve their ovaries for fertility reasons, concurrent salpingectomy should be discussed. There is a proposed theory that certain types of ovarian cancer, such as serous, endometrioid, and clear cell carcinomas, are derived from the fallopian tubes and the endometrium [43, 44]. Genetic studies have demonstrated that the morphology of high-grade serous carcinomas is related more to fallopian tubes than ovaries. The American College of Obstetrician and Gynecologists has concluded that based on the current understanding of ovarian cancer, salpingectomy at the time of hysterectomy, with ovarian preservation, may offer ovarian cancer risk reduction [45]. While salpingectomy, either at the time of hysterectomy or sterilization, does significantly increase total operation time, it did not result in a significant increase in surgical complications [46].

For cisgender women, studies have shown that ovarian conservation may result in a long-term survival benefit up until age 65 years [47], as there is concern over bone health and cardiovascular disease in women who have had oophorectomies. Despite this, these are not contraindications to concurrent oophorectomy at the time of hysterectomy for transgender men.

In transgender men, the replacement of exogenous testosterone after oophorectomy reduces the impact of estrogen deficiency. In a group of transgender men, after 10 years of testosterone therapy after oophorectomy, there was an increase in radial cortical bone size and decreased cortical volumetric bone density – a result of increased bone formation and intracortical bone remodeling [48]. However, this does mean that after oophorectomy, transgender men would require continuous testosterone replacement therapy not only to maintain secondary sexual characteristics, but also to reduce the risk of bone loss and bone fracture as a result of estrogen deficiency [49].

If the ovaries were left in situ, transgender men on exogenous testosterone are at risk for cystic ovaries akin to cisgender women with polycystic ovarian syndrome [27, 50]. Ovarian cysts may cause pain and may require regular surveillance with transvaginal ultrasounds and gynecologic exams. As mentioned earlier, seeking gynecologic care can result in gender dysphoria for transgender men. In addition, many patients fear having to present to an emergency room for an acute gynecologic condition for fear of being discriminated, or not cared for appropriately, as a result of their transgender status.

Apart from the endocrinological considerations, the above considerations are equally important. Patients should be thoroughly counseled about the risks and benefits of concurrent oophorectomy at the time of hysterectomy. As previously mentioned, fertility counseling is recommended prior to proceeding with oophorectomy. Some patients may not have firm notions of family planning at the time of hysterectomy. For these patients, it is reasonable to offer a staged procedure of hysterectomy followed by oophorectomy at a different time.

Concurrent Vaginectomy +/− Phalloplasty at the Time of Hysterectomy

Vaginectomy is the excision and/or complete obliteration of the vaginal canal. Transgender men who do not participate in penetrative vaginal sex and/or who have dysphoria related to their vagina may request that vaginectomy be performed concurrently with hysterectomy. If patients are interested in proceeding with a phalloplasty in the future, patients should be counseled that a portion of vaginal epithelium is sometimes salvaged at the time of vaginectomy and used for urethral lengthening at the time of metoidioplasty or phalloplasty surgery. Sometimes, vaginectomy with urethral lengthening is performed as a first-stage procedure in the construction of a neophallus depending on the surgical technique used. This is discussed further and in more detail in another chapter of this book.

Patients who do not desire future phalloplasty but are seeking concurrent vaginectomy should be made aware of the risks associated with this procedure. Concurrent vaginectomy extends surgical time and may necessitate an overnight stay before discharge home. The procedure is also associated with more surgical bleeding and a higher risk of postoperative hematoma and abscess formation.

Concurrent Chest Surgery at the Time of Hysterectomy

Chest surgery includes bilateral subcutaneous mastectomy, chest contouring, obliteration of the inframammary fold, and repositioning of the nipple-areola for transgender men [51, 52]. The surgical approach toward mastectomy is dependent on breast size, degree of excess skin, nipple–areola complex size and skin elasticity [51]. This procedure is usually the first and most commonly performed gender confirmation procedure for transgender men [51]. Thirty-six percent of the transgender men surveyed by the National Transgender Discrimination Survey had pursued gender-affirming chest surgery at the time of the survey, and 61% of men surveyed reported desiring the surgery one day [1]. Chest surgery is associated with a very high satisfaction rate [53] and not only do they create a masculinized chest, mastectomies can also reduce the incidence of breast cancer, which is beneficial in this patient population [54].

The incidence of complications is higher with chest surgery compared to hysterectomy. Issues related to chest surgery may prolong a patient's recovery or require them to stay in the hospital overnight for observation. In a series of 184 subcutaneous mastectomies in 92 transgender men, the complication rate was 12.5%, including minor complications such as a contained hematoma (2.8%), hematoma requiring surgical evacuation (3.3%), wound dehiscence (1.1%), and abscess formation (1.1%) [51]. In another retrospective study of 202 patients, the acute reoperation rate for expanding hematomas was 5% and there was a 30% rate of secondary correction surgeries, typically including scar, nipple, and areola revisions [52].

Box 8.4 Principal ERAS Components to Enhance Postoperative Recovery for Transgender Men Undergoing Hysterectomy

Preoperative components
- Optimization of patient physiologic condition
- Preoperative analgesia
- Contemporary fasting guidelines

Intraoperative components
- Fluid optimization
- Regional anesthesia
- Avoidance of use of laparotomy incisions
- Venous thromboembolism prophylaxis
- Antibiotic for surgical site infection prophylaxis
- Short-acting opioid agents/local nerve blocks
- Maintenance of normothermia
- Intraoperative removal of Foley catheter

Postoperative components
- Fluid optimization
- Analgesic optimization
- Early oral nutrition and ambulation
- Defined discharge pathways

(Adapted from Table 2. Yoong et al. [55])

It is possible to perform a concurrent mastectomy at the time of hysterectomy. Typically, chest surgery is performed by plastic surgeons, while the hysterectomy is performed by gynecologic surgeons. While the sequence of the hysterectomy and mastectomy is mostly dependent on surgical scheduling, it is important to ensure that the patient is positioned appropriately at the beginning of the case to allow for both procedures to be performed efficiently. We recommend positioning the patient in a dorsal lithotomy position in hydraulic stirrups. This position permits the vaginal, laparoscopic and abdominal approaches to hysterectomy. In addition, this position will not affect the surgical field for chest surgery. It is important to ensure good communications between the surgical teams to ensure a safe and collaborative surgery. Same day discharges are possible if postoperative milestones are achieved.

Postoperative Considerations

The Enhanced Recovery After Surgery (ERAS) or "fast-track" protocol is a program that facilitates faster recovery after surgery by minimizing the physiologic stress of surgery and facilitating return to functional baseline [55]. This is achieved through pathways to ensure early ambulation, early feeding, and multimodal pain management. Hospitals that have implemented the ERAS protocol have noticed decreased length of stay, improved patient satisfaction, and decreased hospital costs for gynecologic surgeries [53, 55, 56].

In Box 8.4, we propose an ERAS protocol for transgender men (Box 8.4). Most transgender patients undergoing hysterectomy are healthy. As a result, same day discharge by following an ERAS protocol should be strongly considered.

At the conclusion of the hysterectomy, providers should strongly consider intraoperative removal of the Foley catheter in the absence of an indication for continuous bladder drainage. Catheter management and removal while the patient is awake may trigger dysphoria. Along the same lines, patients should be thoroughly counseled to expect vaginal spotting after surgery.

Lastly, if the patients are admitted postoperatively, providers should be mindful of the patient room assignments. Most hospitals, if there are shared rooms, group patients based on gender. Transgender patients should be assigned based on their gender identity, and private rooms should be offered as an option for privacy and comfort [57].

Summary

Overall, hysterectomy is a safe surgical procedure for transgender men. The best surgical approach is the one that the surgeon feels most competent performing, but a minimally invasive approach should almost always be taken. Surgeons offering hysterectomy to transgender patients should be well versed in the WPATH guidelines and incorporate their recommendations into their respective practices. Providers should be aware of the special perioperative considerations that exist for transgender men undergoing hysterectomy, and they should ensure that their patients receive appropriate fertility counseling. If the patient desires concurrent procedures, a multidisciplinary approach is needed to achieve optimal outcomes.

Key Points

- Hysterectomy may be medically necessary for the treatment of pain, abnormal uterine bleeding, uterine fibroids, and gender dysphoria for transgender men.
- Minimally invasive approach to hysterectomy should be considered as the first option.
- Prior to surgery, discuss patients' desire for concurrent procedures, and their fertility preserving options.
- A multidisciplinary approach is recommended to ensure that the patient is adequately counseled and ready for surgery.

References

1. Grant JM, Mottet LA, Justin Tanis J, with Jack Harrison Jody Herman DmL, Keisling M. Injustice at every turn A report of the National Transgender Discrimination Survey. 2011. https://www.hivlawandpolicy.org/sites/default/files/InjusticeatEveryTurn.pdf. Accessed 26 Nov 2018.
2. Gonzales G, Henning-Smith C. Barriers to care among transgender and gender nonconforming adults. Milbank Q. 2017;95(4):726–48.
3. Chang OH, Haviland MJ, Von Bargen E, Gomez-Carrion Y, Hacker MR, Li J. Female pelvic medicine and reconstructive surgery fellows' exposure to transgender health care. Am J Obstet Gynecol. 2018;219(6):625–6.
4. Bretschneider CE, Sheyn D, Pollard R, Ferrando CA. Complication rates and outcomes after hysterectomy in transgender men. Obstet Gynecol. 2018;132(5):1265–73.
5. Hage JJ, Karim RB. Ought GIDNOS get nought? Treatment options for nontranssexual gender dysphoria. Plast Reconstr Surg. 2000;105(3):1222–7. http://www.ncbi.nlm.nih.gov/pubmed/10724285. Accessed 7 Dec 2018.
6. Obedin-Maliver J, Light A, de Haan G, Jackson RA. Feasibility of vaginal hysterectomy for female-to-male transgender men. Obstet Gynecol. 2017;129(3):457–63.
7. O'Hanlan KA, Dibble SL, Young-Spint M. Total laparoscopic hysterectomy for female-to-male transsexuals. Obstet Gynecol. 2007;110(5):1096–101.
8. WPATH World Professional Association for Transgender Health. Standards of care for the health of transsexual, transgender, and gender nonconforming people. Version 7. https://www.wpath.org/publications/soc.

9. Baggish M, Karram M. Atlas of pelvic anatomy and gynecologic surgery. 4th ed. Philadelphia: Elsevier; 2016.

10. Valea F. Reproductive anatomy: gross and microscopic, clinical correlations, chap. 3. In: Comprehensive gynecology. 7th ed. Philadelphia: Elsevier; 2017. p. 48–76.e1.

11. Irwig MS. Testosterone therapy for transgender men. Lancet Diabetes Endocrinol. 2017;5(4):301–11.

12. Berli JU, Knudson G, Fraser L, et al. What surgeons need to know about gender confirmation surgery when providing care for transgender individuals. JAMA Surg. 2017;152(4):394.

13. Cahill S, Singal R, Grasso C, et al. Do ask, do tell: high levels of acceptability by patients of routine collection of sexual orientation and gender identity data in four diverse American Community Health Centers. Prestage G, ed. PLoS One. 2014;9(9):e107104.

14. Cahill S, Makadon H. Sexual orientation and gender identity data collection in clinical settings and in electronic health records: a key to ending LGBT health disparities. LGBT Health. 2014;1(1):34–41.

15. Moravek MB. Gender-affirming hormone therapy for transgender men. Clin Obstet Gynecol. 2018;61(4):1.

16. Velho I, Fighera TM, Ziegelmann PK, Spritzer PM. Effects of testosterone therapy on BMI, blood pressure, and laboratory profile of transgender men: a systematic review. Andrology. 2017;5(5):881–8.

17. Van Caenegem E, Verhaeghe E, Taes Y, et al. Long-term evaluation of donor-site morbidity after radial forearm flap phalloplasty for transsexual men. J Sex Med. 2013;10(6):1644–51.

18. Ott J, Kaufmann U, Bentz E-K, Huber JC, Tempfer CB. Incidence of thrombophilia and venous thrombosis in transsexuals under cross-sex hormone therapy. Fertil Steril. 2010;93(4):1267–72.

19. Elamin MB, Garcia MZ, Murad MH, Erwin PJ, Montori VM. Effect of sex steroid use on cardiovascular risk in transsexual individuals: a systematic review and meta-analyses. Clin Endocrinol. 2010;72(1):1–10.

20. Auer MK, Fuss J, Nieder TO, et al. Desire to have children among transgender people in Germany: a cross-sectional multi-center study. J Sex Med. 2018;15(5):757–67.

21. Wierckx K, Van Caenegem E, Pennings G, et al. Reproductive wish in transsexual men. Hum Reprod. 2012;27(2):483–7.

22. De Roo C, Lierman S, Tilleman K, et al. Ovarian tissue cryopreservation in female-to-male transgender people: insights into ovarian histology and physiology after prolonged androgen treatment. Reprod Biomed Online. 2017;34(6):557–66.

23. De Sutter P. Gender reassignment and assisted reproduction: present and future reproductive options for transsexual people. Hum Reprod. 2001;16(4):612–4. http://www.ncbi.nlm.nih.gov/pubmed/11278204. Accessed 29 Nov 2018.

24. Maxwell S, Noyes N, Keefe D, Berkeley AS, Goldman KN. Pregnancy outcomes after fertility preservation in transgender men. Obstet Gynecol. 2017;129(6):1031–4.

25. Chen D, Bernardi LA, Pavone ME, Feinberg EC, Moravek MB. Oocyte cryopreservation among transmasculine youth: a case series. J Assist Reprod Genet. 2018;35(11):2057–61.

26. Ikeda K, Baba T, Noguchi H, et al. Excessive androgen exposure in female-to-male transsexual persons of reproductive age induces hyperplasia of the ovarian cortex and stroma but not polycystic ovary morphology. Hum Reprod. 2013;28(2):453–61.

27. Caanen MR, Schouten NE, Kuijper EAM, et al. Effects of long-term exogenous testosterone administration on ovarian morphology, determined by transvaginal (3D) ultrasound in female-to-male transsexuals. Hum Reprod. 2017;32(7):1457–64.

28. Armuand G, Dhejne C, Olofsson JI, Rodriguez-Wallberg KA. Transgender men's experiences of fertility preservation: a qualitative study. Hum Reprod. 2017;32(2):383–90.

29. Fasano G, Moffa F, Dechène J, Englert Y, Demeestere I. Vitrification of in vitro matured oocytes collected from antral follicles at the time of ovarian tissue cryopreservation. Reprod Biol Endocrinol. 2011;9(1):150.

30. Abir R, Ben-Aharon I, Garor R, et al. Cryopreservation of in vitro matured oocytes in addition to ovarian tissue freezing for fertility preservation in paediatric female cancer patients before and after cancer therapy. Hum Reprod. 2016;31(4):750–62.

31. Huang JYJ, Tulandi T, Holzer H, et al. Cryopreservation of ovarian tissue and in vitro matured oocytes in a female with mosaic Turner syndrome: Case Report. Hum Reprod. 2007;23(2):336–9.

32. Ethics Committee of the American Society for Reproductive Medicine. Access to fertility services by transgender persons: an Ethics Committee opinion. Fertil Steril. 2015;104(5):1111–5.

33. Hembree WC, Cohen-Kettenis P, Delemarre-van de Waal HA, et al. Endocrine treatment of transsexual persons:an Endocrine Society Clinical Practice Guideline. J Clin Endocrinol Metab. 2009;94(9):3132–54.

34. Coleman E, Bockting W, Botzer M, et al. Standards of care for the health of transsexual, transgender, and gender-nonconforming people, version 7. Int J Transgenderism. 2012;13(4):165–232.

35. American College of Obstetricians and Gynecologists. *Committee Opinion Number 701:* Choosing the route of hysterectomy for benign disease: American College of Obstetricians and Gynecologists; 2017.

36. Aarts JW, Nieboer TE, Johnson N, et al. Surgical approach to hysterectomy for benign gynaecological disease. Cochrane Database Syst Rev. 2015;(8):CD003677.

37. Miller N, Bédard YC, Cooter NB, Shaul DL. Histological changes in the genital tract in transsexual women following androgen therapy. Histopathology. 1986;10(7):661–9. http://www.ncbi.nlm.nih.gov/pubmed/2427430. Accessed 23 Nov 2018.

38. Albright BB, Witte T, Tofte AN, et al. Robotic versus laparoscopic hysterectomy for benign disease: a systematic review and meta-analysis of randomized trials. J Minim Invasive Gynecol. 2016;23(1):18–27.

39. Nygaard I, Barber MD, Burgio KL, et al. Prevalence of symptomatic pelvic floor disorders in US women. JAMA. 2008;300(11):1311.

40. Harris RL, Cundiff GW, Coates KW, Bump RC. Urinary incontinence and pelvic organ prolapse in nulliparous women. Obstet Gynecol. 1998;92(6):951–4. http://www.ncbi.nlm.nih.gov/pubmed/9840556. Accessed 27 Nov 2018.

41. Vergeldt TFM, Weemhoff M, IntHout J, Kluivers KB. Risk factors for pelvic organ prolapse and its recurrence: a systematic review. Int Urogynecol J. 2015;26(11):1559–73.

42. Alperin M, Weinstein M, Kivnick S, Duong TH, Menefee S. A randomized trial of Prophylactic Uterosacral Ligament Suspension at the time of hysterectomy for Prevention of Vaginal Vault Prolapse (PULS): design and methods. Contemp Clin Trials. 2013;35(2):8–12.

43. Kurman RJ, Shih I-M. The origin and pathogenesis of epithelial ovarian cancer: a proposed unifying theory. Am J Surg Pathol. 2010;34(3):433–43.

44. Erickson BK, Conner MG, Landen CN. The role of the fallopian tube in the origin of ovarian cancer. Am J Obstet Gynecol. 2013;209(5):409–14.

45. American College of Obstetricians and Gynecologists. Acog Committee Opinion: Salpinigectomy for Ovarian Cancer Prevention. American College of Obstetricians and Gynecologists; 2015. https://www.acog.org/Clinical-Guidance-and-Publications/Committee-Opinions/Committee-on-Gynecologic-Practice/Salpingectomy-for-Ovarian-Cancer-Prevention#here. Accessed 26 Nov 2018.

46. McAlpine JN, Hanley GE, Woo MMM, et al. Opportunistic salpingectomy: uptake, risks, and complications of a regional initiative for ovarian cancer prevention. Am J Obstet Gynecol. 2014;210(5):471.e1–471.e11.

47. Parker WH, Broder MS, Liu Z, Shoupe D, Farquhar C, Berek JS. Ovarian conservation at the time of hysterectomy for benign disease. Obstet Gynecol. 2005;106(2):219–26.

48. Van Caenegem E, Wierckx K, Taes Y, et al. Bone mass, bone geometry, and body composition in female-to-male transsexual persons after long-term cross-sex hormonal therapy. J Clin Endocrinol Metab. 2012;97(7):2503–11.

49. Adelman MR, Sharp HT. Ovarian conservation vs removal at the time of benign hysterectomy. Am J Obstet Gynecol. 2018;218(3):269–79.

50. Loverro G, Resta L, Dellino M, et al. Uterine and ovarian changes during testosterone administration in young female-to-male transsexuals. Taiwan J Obstet Gynecol. 2016;55(5):686–91.

51. Monstrey S, Hoebeke P, Selvaggi G, et al. Penile reconstruction: is the radial forearm flap really the standard technique? Plast Reconstr Surg. 2009;124(2):510–8.

52. Cregten-Escobar P, Bouman MB, Buncamper ME, Mullender MG. Subcutaneous mastectomy in female-to-male transsexuals: a retrospective cohort-analysis of 202 patients. J Sex Med. 2012;9(12):3148–53.

53. Scheib SA, Thomassee M, Kenner JL. Enhanced Recovery After Surgery (ERAS) in gynecology: a review of the literature. J Minim Invasive Gynecol. 2019;26(2):327–43.

54. Gooren LJ. Care of transsexual persons. N Engl J Med. 2011;364(13):1251–7.

55. Yoong W, Sivashanmugarajan V, Relph S, et al. Can enhanced recovery pathways improve outcomes of vaginal hysterectomy? Cohort control study. J Minim Invasive Gynecol. 2014;21(1):83–9.

56. Modesitt SC, Sarosiek BM, Trowbridge ER, et al. Enhanced recovery implementation in major gynecologic surgeries: effect of care standardization. Obstet Gynecol. 2016;128(3):457–66.

57. Tollinche LE, Walters CB, Radix A, et al. The perioperative care of the transgender patient. Anesth Analg. 2018;127(2):359–66.

Surgical Anatomy: Metoidioplasty

Borko Stojanovic, Marta Bizic,
and Miroslav L. Djordjevic

Introduction

Reconstruction of the neophallus is one of the most challenging tasks in transgender male gender affirmation surgery. There is a variety of available surgical techniques, but their outcomes are not equally acceptable to all patients. Metoidioplasty is a variant of phalloplasty for transgender male patients, wherein a small neophallus is created from a hormonally enlarged clitoris. It results in male appearance of genitalia, with completely preserved erogenous sensation and voiding in standing position, but without the possibility for penetrative sexual intercourse. The latest refinements in metoidioplasty technique are based on the advances in urethroplasty, perioperative care and the knowledge of the female genital anatomy, as well as the changes that occur to this anatomy with preoperative hormonal changes in the transgender population [1, 2].

Clear understanding of female genital anatomy and embryology is very important in male gender-affirming surgery. The human penis and clitoris develop from the same ambisexual genital tubercle, and the major anatomical difference is that clitoris becomes separated from the urethra. The clitoris plays a fundamental role in female sexual functioning, and its main characteristics – position, structure, and innervation – have been greatly clarified in recent studies on human cadavers and magnetic resonance imaging [3–5]. The possibility of using the clitoris for penile substitution in transgender male patients was originally reported by Durfee and Rowland in 1973 [6]. Since then, the techniques have been greatly improved, defining this procedure as metoidioplasty, the term derived from the Greek words "meta" – "toward" and "oidion" – "male genitalia" [7]. Today, metoidioplasty represents a one-stage procedure wherein a hormonally enlarged clitoris is used to create a small penis, simultaneously with urethral lengthening and scrotoplasty.

Anatomical Considerations

All parts of female external genitalia are used for complex reconstruction in metoidioplasty. The clitoris is transformed into the neophallus; urethral plate and both labia minora are used for urethral lengthening and neophallic skin reconstruction; periurethral tissue, vaginal flap, and bulbospongious muscle cover the neourethra; labia majora are used to form the scrotum. Successful outcome is based on the high proficiency in surgical anatomy of female genitalia.

B. Stojanovic (✉) · M. Bizic · M. L. Djordjevic
Belgrade Center for Urogenital Reconstructive
Surgery, School of Medicine, University of Belgrade,
Belgrade, Serbia
e-mail: stojanovic@uromiros.com

© Springer Nature Switzerland AG 2021
D. Nikolavsky, S. A. Blakely (eds.), *Urological Care for the Transgender Patient*,
https://doi.org/10.1007/978-3-030-18533-6_9

The Clitoris

The clitoral anatomy was an enigma for decades, but recent literature has documented its anatomical features and components. Clitoris is the erectile organ located medial and inferior to the pubic arch and symphysis, with a boomerang-shaped appearance. The anatomy of the clitoris is best understood when divided into its components: glans, prepuce, body, crura, bulbs, suspensory ligaments, and root [8] (see Fig. 9.1).

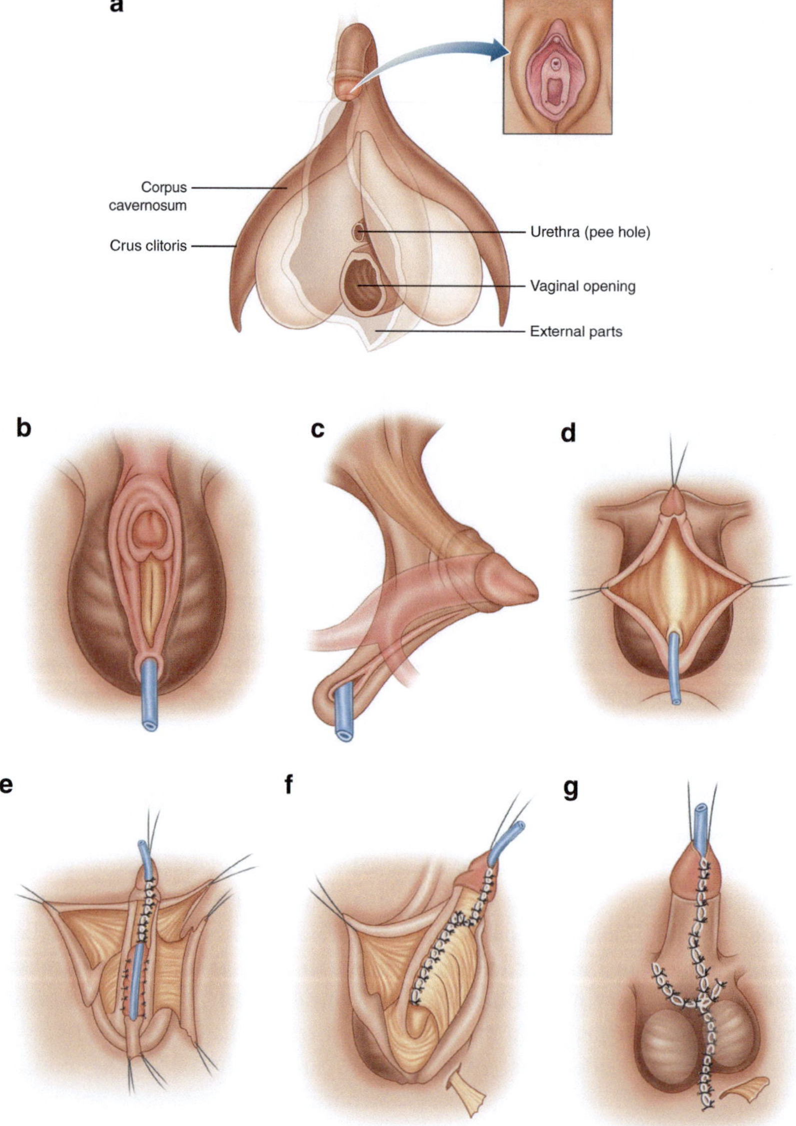

Fig. 9.1 Schematic presentation of normal clitoris and clitoral anatomy in metoidioplasty. (**a**) Normal clitoris. (**b**) Ventral aspect of hormonally enlarged clitoris; labia majora appear as scrotums. (**c**) Clitoral bodies are curved due to dorsal ligamentous support and short urethral plate. (**d**) Urethral plate is wide and adherent, with visible demarcation to labia minora. (**e**) Urethroplasty – buccal mucosa graft, previously quilted, combined with well-vascularized labia minora flap. (**f**) Flap is joined with buccal mucosa graft to create neourethra. (**g**) Final appearance of the neophallus

Clitoral glans and prepuce are the visible parts of the clitoral complex and lie at the superior apex of the vestibule. The prepuce or clitoral hood is formed out of fused labia minora anterior borders, at the level of the glans. The glans is a midline, densely neural, nonerectile structure that is the only external manifestation of the clitoris. According to the study performed on 200 premenopausal women with no hormonal disbalance, the mean transverse diameter of the clitoral glans was found to be 3.4 ± 1 mm, while the longitudinal diameter was 5.1 ± 1.4 mm, and the total length was 16 ± 4.3 mm [9]. Clitoral bulbs are located on the superficial aspect of the vaginal wall. The bulbs engorge during arousal, increasing the vaginal rigidity. In cadaveric studies, clitoral bulbs were found to be 3–4 cm in length when flaccid and up to 7 cm in length when erect. Clitoral body is composed of paired corpora cavernosa that diverge, forming two crura, which are attached to the pubic bones. The clitoral body measures 1–2 cm in width and 0.5–3.5 cm in length, while the crura, the internal and hidden parts of the corpora, measure 5–9 cm in length [9]. With testosterone therapy, the clitoris could be lengthened between 2 and 6 cm preoperatively. The clitoral glans, although attached to the labia minora inferiorly, can attain a size of 2 cm in diameter.

Clitoral body is secured to the fascia of the mons pubis, pubic symphysis, and labia by the suspensory ligaments that have superficial and deep portion. The superficial part attaches the clitoral body and glans to the mons pubis and extends into the medial aspect of the labia majora. It is a 7–8 cm wide, thick, fibro-fatty structure. The deep part connects the clitoral body to the pubic bones. The suspensory ligaments are different in shape, orientation, and composition between the genders. The role of the penile suspensory ligament is to stabilize the erect penis and to maintain the adequate angle to the abdominal wall during coitus. The clitoral suspensory ligaments play an important role in preventing the straightening of the clitoris during the erection, keeping it in curved position maintaining its stability during sexual activity [10].

Baskin et al. [11] found anatomical analogy between fetal penis and clitoris by anatomical dissection of the clitoris. The innervation of the clitoris is found to originate from the dorsal nerve of the clitoris, branches of the pudendal nerve and cavernous nerves with the position at the 11 and 1 o'clock along the clitoral body. The authors also emphasized the absence of the nerves at 12 o'clock position with the lowest nerve density on the ventral aspect of the glans, while the top and dorsal portions of the clitoral glans were abundantly innervated. Vaze et al. [12] also researched the course of the dorsal nerve of the clitoris. In this study on six adult cadavers, their findings were similar to those of Baskin et al. [11], but the exact function of the dorsal clitoral nerve remained uncertain. These findings point out the importance of cautious dissection of these nerves during clitoral surgery in order to prevent their intraoperative injury, as well as postoperative consequences. Vascular supply of the clitoris originates from the dorsal clitoral arteries, perineal arteries, deep arteries, and external pudendal artery, while the venous drainage is provided by the deep dorsal vein into the vesical venous plexus. The relationship between the clitoris and surrounding structures has also been analyzed. Recent research has demonstrated a close relationship between the clitoris, urethra, and vagina in both anatomical and functional aspects [13].

Labia Minora and Majora

Labia minora are paired, pigmented, hairless mucocutaneous folds rich in nerve endings and sensory receptors. They surround the vestibule and spread toward labia majora laterally. Labia minora separate anteriorly in two folds: superior, that forms the clitoral hood, and inferior, that forms the clitoral frenulum. Posteriorly, labia minora merge and form posterior fourchette. The Hart line defines the border between labia minora and vaginal vestibule. The dermis of labia minora is rich in elastic fibers and small blood vessels, making it similar to the corpus spongiosum of the penis. Labia minora are innervated along their edge and inner side, with branches originating from internal pudendal nerve, ilio-inguinal and genitofemoral nerves [14]. Free nerve endings, Pacinian and Meissner's corpuscles, are present in labia minora skin, suggesting their important role in stimulus energy transmission to the spinal cord and brain [15]. Awareness of these anatomical features is of the utmost importance in metoidioplasty, in order to preserve the sensation and sexual stimuli in the neophallus. Labia minora are perfused by small arteries that run perpendicular to the long axis of the labia with the confluence under the edge of labia. Two posterior thirds of the labia minora are supplied by internal pudendal artery, while the anterior third is perfused by small arteries deriving from external pudendal artery. The venous blood is drained by internal pudendal vein and vaginal venous plexus [16]. There is a large variation in length of labia minora, from 2 to 10 cm (from the clitoral hood to the posterior fourchette), while the width varies from 0.7 to 5 cm [17].

Labia majora are paired lateral folds of hair-bearing skin and adipose tissue that extend inferiorly from the mons pubis and merge with the neighboring skin, forming the posterior fourchette. Besides the hair follicles and adipose tissue, labia majora contain distal ends of round ligaments, and sebaceous and apocrine and eccrine sweat glands. The lateral side of the labia majora in adults is usually pigmented and contains hair follicles, while the internal is smooth, pink, and hairless. Labia majora match the scrotum in males, which is why they are used for scrotoplasty in male gender affirmation surgery. The composition of labia majora is very important in postoperative follow-up, as Camper's and Colles fascia form the superficial and deep layers of labia majora. The Colles fascia is inferiorly attached to the ischiopubic rami and posteriorly to the urogenital diaphragm, but without the anterior attachment, which allows the distribution of possible hematomas toward the perineum and anterior abdominal wall. The innervation of labia majora originates from the pudendal nerve, but there are also small branches from ilio-inguinal and posterior femoral cutaneous nerve. Vascular supply originates from internal pudendal arteries and from external pudendal arteries creating the net inside the labia majora. Venous drainage goes through the pudendal veins. The average length of labia majora ranges from 7 to 12 cm [17].

The Urethra

The urethral meatus opens inside the vestibule, above the vaginal opening and approximately 2 cm below the clitoris. The average length of the female urethra is 3.5 cm (ranging from 3 to 4 cm). Paired paraurethral glands (Skene glands) encircle urethral meatus and produce mucus during arousal. The bulbospongiosus muscle arises from the perineal centrum tendineum, covering vestibular bulb and ending on clitoris. Posterior urethra is innervated with more small nerves than the anterior urethra, and contains significantly larger blood vessels comparing to the anterior urethra [18].

Metoidioplasty Techniques

All patients are required to fulfill criteria according to WPATH Standards of Care prior to surgery [19]. Hormonal (testosterone) treatment causes hypertrophy of the clitoris and labia. Additional clitoral enlargement is achieved by applying dihydrotestosterone gel locally and using vacuum device twice daily, for a period of 3 months before surgery [20] (Fig. 9.2a). Patients are advised to stop hormonal therapy 2 weeks before surgery to avoid excessive intraoperative bleeding. Metoidioplasty can be performed as a multistaged surgery, or combined with hysterectomy, vaginectomy, and scrotoplasty as a single-stage procedure [21]. The most commonly used metoidioplasty techniques are simple metoidioplasty, ring metoidioplasty and Belgrade metoidioplasty.

Simple Metoidioplasty

The simple metoidioplasty starts with clitoral skin incision, followed by clitoral degloving and division of suspensory ligaments, dorsally.

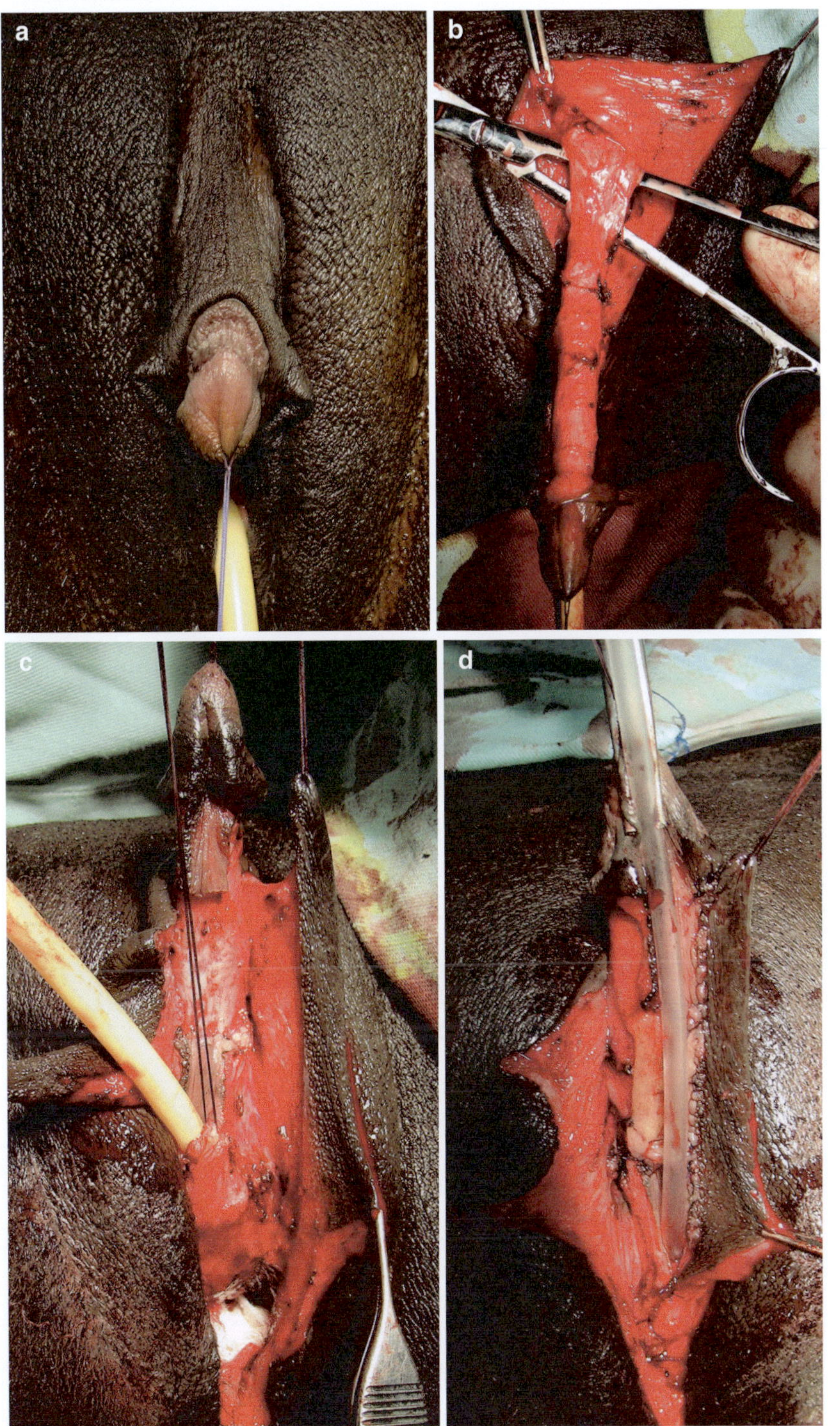

Fig. 9.2 (**a**) Preoperative appearance. Clitoris is enlarged due to hormonal treatment. (**b**) Clitoral ligaments are completely dissected up to the bone attachment, with preservation of neurovascular bundle, to enable maximal lengthening of the clitoris. (**c**) Bulbar part of the neourethra is created. Short urethral plate is divided. Vascularized flap is harvested from the left labia minora. (**d**) Buccal mucosa graft is fixed and quilted to cover the gap after division of urethral plate. Labia minora flap is joined with the new urethral plate to create neourethra. (**e**) Neourethra is covered with additional layer of well-vascularized tissue. (**f**) Scrotoplasty is done using both labia majora. Testicular implants are inserted into the new scrotum. (**g**) Final result after metoidioplasty

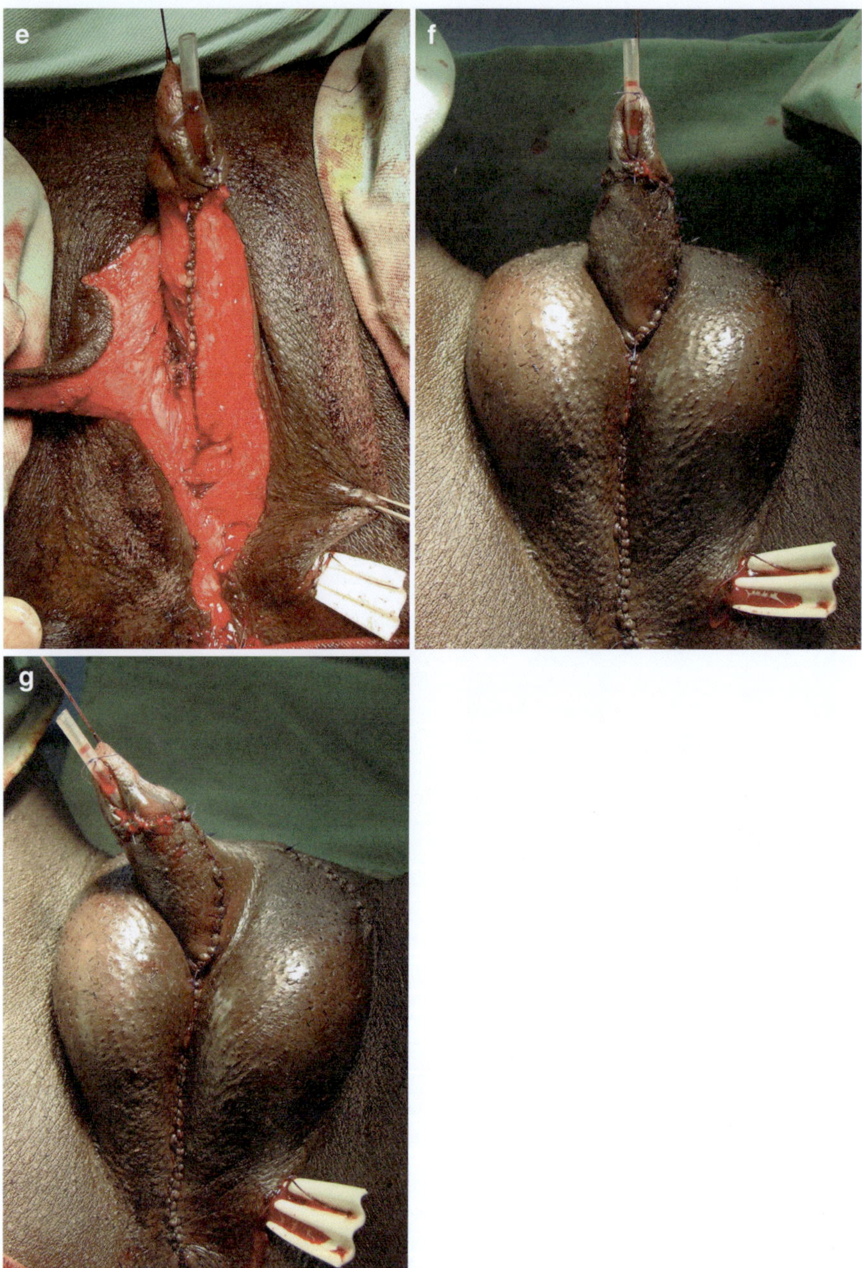

Fig. 9.2 (continued)

Ventrally, urethral plate is dissected and divided for additional straightening of the clitoris. The remaining clitoral skin with labia minora and majora is used to cover the shaft of the neophallus. Levator muscles are also dissected and used for additional support and enlargement of the neophallus. Urethral opening remains intact. A 14Fr Foley catheter is placed into the bladder.

Urethral lengthening is performed in the second stage to enable voiding in standing position. Despite its limitations, simple metoidioplasty provides a complication-free procedure at relatively low cost, in an outpatient setting [22].

In order to improve outcomes, modifications of simple metoidioplasty were reported [23]. A very long flap of anterior vaginal wall (5–7.5 cm) was used to create bulbar urethra. Additional support was provided by one labia minora flap, used to cover suture lines. Penile neourethra was created from a labia minora flap and the urethral plate, which was divided at the level of the female urethral opening. As the course of dissection was from proximal to distal, it could compromise the vascularization of the mobilized urethral plate. The same authors reported long-term results of this technique, with complication rate of 85% [24]. They stated that an average of 2.6 procedures per patient were performed in their series to complete genital reconstruction. Perovic et al. [25] reported good results of simple metoidioplasty combined with urethral lengthening in 22 patients. The main complications were related to urethral reconstruction, in 23% of cases.

Ring Metoidioplasty

This technique is the same as simple metoidioplasty, but it includes extending the urethral plate as well. Special dorsal urethral ring flap is harvested from introital vaginal mucosa. The ring flap is attached to the underlying clitoral bodies, allowing its tubularization without tension. Originally described by Takamatsu [26], this technique allows creation of the posterior urethral plate extension that is necessary for urethral lengthening. The ventral part of the urethra is created from long vaginal flap. Remaining labial skin is used to cover the shaft of the neophallus. Scrotoplasty is performed in the second stage, with good aesthetic result in almost all individuals. The ability to void in standing position is possible in minority of patients, and presents the main disadvantage [26]. The most common complications are urethral fistula (10–26%) and stricture (3–5%).

Belgrade Metoidioplasty

Belgrade center reported their original technique of metoidioplasty based on the repair of most severe forms of hypospadias [25]. The same surgical principles are used due to the similarities in surgical anatomy of penis and clitoris. Many refinements of the procedure have been reported in order to improve results of urethral reconstruction and minimize complication rate, in one-stage surgery [27–29]. Crucial steps of the procedure are straightening and lengthening of the clitoris by division of suspensory clitoral ligaments and short urethral plate; urethral lengthening from the native meatus to the top of the neophallus to enable voiding in standing position; reconstruction of the penile shaft skin, scrotum, and perineum with insertion of testicular implants [30].

Creation of the Neophallus

Creation of the neophallus starts with a circular incision beneath the glans, at the border between the inner and outer layer of the clitoral prepuce and continues around the urethral plate and native urethral orifice. Clitoral degloving is performed to expose clitoral body and suspensory ligaments. Suspensory ligaments are then detached from the pubic bone by thermocautery to lengthen the clitoris maximally (Fig. 9.2b). Care must be taken to avoid injury of the neurovascular structures during this maneuver. Paired clitoral neurovascular bundle originates from pudendal neurovascular bundle and ascends to the upper part of the clitoral body where the crura unite. The dorsal clitoral nerves pass in large fibers to enter the deep layers of the glans, without visible distal branches that reach the tip of the clitoris. Analogously to glans penis innervation, the innervation of the glans clitoris is rich, particularly in its dorsal part [2]. The urethral plate is short, causing ventral curvature of the clitoris, and therefore has to be divided. It is carefully dissected from the clitoral body, to prevent injury to the spongiosal tissue around the urethral plate and vigorous bleeding. Dissection includes bulbar part of the urethral plate, around the native meatus, to enable its good mobility for urethral reconstruction, but also to preserve the blood supply to the urethral plate. In this way, complete straightening and lengthening of the clitoris are achieved. However, it leaves a defect in urethral plate, which needs to be replaced with another tissue.

Urethral Reconstruction

Reconstruction of the urethra starts with reconstruction of its bulbar part. A well-vascularized periurethral flap is harvested from the anterior vaginal wall, with the base enclosing the urethral meatus. This flap is joined with the proximal part of the divided urethral plate using interrupted sutures, forming the bulbar part of the neourethra (Fig. 9.2c). Further urethral lengthening is performed by using buccal mucosa or skin graft and vascularized genital flaps (labia minora flap or clitoral skin flap). Buccal mucosa graft has become the gold standard material in urethral reconstruction, especially due to its histological attributes. Graft harvesting from the inner cheek is a safe procedure without morbidity of the donor site. Ellipse-shaped graft of appropriate size is designed, keeping the margin away from Stenson's duct and at least 10 mm away from the vermillion border [27]. Size of the graft depends on the size of the defect created after division of urethral plate. Buccal mucosa graft is harvested superficially to the buccinator muscle and prepared. After proper hemostasis is carried out, donor site is closed with a running suture. Split-thickness skin graft can be used as an alternative, harvested from hairless surface of labia minora. The graft is properly oriented and anastomosed to the proximal and distal margin of divided urethral plate to cover the gap. Additional quilting of the graft to the corporeal bodies, with interrupted sutures, is very important for better survival of the graft (Fig. 9.2d). The dorsal urethral plate is constituted in this way. The ventral part of the neourethra is created using a labia minora flap or dorsal clitoral skin flap. Labia minora has a very rich blood supply and represents a method of choice. Its dissection starts from the vaginal vestibulum and rises toward the clitoral glans. The lateral margin of the flap is created along the border between the inner and outer labial surface. The flap is harvested by de-epithelialization of the outer labial skin to preserve abundant vascularization. Pedicle of the flap is additionally mobilized from the subcutaneous tissue of labia majora to enable tension-free anastomosis with

buccal mucosa graft. An alternative option is to harvest longitudinal dorsal clitoral skin flap, and transpose it on the ventral side using buttonhole maneuver. The margins of labia minora or clitoral skin flap are then joined to the margins of the buccal mucosa graft by two lateral running sutures, to form penile neourethra [28]. The glans is then opened by two vertical parallel incisions, and both glans wings are dissected extensively. The distal part of the urethral plate and glans wings are used to form glandial neourethra and to create urethral meatus at the top of the neophallus.

Neourethra is covered with additional layers of well-vascularized genital tissue in all cases, in order to prevent superposition of the suture lines and urethral fistula (Fig. 9.2e). The bulbar urethra suffers the highest urinary stream pressure and therefore represents a weak point for postoperative fistula formation. The joining of the clitoral bulbs over the neourethra and the covering with vascularized surrounding tissue are considered key to successful fistula prevention at the place of anastomosis with native urethral orifice. A perforated 10-12Fr silicone tube is placed into the neourethra to maintain its lumen. Available clitoral and labia minora skin is used to cover the shaft of the neophallus.

Scrotoplasty

Both labia majora are joined in the midline to form the scrotum. Subcutaneous pockets for testicular prosthesis are created through incision made at the top of each labia majora. Silicone testicular implants of appropriate size are inserted, irrigated with antibiotic solution, and the pockets are closed in two layers, finalizing the scrotoplasty (Fig. 9.2f). Perineum and penoscrotal angle are reconstructed to have male appearance. Penrose drain is inserted in perineal region (Fig. 9.2g).

In certain cases, with well-developed urethral plate, urethral lengthening can be performed by simple tubularization of the wide plate over a catheter (Fig. 9.3a–f). The choice of this procedure is based on excellent width and extreme mobility of the urethral plate that enables tubularization urethroplasty without affecting neophallic length.

Perioperative Care

Suprapubic tube is inserted into the bladder for urine diversion. A 10–12Fr catheter is left in the neourethra as a urethral stent, which is used for buccal mucosa moisturizing for the first 72 h after surgery. Broad-spectrum antibiotics and oxybutynin are prescribed while the catheter is in place. The urethral stent is removed 10 days after surgery, and neourethra irrigated with 5 ml of saline every day until beginning of voiding. Patient starts to void 3 weeks after surgery, and suprapubic tube is removed safely the next day. Postoperative use of the vacuum pump for at least 6 months is necessary to prevent retraction of the neophallus, combined with a phosphodiesterase type-5 inhibitors treatment.

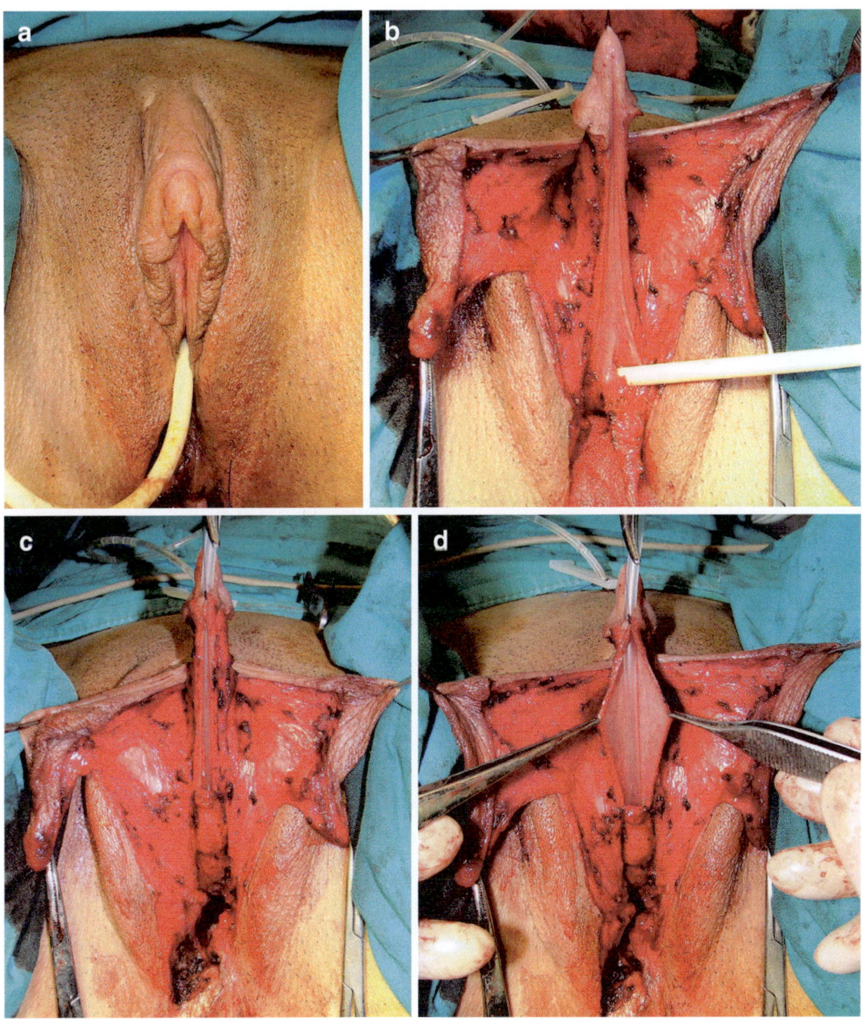

Fig. 9.3 (**a**) Preoperative appearance of hormonally enlarged clitoris. (**b**) Urethral plate is elastic and wide. Both labia minora are harvested as a good vascularized flaps. (**c**) Bulbar urethra is formed and covered with surrounding tissue to prevent postoperative fistula. (**d**) Urethral plate is tubularized to create neourethra. (**e**) Final outcome. Two testicular implants are inserted into the scrotum created from both labia majora. (**f**) Appearance at the end of surgery

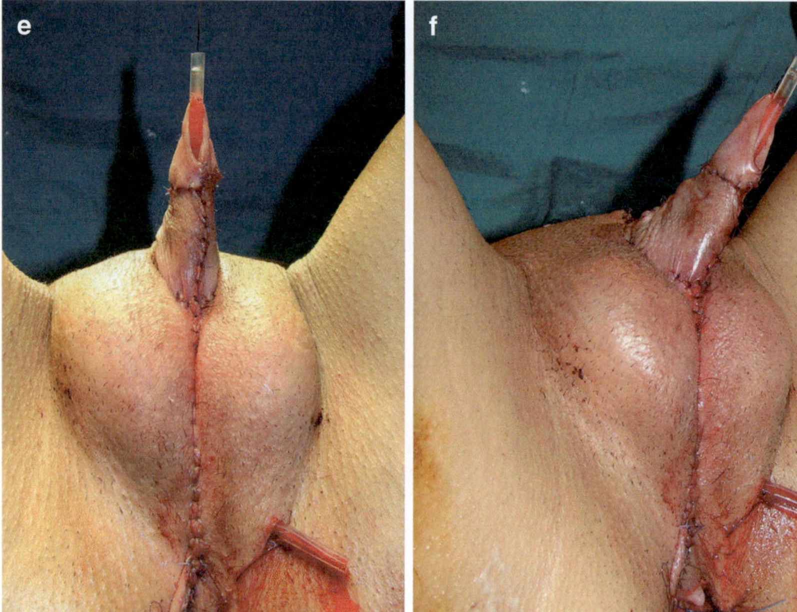

Fig. 9.3 (continued)

Outcomes and Complications

Outcomes

The goals of metoidioplasty are good aesthetic, functional, and psychosexual outcomes. It includes male appearance of genitalia with naturally positioned neophallus and scrotum, voiding while standing, and completely preserved erogenous sensation of the neophallus. Preoperative counseling plays a very important role, because the main criterion for successful outcome is patients' satisfaction. According to patient-reported outcome measures, metoidioplasty has good cosmetic result, and voiding in standing position is achieved in almost all cases. Although length of the neophallus is inadequate for full penetration, majority of patients report satisfaction with quality of erection, sensation of the neophallus, and sexual arousal, confirming overall sexual satisfaction and good psychosexual outcome [21, 31]. Preserved sensation of the neophallus guarantees a satisfying functional and psychosexual quality of life for these patients. A person who is not completely satisfied with metoidioplasty results can always require total phalloplasty. It is reported that 12–15% of patients with metoidioplasty eventually proceed with total phalloplasty [21]. However, complete assessment of patients' quality of life is possible only in long-term follow-up.

Complications

Postoperative complications can be classified as minor, which can be managed nonoperatively; and major, which require surgical repair. Minor postoperative complications include hematomas, wound infections, urinary tract infections, and minor urethral (dribbling, spraying, urethral fistula). These complications are reported in approximately 30% of patients, and resolve spontaneously 3–6 months after surgery. Major complications require revision surgery, and are most frequently related to urethroplasty (urethral fistula, stricture, diverticulum, dehiscence of the neourethra). Urethral fistula is reported in 7–25%, and stricture in 3–12% of cases [32]. Refinements in urethroplasty techniques reduced previously reported incidence of urethral fistula of almost 50% to less than 10% [24, 32]. Urethral fistula repair is performed by excision and covering with local vascularized flap. Urethral stricture is repaired by anastomotic or buccal mucosa graft urethroplasty. Other major complications include testicular implant rejection and dislocation, reported in 2–3% of patients. In case of dislocated testicular implant, repositioning and fixation of the implant into the proper place, with the creation of a new capsule is indicated [32].

Take-Home Points
- Metoidioplasty is a variant of transmasculine gender affirmation phalloplasty, where hormonally enlarged clitoris is used to create a neophallus.
- New insights in clitoral anatomy, advances in urethroplasty and perioperative care have improved outcomes of metoidioplasty.
- Goals of metoidioplasty are: male appearance of genitalia, voiding in standing position and preserved erogenous sensation of the neophallus; achieved in a one-stage surgery.
- Straightening and lengthening of the clitoris is performed by division of suspensory clitoral ligaments and short urethral plate, while preserving neurovascular bundle.
- Combined buccal mucosa graft and well-vascularized labia minora flap presents the best option for one-stage urethral lengthening from the native meatus to the tip of the neophallus.
- Metoidioplasty procedure has good aesthetic, functional, and psychosexual outcome.
- The main disadvantage of the procedure is the length of the neophallus, which is inadequate to allow penetrative sexual intercourse.

Conclusions

Metoidioplasty represents a surgical option of neophalloplasty for transgender males, where neophallus is created from hormonally hypertrophied clitoris. The main goal is to create male-appearance genitalia that enable voiding in standing position, satisfactory aesthetic result, and good sexual function. Since the publication of original procedure almost 50 years ago, the techniques of metoidioplasty have evolved significantly, mostly due to improved knowledge in surgical anatomy of female genitalia.

Transection of all layers of suspensory ligament, followed by dissection of short urethral plate, is necessary for complete straightening and lengthening of the clitoris. Preservation of the neurovascular supply and dorsal aspect of the glans, during dissection, is essential for maintaining sexual function. This recognition in surgical anatomy, combined with our previous observations and experience in genital reconstructive surgery, improved surgical outcomes. Metoidioplasty has established as a one-stage procedure, with low complication rate and high level of patient satisfaction. The main disadvantage is the size of the neophallus, which is inadequate for penetrative sexual intercourse, and all patients should be informed of this fact prior to surgery. However, majority of patients report satisfaction with surgical results.

Acknowledgments This work is supported by the Ministry of Science and Technical Development, Republic of Serbia, Project No. 175048.

References

1. Bizic MR, Stojanovic B, Djordjevic ML. Genital reconstruction for the transgendered individual. J Pediatr Urol. 2017;13:446–52.
2. Stojanovic B, Djordjevic ML. Anatomy of the clitoris and its impact on neophalloplasty (metoidioplasty) in female transgenders. Clin Anat. 2015;28(3):368–75.
3. Baskin L, Shen J, Sinclair A, et al. Development of the human penis and clitoris. Differentiation. 2018;103:74–85.

4. Oakley SH, Mutema GK, Crisp CC, et al. Innervation and histology of the clitoral-urethal complex: a cross-sectional cadaver study. J Sex Med. 2013;10:2211–8.

5. Agarwal MD, Resnick EL, Mhuircheartaigh JN, et al. MR imaging of the female perineum: clitoris, labia, and introitus. Magn Reson Imaging Clin N Am. 2017;25:43555.

6. Durfee R, Rowland W. Penile substitution with clitoral enlargement and urethral transfer. In: Laub DR, Gandy P, editors. Proceedings of the second interdisciplinary symposium on gender dysphoria syndrome. Palo Alto: Stanford University Press; 1973. p. 181–3.

7. Lebovic GS, Laub DR. Metoidioplasty. In: Ehrlich RM, Alter GJ, editors. Reconstructive and plastic surgery of the external genitalia. Philadelphia: WB Saunders Co; 1999. p. 355–60.

8. O'Connell HE, Sanjeevan KV, Hutson JM. Anatomy of the clitoris. J Urol. 2005;174:1189–95.

9. Mazloomdoost D, Pauls RN. A comprehensive review of the clitoris and its role in female sexual function. Sex Med Rev. 2015;3:245–63.

10. Rees MA, O'Connell HE, Plenter RJ, et al. The suspensory ligament of the clitoris: connective tissue supports of the erectile tissues of the female urogenital region. Clin Anat. 2000;13:397–403.

11. Baskin LS, Erol A, Li YW, et al. Anatomical studies of the human clitoris. J Urol. 1999;162:1015–20.

12. Vaze A, Goldman H, Jones JS, et al. Determining the course of the dorsal nerve of the clitoris. Urology. 2008;72:1040–3.

13. Puppo V. Anatomy and physiology of the clitoris, vestibular bulbs, and labia minora with a review of the female orgasm and the prevention of female sexual dysfunction. Clin Anat. 2013;26:134–52.

14. Clerico C, Lari A, Mojallal A, et al. Anatomy and aesthetics of the labia minora: the ideal vulva? Aesthet Plast Surg. 2017;41:714–9.

15. Schober J, Aardsma N, Mayoglou L, et al. Terminal innervation of female genitalia, cutaneous sensory receptors of the epithelium of the labia minora. Clin Anat. 2015;28:392–8.

16. Georgiou CA, Benatar M, Dumas P, et al. A cadaveric study of the arterial blood supply of the labia minora. Plast Reconstr Surg. 2015;136:167–78.

17. Yeung J, Pauls RN. Anatomy of the vulva and the female sexual response. Obstet Gynecol Clin N Am. 2016;43:27–44.

18. Mazloomdoost D, Westermann LB, Mutema G, et al. Histologic anatomy of the anterior vagina and urethra. Female Pelvic Med Reconstr Surg. 2017;23:329–35.

19. Coleman E, Bockting W, Botzer M, et al. Standards of care for the heatlth and transsexuals, transgender, and gender-nonconforming people, version 7. Int J Transgendr. 2011;13:165–232.

20. Djordjevic ML, Stanojevic D, Bizic M, et al. Metoidioplasty as a single stage sex reassignment surgery in female transsexuals: Belgrade experience. J Sex Med. 2009;6:1306–13.

21. Stojanovic B, Bizic M, Bencic M, et al. One-stage gender-confirmation surgery as a viable surgical procedure for female-to-male transsexuals. J Sex Med. 2017;14:741–6.

22. Bowers ML, Stojanovic B, Bizic M. Female-to-male gender affirmation metoidioplasty. In: Salgado CJ, Monstrey SJ, Djordjevic ML, editors. Gender affirmation: medical and surgical perspectives. New York: Thieme Medical Publishers Inc; 2017. p. 109–18.

23. Hage JJ. Metaidoioplasty: an alternative phalloplasty technique in transsexuals. Plast Reconstr Surg. 1996;97:161–7.

24. Hage JJ, van Turnhout AA. Long-term outcome of metaidoioplasty in 70 female-to-male transsexuals. Ann Plast Surg. 2006;57:312–6.

25. Perovic SV, Djordjevic ML. Metoidioplasty: a variant of phalloplasty in female transsexuals. BJU Int. 2003;92:981–5.

26. Takamatsu A, Harashina T. Labial ring flap: a new flap for metaidoioplasty in female-to-male transsexuals. J Plast Reconstr Aesthet Surg. 2009;62:318–25.

27. Djordjevic ML, Bizic M, Stanojevic D, et al. Urethral lengthening in metoidioplasty (female-to-male sex reassignment surgery) by combined buccal mucosa graft and labia minora flap. Urology. 2009;74:349–53.

28. Djordjevic ML, Bizic MR. Comparison of two different methods for urethral lengthening in female to male (metoidioplasty) surgery. J Sex Med. 2013;10:1431–8.

29. Vukadinovic V, Stojanovic B, Majstorovic M, et al. The role of clitoral anatomy in female to male sex reassignment surgery. ScientificWorldJournal. 2014;437378:2014.

30. Djordjevic ML, Stojanovic B. Metoidioplasty. In: Tran TA, Panthaki ZJ, Hoballah JJ, Thaller SR, editors. Operative dictations in plastic and reconstructive surgery. Cham: Springer International Publishing AG; 2017. p. 573–7.

31. Frey JD, Poudrier G, Chiodo MV, et al. A systematic review of metoidioplasty and radial forearm flap phalloplasty in female-to-male transgender genital reconstruction: is the "ideal" neophallus an achievable goal? Plast Reconstr Surg Glob Open. 2016;4(12):e1131.

32. Djordjevic ML. Novel surgical techniques in female to male gender confirming surgery. Transl Androl Urol. 2018;7:628–38.

Surgical Anatomy: Phalloplasty

10

Loren S. Schechter and Alexander R. Facque

Introduction

Motivated initially by oncologic and traumatic tissue losses, modern phalloplasty was introduced in 1936 through the pioneering work of the Russian surgeon Nicolaj Bogoraz [1]. Following World War II, these concepts were later applied to persons of transgender experience by Sir Harold Gillies [2]. Performed on a fellow physician in 1946, Dr. Gillies completed the first transgender male phalloplasty. This involved a series of steps, first advancing tubed abdominal tissue to the perineum in order to create an elongated urethra [2]. The urethral segment was then placed within another adjacent segment of tubed tissue, establishing the tube-within-a-tube technique. With the advent and advances in microsurgery, the radial forearm free flap, first described for use in phalloplasty by Chang and Hwang 1984 [3], emerged as the most common technique for phalloplasty [4]. Since that time, there have been a number of modifications designed to improve urethral reconstruction and reduce prosthetic complications [5]. This chapter reviews the surgical anatomy of the most commonly used flaps; the fasciocutaneous radial forearm free flap (RFFF) as well as the fasciocutaneous anterolateral fasciocutaneous thigh flap (ALT). Other, less commonly used techniques, such as the superficial circumflex iliac perforator flap (SCIP) and the gracilis muscle flap are also discussed. (See Table 10.1.)

Goals of Reconstruction

In general, the goals of phalloplasty include: creation of an aesthetically pleasing phallus (size and contour), capacity for standing urination, ability to achieve rigidity for penetrative intercourse, and both protective and erogenous sensation [6, 7]. Each patient's goals should be discussed prior to surgery so as to personalize the surgical approach and technique.

(a) *Selection of Flap/Donor Site* Donor site selection is an important consideration in surgical planning. In the case of the RFFF, with the forearms uncovered, the donor site will be evident at conversational distance. When contemplating a thigh-based flap, the amount of subcutaneous fat at the donor site should be considered. The amount of subcutaneous fat has implications regarding the circumference of the reconstructed phallus as well as the ability to perform a urethral reconstruction using a tube-within-a-tube technique.

L. S. Schechter (✉)
Clinical Professor of Surgery, The University of Illinois at Chicago Attending Surgeon Rush University, Director, The Center for Gender Confirmation Surgery Weiss Memorial Hospital,, Morton, IL, USA
e-mail: lss@univplastics.com

A. R. Facque
Gender Confirmation Center of San Francisco, Morton, IL, USA

© Springer Nature Switzerland AG 2021
D. Nikolavsky, S. A. Blakely (eds.), *Urological Care for the Transgender Patient*,
https://doi.org/10.1007/978-3-030-18533-6_10

Table 10.1 Phalloplasty flaps. The most common flaps are categorized by their (neuro) vascular pedicles

	Arterial pedicle	Venous pedicle	Nerve pedicle	Flap size	Pedicle length	Artery size
RFFF	Radial artery	Vena comitantes [2], cephalic vein	Lateral antebrachial cutaneous nerve	13 cm at wrist, 15–18 cm in length	Up to 15 cm	1.5–2.5 mm
ALT	Descending branch of lateral femoral circumflex artery	Vena comitantes [2]	Lateral femoral cutaneous nerve of the thigh	Up to 8 × 25 cm	7 cm or longer	1.5–2.5 mm
SCIP	Superficial circumflex iliac artery	Vena comitantes, superficial circumflex iliac vein, superficial epigastric vein	Not typically sensate, possible to include lateral cutaneous branch of T12	10 × 15 cm	2–5 cm	1–2 mm
Gracilis	Medial femoral circumflex artery	Vena comitantes [2]	Branch from the obturator nerve to gracilis	If taken with skin paddle (TUG) 11 cm wide up to 25 cm long	6–8 cm	1–2 mm

If a patient requests urethral lengthening and has thick subcutaneous thigh tissue, the radial forearm may be a better option to achieve an anatomically appropriately sized phallus with an inner-lined urethra capable of standing urination.

(b) *Sexual Function* If the patient anticipates performing insertive intercourse with his phallus, an implantable penile prosthesis is required. This is typically performed concurrent with testicular implant(s) and generally awaits return of protective sensation in the flap (9–12 months following the phalloplasty).

Preoperative Considerations/ Indications

Prior to surgery, in accordance with the *Standards of Care* (World Professional Association for Transgender Health, SOC, V. 7), two mental health assessments are obtained. A history of bleeding/clotting disorders and vascular disease is assessed. If an RFFF is chosen, a preoperative Allen's test is conducted (although this may be of limited value). Additionally, electrolysis of the donor site (either forearm or thigh) may be required so as to reduce the density of intra-urethral hair growth. A complete blood count is obtained, as the hemoglobin/hematocrit may be elevated as a result of testosterone therapy. If the patient is polycythemic, testosterone may need to be discontinued preoperatively.

Reconstructive Options

The most common donor site is the radial forearm [4]. The tissue is thin, relatively hairless on the volar/ulnar border (urethral portion) of the flap, and has reliable neurovascular anatomy. The forearm flap typically allows a phalloplasty with simultaneous construction of the shaft and urethra using a tube-within-a-tube technique [4]. Additionally, if desired, a glansplasty can often be performed at the time of the phalloplasty. The primary drawback of the forearm flap is the conspicuous donor site. An alternative donor site is the anterolateral thigh flap. Most often, this flap is performed as a pedicled flap. The vascular anatomy is somewhat more variable than the RFFF (either septocutaneous or musculocutaneous perforators), and the subcutaneous tissue is typically thicker than the RFFF. This may preclude the use of a tube-within-a-tube technique and may necessitate secondary debulking procedures (Fig. 10.1). Also, a glansplasty, if desired, is performed at a later date. Additional phalloplasty

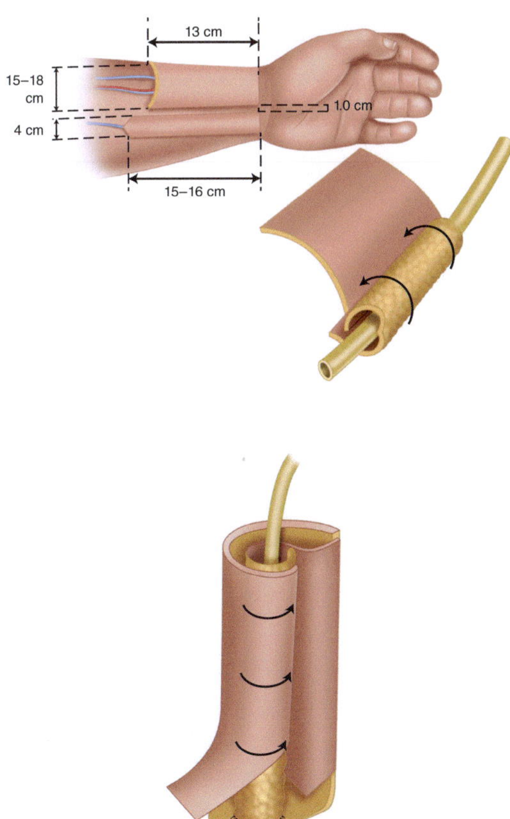

Fig. 10.1 Tube-within-a-tube technique for phalloplasty with urethral lengthening. The radial forearm free flap (RFFF) is raised on perforators from the radial artery. After elevation, a bridge of skin between the radial and ulnar portions of the flap is de-epithelialized. The flap is double tubed in order to provide skin lining for the neourethra and external phallic skin

options include the use of combined flaps, such as a superficial circumflex iliac perforator flap or RFFF for urethral reconstruction and an ALT flap for shaft reconstruction (Fig. 10.2). Less common options include regional flaps, such as gracilis muscle flaps, used either for phalloplasty or as a treatment for urethral stricture/fistula.

Surgical Anatomy

(a) *Donor site anatomy*
   (i) *Radial forearm*
       1. *Radial artery course* The radial forearm flap, supplied by the radial artery, has a long, large caliber, and reliable arterial pedicle. The radial and ulnar arteries of

the forearm arise as terminal branches from the bifurcation of the brachial artery in the distal portion of the antecubital fossa. The radial artery is typically the more diminutive of the two. In the proximal forearm, the radial artery lies deep to the brachioradialis muscle as it runs medial to the neck of the radius. In this location, deep to the artery, is the common tendon of the biceps brachii. Further distally, the radial artery is located between the brachioradialis and the pronator teres, supinator, and flexor digitorum superficialis (FDS) as it travels toward the styloid process of the radius. In the mid and distal wrist, the radial artery is located between the brachioradialis and the tendon of the flexor carpi radialis (Fig. 10.2).

In the wrist, the radial artery travels along the floor of the anatomic snuff box before entering the hand. In the hand, the radial artery forms a connection with the superficial palmar arch (typically supplied predominately by the ulnar artery) before continuing as the predominate supply to the deep palmar arch (which is also in continuity with the ulnar artery).

2. *Venous anatomy* The forearm has both deep (vena comitantes) and superficial venous networks with communications between them (recognizing that there is anatomic variability regarding the superficial venous network). The deep veins accompany the arterial pedicle, and the sensory nerves accompany the superficial veins. Most often, there are two valved vena comitantes traveling with the radial artery. The vena comitantes have numerous valveless connections, allowing the flap to survive on retrograde flow. Most of the superficial veins drain to the cephalic or basilic veins (named for their relative embryologic positions, cephalic being toward the head and basilic toward the "base"). The cephalic vein arises from the lateral aspect of the dorsal venous network,

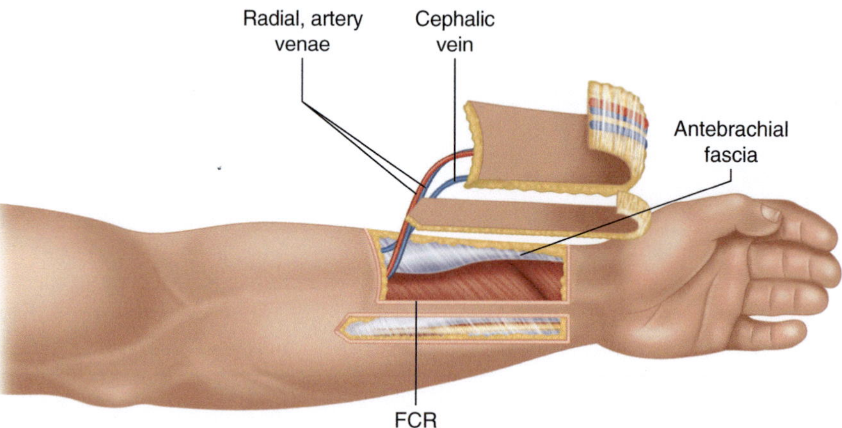

Fig. 10.2 Radial forearm free flap (RFFF) arterial and venous pedicle. Fasciocutaneous perforators from the radial artery supply the RFFF. Proximally, the radial artery lies deep to the brachioradialis muscle as it runs medial to the neck of the radius. In the mid and distal wrist, the radial artery is located between the brachioradialis and the tendon of the flexor carpi radialis. Venous drainage of the flap is provided by both deep and superficial systems comprised of the cephalic vein and paired vena comitantes accompanying the artery, respectively. (Note: for purposes of simplification, in figure 10.2 the de-epithelialized segment adjoining the urethral and outer cutaneous portions of the flap is not shown)

continuing to collect tributaries, as it courses proximally on the anterolateral aspect of the forearm. Due to its superficial position, the cephalic vein is often visible. The cephalic vein joins the medial cubital vein at the cubital fossa before continuing proximally along the lateral aspect of the arm. It then runs between the deltoid and pectoralis muscles within the delto-pectoral groove before piercing the clavipectoral fascia and draining into the terminal portion of the axillary vein.

The basilic vein is formed from the dorsal venous network along the medial aspect of the wrist. Proximally, it ascends parallel to the brachial artery and the medial cutaneous nerve of the forearm to the axilla.

3. *Sensory innervation* Cutaneous sensation of the radial forearm flap is provided primarily by the anterior branch of the lateral antebrachial cutaneous nerve (LABC) of the forearm. This nerve is the terminal sensory branch of the musculocutaneous nerve (nerve roots C6 and C7) and is found adjacent to the cephalic vein in the lateral aspect of the forearm. The anterior branch supplies cutaneous innervation to the more lateral aspect of the volar forearm, whereas the posterior branch carries the sensory impulses from the dorsolateral forearm.

Similarly, the anterior branch of the medial antebrachial cutaneous nerve (MABC) caries sensory innervation from the ulnar, volar aspect of the forearm. In the RFFF, this nerve supplies sensation to what will typically become the urethra. The MABC travels along the medial aspect of the forearm adjacent to the basilic vein. It courses through the cubital fossa before joining the medial cord of the brachial plexus (nerve roots C8 and T1).

(ii) *ALT*

1. *Descending branch of lateral femoral circumflex course* The arterial supply of the anterolateral thigh flap is the descending branch of the lateral femoral circumflex artery (DBLC). The lateral femoral circumflex artery arises from the profunda femoris and gives off ascending, transverse, and descend-

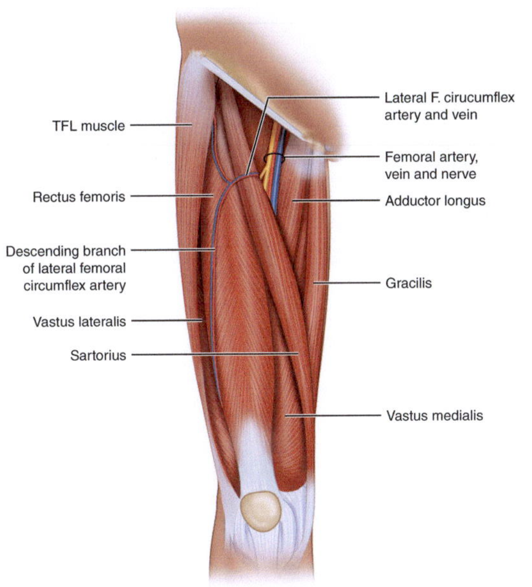

Fig. 10.3 Pedicle and perforators of the anterolateral thigh (ALT) flap. The perforators of the ALT flap arise from the descending branch of the lateral circumflex artery. Musculocutaneous perforators may be found within the substance of the vastus lateralis muscle, although more proximal fasciocutaneous perforators within the intermuscular septum may also be present

ing branches. The descending branch supplies the muscles and skin of the anterolateral thigh. The vessel descends between the rectus femoris and vastus lateralis muscles, on the surface of the vastus intermedius. The DBLC is often found deep within the septal plane, and, on occasion, enters the substance of the vastus lateralis muscle as it travels distally (Fig. 10.3).

The perforators supplying the flap are most commonly found within the middle third of a line drawn between the ASIS and the lateral patella.

The arterial pedicle is often between 7 and 8 cm long (or longer) and, if used as a free flap, has a diameter of 1–3 mm. When using the ALT in a pedicled fashion, the more distal perforators (typically musculocutaneous) are selected. Although septocutaneous perforators may occur more proximally (and facili-

tate flap dissection), they shorten the effective flap pedicle length and thus limit the excursion of the flap.

2. *Venous anatomy* The venous drainage of this flap is through two accompanying vena comitantes. Usually one of the comitantes is dominant, with a caliber similar to that of the artery.

3. *Sensory innervation* The lateral femoral cutaneous nerve of the thigh provides cutaneous sensation. This nerve arrives from the dorsal divisions of the L2-L3 nerve roots and exits the abdominal cavity under the inguinal ligament. The nerve then travels over the sartorius muscle, where it splits into anterior and posterior divisions. The anterior division is located approximately 10 cm inferior to the inguinal ligament. This division has anterior and lateral branches that innervate the skin inferiorly to the knee.

(iii) *Gracilis* This long, thin thigh muscle can be harvested bilaterally to perform phalloplasty. More commonly, it may be used to repair refractory urethral strictures/fistula. The gracilis muscle has a dominant vascular pedicle, the medial circumflex femoral artery, with additional minor pedicles (Fig. 10.4). While a skin island can be harvested with the gracilis muscle, a skin paddle is not commonly used in phalloplasty procedures.

1. *Arterial anatomy* While retracting the adductor longus muscle, the medial femoral circumflex artery is located on the surface of the adductor magnus muscle.

2. *Venous anatomy* The venous drainage of this flap parallels the arterial system.

3. *Innervation* The gracilis muscle receives motor innervation from a branch of the obturator nerve.

(iv) *Superficial circumflex iliac artery perforator flap (SCIP)* This flap is used primarily as a pedicled flap to reconstruct the urethra. Most often, this flap is used in conjunction with an ALT flap (which is

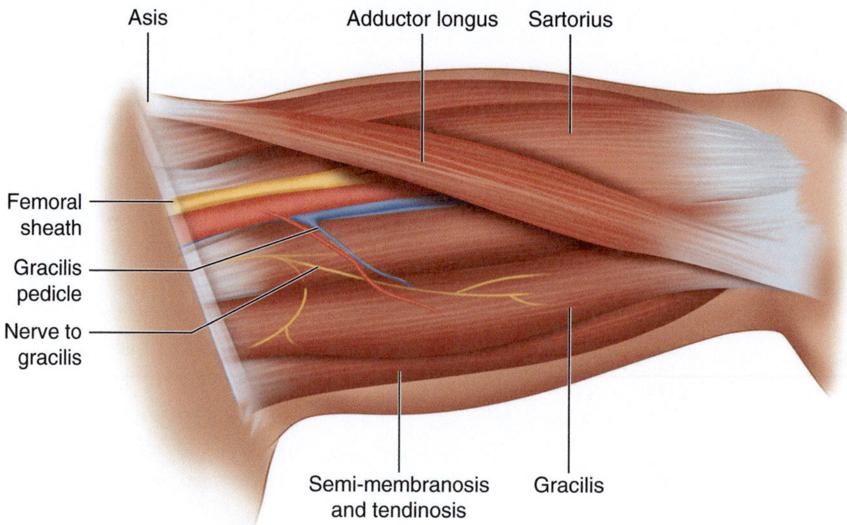

Fig. 10.4 Vascular supply to the gracilis muscle. The gracilis muscle has a dominant vascular pedicle, the medial circumflex femoral artery. This flap is most frequently employed to repair refractory urethral strictures or fistulae

Fig. 10.5 The superficial circumflex iliac perforator (SCIP) or "groin" flap. The SCIP flap is primarily used in urethral reconstruction in conjunction with a second flap. The arterial pedicle originates from the femoral artery and pierces the fascia of the sartorius muscle inferior to the inguinal ligament. The pedicle length is short, often 2–5 cm

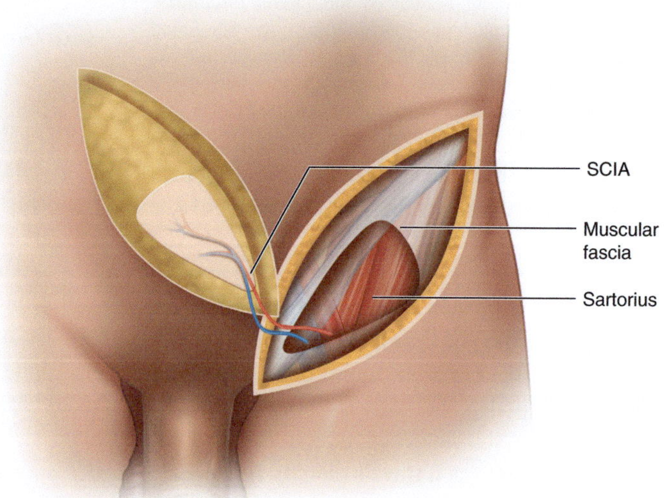

used to construct the shaft of the phallus).

1. *Arterial anatomy* This flap, also referred to as the "groin flap," is supplied by the superficial circumflex iliac artery (SCIA), a branch of the superficial femoral artery. The artery pierces the fascia of the sartorius muscle inferior to the inguinal ligament on its medial aspect. The artery is small caliber, 1–2 mm, and provides a pedicle length of approximately 2–5 cm (Fig. 10.5).

2. *Venous anatomy* The venous drainage is provided by a cutaneous vein travelling with the artery. This vein is typically larger than the artery and drains into the saphenous system before draining into the femoral vein.

(b) *Perineal regional anatomy*

   (i) *Perineal arteries* The primary blood supply to the perineum is the internal pudendal artery, a branch of the internal iliac. This artery exits the pelvis through the greater sciatic foramen inferior to the piriformis and enters the perineum at the lesser sciatic foramen. It then passes through the pudendal canal to the urogenital triangle running medial to the ischial tuberosity. The artery divides into its terminal branches, the perineal and the dorsal arteries of the penis or clitoris.

   (ii) *Venous anatomy* The internal pudendal veins run with the internal pudendal artery along the course described above.

   (iii) *Sensory innervation* The primary nerve of the perineum is the pudendal nerve, which contains both motor and sensory components. This nerve is part of the sacral plexus (nerve roots S2-S4) and follows the course of the pudendal artery as described above. Inside the pudendal canal, the pudendal nerve divides into inferior rectal and perineal branches before continuing as the dorsal nerve of the clitoris (or penis).

   (iv) *Erogenous sensation* The dorsal nerves (clitoris/penis) are terminal branches of the pudendal nerve, providing afferent sensation from the clitoris/penis to the sacral plexus (S2-S4).

(c) *Groin anatomy* Knowledge of the femoral triangle and groin is relevant in recipient site neurovascular exposure. The femoral triangle is bordered by the inguinal ligament superiorly, medially by the border of the adductor longus, and laterally by the sartorius muscle.

   1. *Arterial anatomy* Within the femoral triangle, the contents of the femoral sheath include: the femoral nerve, artery, and vein (from lateral to medial). These structures emerge beneath the inguinal ligament and continue into the adductor canal, an intermuscular space between the sartorius and adductor longus muscles. The superficial epigastric artery, superficial (and sometimes the deep) circumflex iliac arteries (the arterial supply of the SCIA flap), and the superficial and deep external pudendal arteries arise from the anterior aspect of the proximal part of the femoral artery. Approximately 1–5 cm inferior to the inguinal ligament, before entering the adductor canal, the femoral artery gives off the profunda femoris artery. This artery passes posterior to the adductor longus before giving off medial and lateral circumflex arteries, branches of which supply the gracilis and ALT flaps, respectively. The femoral artery continues inferiorly through the adductor canal toward the popliteal space, giving off branches to supply the muscles of the anterior compartment before continuing as the popliteal artery.

   2. *Venous anatomy* The femoral vein is the continuation of the popliteal vein of the leg. As it ascends in the adductor canal, the femoral vein lies posterolateral, and later posterior, to the femoral artery before continuing deep to the inguinal ligament where it becomes the external iliac vein. Within the femoral triangle, the femoral vein receives tributaries from the profunda femoris vein, as well as superficial epigastric vein (draining the anterior, superficial abdominal wall) and the superficial circumflex iliac vein (draining the groin as well as the lateral, superficial abdominal wall). The superficial epigastric vein and superficial circumflex iliac veins are options for secondary venous anastomoses providing additional drainage for the RFF flap.

   3. *Sensory innervation* The skin overlying the femoral triangle, the inner thigh, and the skin of the labia and scrotum are supplied by the genitofemoral and ilioinguinal nerves (L1 and L1/L2, respectively). After providing sensation to the more midline labial or scrotal skin, the labial branches of the ilioinguinal nerve coalesce and pass through the superficial inguinal ring, traveling with either the spermatic cord, or the round ligament. The nerve

then pierces the internal oblique and transversus abdominis to enter the pelvis, where it is joined by the iliohypogastric nerve to form the first lumbar nerve root. The ilioinguinal nerve can be identified within the inguinal canal by incising the external oblique aponeurosis, superior and lateral to the pubic tubercle. In contrast to the ilioinguinal nerve, the genital branch of the genitofemoral nerve travels through both the deep and superficial inguinal rings and hence the entire course of the inguinal canal. This nerve supplies sensation to the more lateral labial or scrotal skin, as well as the innermost aspect of the upper thigh. The femoral branch of the genitofemoral nerve supplies sensation to the skin over the femoral triangle. This nerve courses through the femoral canal to enter the pelvis where it then joins the genital branch, forming the genitofemoral nerve.

Operative Technique

(a) *Surgical staging* In general, phalloplasty involves construction of the phallus (+/− glansplasty), urethra, scrotum, colpectomy/colpocleisis, and subsequent placement of implantable penile and testicular prostheses. As noted, the approach is individualized based upon the goals, body habitus, and medical condition of the patient.

The RFF typically allows simultaneous construction of the penile shaft and urethra using a tube-within-a-tube technique. The prostheses are typically placed 9–12 months later, following return of protective sensation.

(i) *Primary phallopasty*

1. *Radial forearm* A preoperative Allen's test is performed to confirm patency of the palmar arch. Most commonly, the nondominant forearm is chosen, although this is left to the discretion of the patient (and based upon the Allen's test). Depending upon hair growth, preoperative depilation of the forearm may be required. The flap design includes the neurovascular structures (radial artery, cephalic vein, lateral antebrachial cutaneous nerve, and, at times, the anterior branch of the medial antebrachial cutaneous nerve). The shaft is typically designed between 13 and 15 cm in length, with a urethral extension of an additional 2–3 cm in length (15–18 cm). The urethral width is approximately 4 cm, and the flap

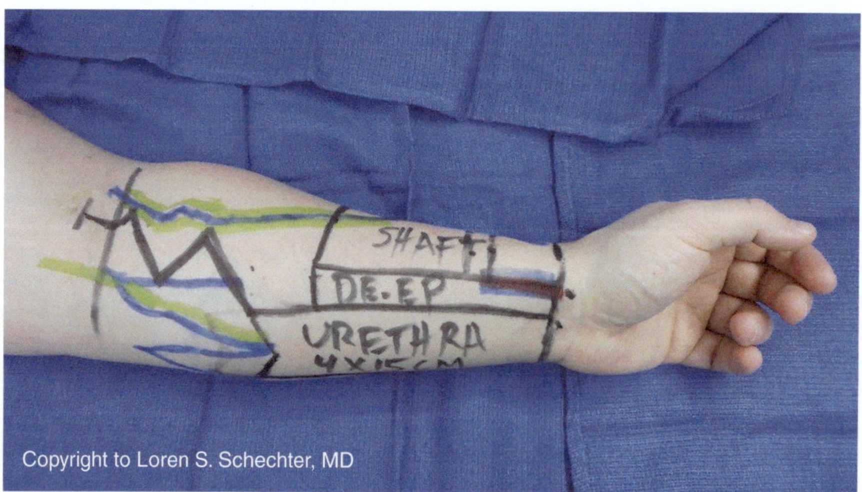

Copyright to Loren S. Schechter, MD

Fig. 10.6 Preoperative markings for radial forearm free flap phalloplasty with urethral lengthening. The ulnar portion of the flap corresponds to the urethra, and the radial portion of the flap represents the penile shaft. The intervening skin is de-epithelialized

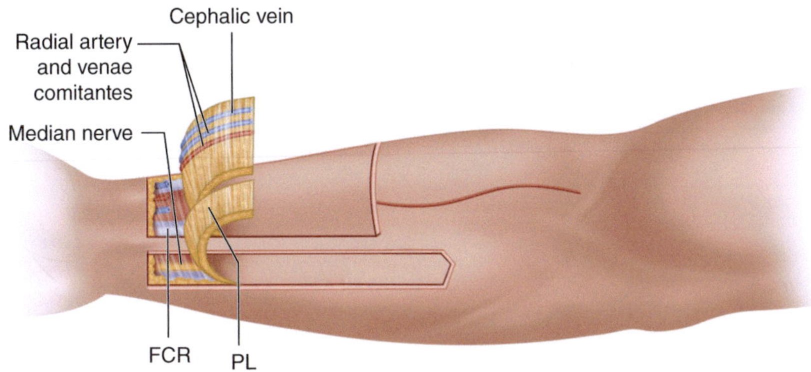

Fig. 10.7 Radial forearm flap pedicle and elevation. The pedicle is first identified distally. Prior to division of the radial artery, and Allen's test is performed. The flap may be raised above or below the fascia, with care taken to preserve the radial nerve. (Note: for purposes of simplification, as in figure 10.2 the de-epithelialized segment adjoining the urethral and outer cutaneous portions of the flap is not shown

width may be 13–14 cm at the wrist, and widened proximally based upon the individual's body habitus (Fig. 10.6).

The flap dissection begins proximally so as to identify the cephalic vein, the lateral antebrachial cutaneous nerve, and, if possible, another superficial vein on the ulnar border of the flap. The flap may be harvested either supra- or subfascially. The radial nerve is identified and protected during pedicle dissection (Fig. 10.7). A second surgical team may be performing the perineal portion of the procedure (colpectomy/colpocleisis, construction of the pars fixa, and scrotoplasty), as well as subsequent recipient vessel (femoral artery, saphenous vein, ilioinguinal nerve) dissection. The flap is shaped in situ on the forearm. Subsequently, the phallus is transferred to the perineum, and the urethral and neurovascular anastomoses are performed (Fig. 10.8). The femoral artery is the most common recipient vessel (other recipient options include the deep inferior epigastric artery or the descending branch of the lateral femoral cutaneous artery). The arterial anastomosis may be performed between the radial artery and the femoral artery in an end-to-side fashion. Alternatively, in order to lengthen the vascular pedicle, an arteriovenous loop may be created between the saphenous vein and the femoral artery. In this technique, the saphenous vein is divided distally and anastomosed to the femoral artery. The flap vessels are anastomosed to the appropriate portion of the arteriovenous loop. From a technical perspective, the loop effectively lengthens the vascular pedicle (Fig. 10.9). The venous anastomosis is performed between the cephalic vein and the saphenous vein (or the venous limb of the AV loop described above). Additional venous anastomoses may be performed between additional superficial veins of the forearm and the SIEV and SCIV (the vena comitantes of the RFF flap are dissected proximally, to include the communicating venous branch between the vena comitantes and the cephalic vein. This allows a single venous anastomosis to drain both the superficial and deep venous systems). For protective sensation, the lateral antebrachial cutaneous nerve is typically coapted to the ilioinguinal nerve.

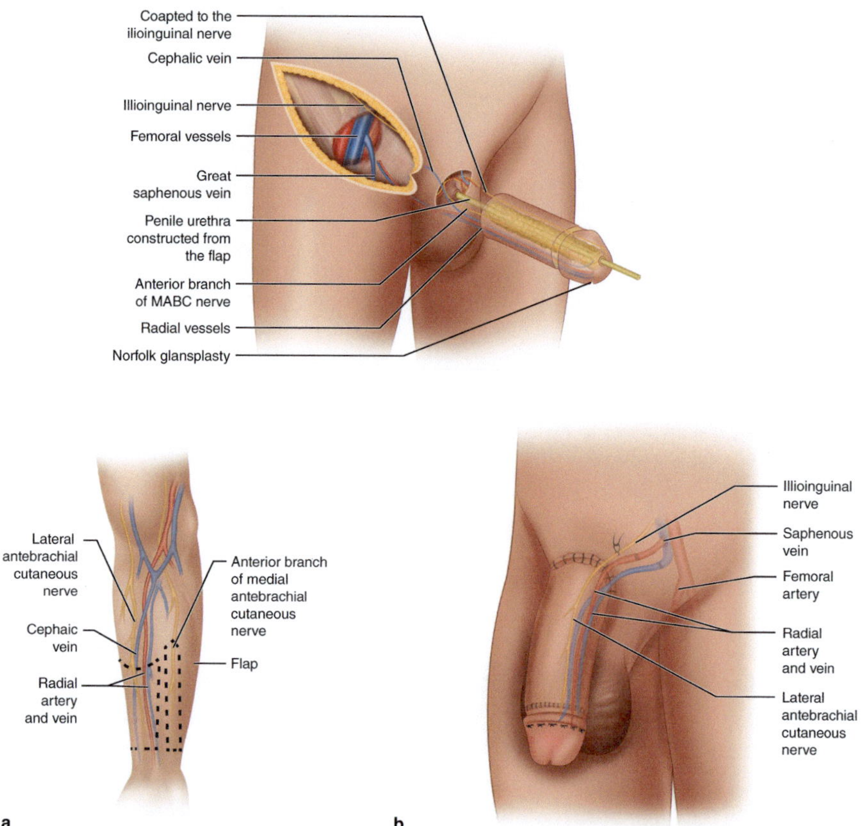

Fig. 10.8 Flap transfer. The flap is shaped in situ on the forearm and then transferred to the groin. (**a**) flap anatomy, prior to elevation, including sensory contributions of the MABC and LABC. (**b**) RFFF after inset, with nerve, arterial, and venous anastomosis. A glansplasty has also been performed

2. *ALT* A line is drawn between the anterior superior iliac spine (ASIS) and the lateral patella, identifying the septum between the rectus femoris and the vastus lateralis. The cutaneous perforators are most commonly found at the junction of the proximal and middle thirds of this line and are confirmed using a handheld Doppler (Fig. 10.10). Once the perforators are identified, the flap dimensions are outlined as noted above. Dissection of the flap begins medially by retracting the rectus femoris, thereby allowing identification of the descending branch of the lateral femoral circumflex artery and relevant cutaneous perforators. Most often, musculocutaneous perforators (through the vastus lateralis) are identified and dissected in a retrograde fashion to the descending branch of the lateral femoral circumflex artery. The lateral femoral cutaneous nerve is identified at the proximal aspect of the flap and dissected for a length of 7–10 cm. Following elevation, the flap is passed beneath the rectus femoris and sartorius muscle to its position in the pubic region (the arterial branch to the rectus femoris is divided if additional pedicle length is required).

(ii) *Urethral reconstruction* Urethral lengthening can take place at the time of primary phalloplasty using the "tube within a tube" technique, through urethral pre-lamination, or with additional flap transfer, such

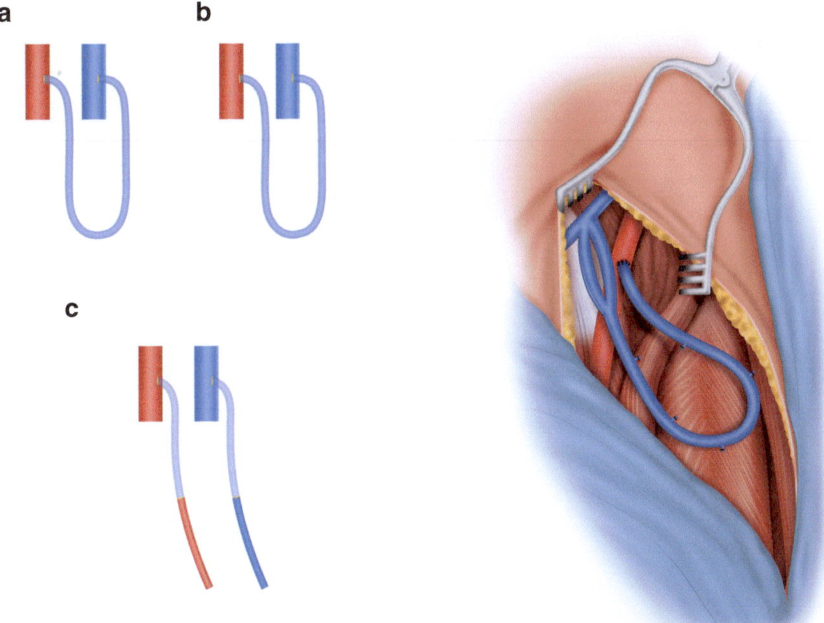

Fig. 10.9 (**a**, **b**, **c**) Arteriovenous loop demonstration. The saphenous vein is divided distally and anastomosed (end-to-side) to the femoral artery (**a**, **b**). The AV loop is divided (**c**), effectively lengthening the pedicle length. The flap vessels are anastomosed to the arterial and venous limbs of the loop

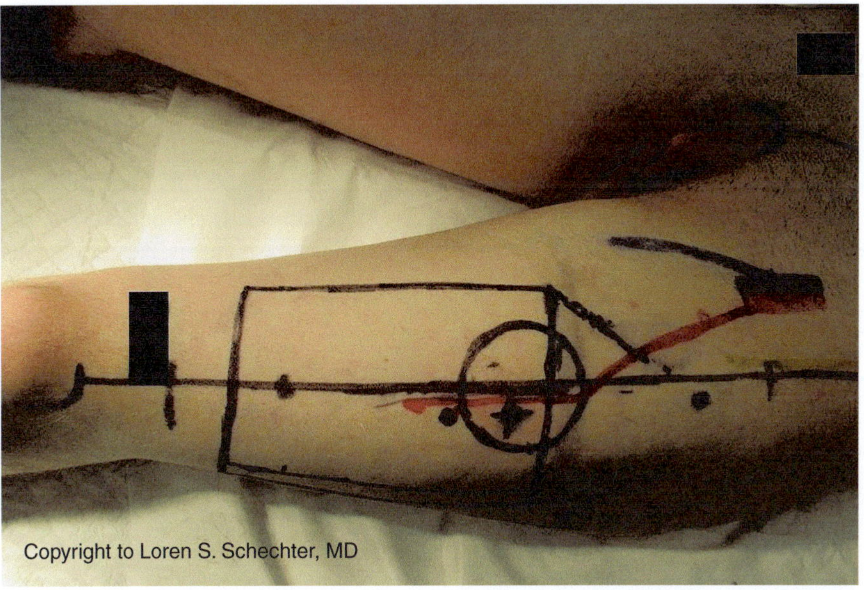

Fig. 10.10 Preoperative markings for anterolateral thigh phalloplasty. The cutaneous perforators arise from the descending branch of the lateral circumflex artery. They are most commonly found at the junction of the proximal and middle thirds of a line connecting the anterior superior iliac spine (ASIS) and the lateral patella. Perforator position is confirmed using a handheld Doppler

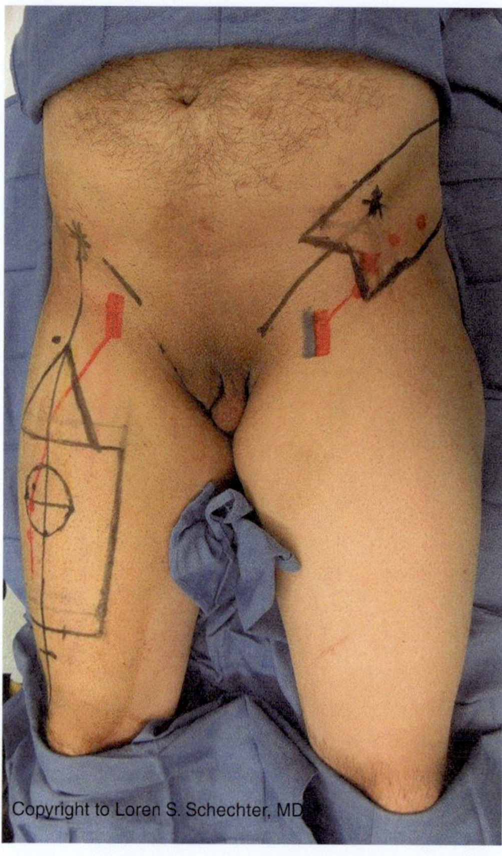

Fig. 10.11 Combined superficial circumflex iliac and anterolateral thigh flaps for phalloplasty with urethral lengthening. The superficial circumflex iliac artery perforator flap (SCIP) represents the urethral segment while the anterolateral thigh flap (ALT) forms the shaft of the phallus

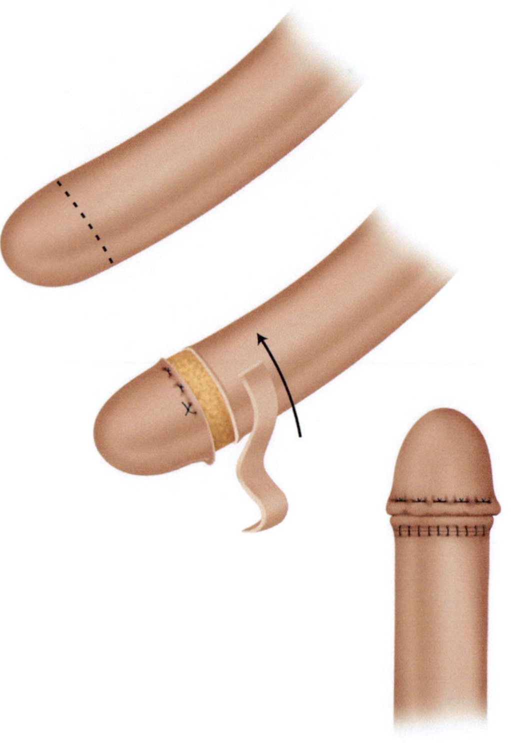

Fig. 10.12 Glansplasty. Depending on flap choice and patient preference, glansplasty is performed either at the time of the initial phalloplasty, or as a staged, secondary procedure. In this technique, a skin flap is elevated distally and folded on itself. The resultant defect is skin grafted

as the SCIP or "groin" flap (Fig. 10.11). It is the senior author's preference to avoid pre-lamination as this is believed to result in increased urethral complications compared with a vascularized urethral lining. Urethral stricture and fistula are not uncommon, and techniques for repair are discussed in other chapters [8].

(iii) *Placement of clitoris* The paired dorsal clitoral nerves provide primary erogenous sensation to the clitoris. One of the nerves can be dissected and coapted to a cutaneous nerve in the forearm flap. Alternatively, the innervation to the clito-

ris is left intact, and the clitoris is de-epithelialized and buried at the base of the phallus [9]. The benefit of leaving clitoral nerves intact is that erogenous stimulation via the clitoral nerves may be reliably maintained and orgasm achieved through manipulation of the base of the phallus during insertive intercourse. Coapting both clitoral nerves to the sensory nerves of the flap risks the loss of erogenous sensation should the nerves fail to reinnervate the flap.

(iv) *Glansplasty* Known as the Norfolk technique, creation of the glans penis most commonly involves creation of the coronal ridge with elevation of a distally-based flap. The resultant defect is then skin grafted (Fig. 10.12) [10]. When performing RFF phalloplasty, the glansplasty is most often performed at the time of the initial phalloplasty. When performing ALT phalloplasty, the glansplasty is performed at a secondary setting [10].

(v) *Implant placement*

1. *Malleable vs. hydraulic* If penetrative intercourse is desired, penile implants are placed at a secondary setting, typically 9–12 months following the phalloplasty, upon return of protective sensation. Malleable or semirigid implants provide constant firmness to the phallus and are at increased risk of erosion and exposure. Inflatable or hydraulic implants involve the placement of cylinders within the phallus and a pump placed in the hemi-scrotum. An additional reservoir may also be placed depending upon the type of device [11].

2. *Testicular implants* Testicular implant(s) are typically placed at the time of placement of the penile prosthesis [12].

Hospital Course

(a) Following surgery, patients are admitted to the intensive care unit (or flap monitoring unit), to receive hourly flap checks (assessing arterial inflow and venous return via a hand-held Doppler and clinical examination). If vascular compromise is suspected (typically noted on physical exam with either signs of venous congestion – duskiness, increased turgor, dark/robust bleeding from a pinprick – or arterial insufficiency – pale cool flap, no bleeding from pinprick, loss of Doppler signal), emergent return to the operating room is warranted.

A forced air warmer is placed over the phallus for the first 24 h. Hourly flap checks are performed for 3 days following surgery. During this time, the phallus is positioned perpendicular to the body so as to promote venous drainage and reduce the risk of pedicle kinking. Depending upon the flap type and vascular configuration, patients may remain on bed rest for another 48 h.

Patients frequently travel for surgery and are therefore requested to stay in the area for at least 3 weeks following surgery. Post-discharge follow-up with a local urologist is recommended.

(b) *Catheter management* At the time of phalloplasty with concomitant urethral reconstruction, a suprapubic tube and a transurethral catheter are placed. Both catheters are left open to gravity drainage.

Outpatient Care

(a) Patients typically convalesce at a skilled nursing facility. The risk of vascular-related complications progressively decreases following surgery; however, delayed flap loss due to arterial or venous insufficiency is possible. Areas of partial-thickness flap loss may be managed with local care. However, secondary procedures, such as a skin graft may be warranted.

(b) *Catheter management* Approximately, 2–4 weeks following surgery, patients are scheduled for cystoscopy with retrograde urethrogram. At this time, a trial of voiding may be performed, and the suprapubic tube may be capped. Post-void residuals are followed and help to guide removal of the SPT. Approximately 4 weeks after transurethral catheter removal, if post-void residuals are low, the SPT is removed.

(c) *Operative precautions* Care is taken with subsequent surgical procedures (i.e., implantation of prostheses). The vascular pedicle remains at risk during these procedures. As such, the surgeon should be aware of the laterality of the vascular pedicle and attempt to avoid dissection in this area, if possible.

Outcomes/Conclusion

Gender-confirming phalloplasty is a multistage procedure. Knowledge of the relevant anatomy is required as this is considered one of the most technically challenging and demanding procedures in reconstructive surgery. While complications are not uncommon, satisfactory long-term results can be achieved [13]. Further directions for the field include the development of prosthetics specifically designed for placement within the flap phalloplasty and techniques designed to minimize donor site visibility and reduce urethral complications. Consideration to staging the phalloplasty (i.e., first-stage pars fixa reconstruction (with staging metoidioplasty) followed by second-stage shaft and penile urethra reconstruction) should be given. While this may not reduce the complication rate, staging may make the procedures more manageable for the patient.

Take-Home Points
- Phalloplasty is an important component in the treatment of some transmasculine individuals with gender dysphoria.
- The most common phalloplasty technique is the radial forearm free flap.
- All phalloplasty are performed in a staged fashion, especially if prosthetic placement is desired.
- Urethral stricture and fistula are common complications following phalloplasty. Other risks include flap- and prosthetic-related complications.
- Following phalloplasty, many patients will experience a urologic complication at some point in their recovery. As many patients travel for surgery, improved knowledge of urologic management will facilitate postoperative care.

References

1. Schultheiss D, Gabouev AI, Jonas U, Nair R, Sriprasad S, Nikolaj A. Bogoraz (1874-1952): pioneer of phalloplasty and penile implant surgery. J Sex Med. 2005;2(1):139–46.
2. 1129 Sir Harold Gillies: Pioneer of phalloplasty and the birth of uroplastic surgery. J Urol. 2010;183(4):e437.
3. Chang TS, Hwang WY. Forearm flap in one-stage reconstruction of the penis. Plast Reconstr Surg. 1984;74:251–8.
4. Morrison SD, Shakir A, Vyas KS, Kirby J, Crane CN. Phalloplasty: a review of techniques and outcomes. Plast Reconstr Surg. 2016;138:594–615.
5. Trombetta C, Liguori G, Bertolotto M. Management of gender dysphoria: a multidisciplinary approach. Springer-Verlag Italia: Milan; 2015.
6. Monstrey S, Hoebeke P, Selvaggi G. Penile reconstruction: is radial forearm really the standard technique? Plast Reconstr Surg. 2009;124(2):510–8.
7. Selvaggi G, Monstrey S, Ceulemans P, T'Sjoen G, De Cuypere G, Hoebeke P. Genital sensitivity after sex reassignment surgery in transsexual patients. Ann Plast Surg. 2007;58(4):427–33.
8. Salgado CJ, Nugent AG, Moody AM, Chim H, Paz AM, Chen HC. Immediate pedicled gracilis flap in radial forearm flap phalloplasty for transgender male patients to reduce urinary fistula. J Plast Reconstr Aesthet Surg. 2016;69(11):1551–7.
9. Song C, Wong M, Wong CH, Ong YS. Modifications of the radial forearm flap phalloplasty for female-to-male gender reassignment. J Reconstr Microsurg. 2011;27(2):115–20.
10. Hage JJ, de Graaf FH, Bouman FG, Bloem JJ. Sculpturing the glans in phalloplasty. Plast Reconstr Surg. 1993;92(1):157–61.
11. Kocjancic E, Iacovelli V. Penile prosthesis. Clin Plast Surg. 2018;4:407–14.
12. Djordjevic ML. Novel surgical techniques in female to male gender confirmation surgery. Transl Androl Urol. 2018;7(4):628–38.
13. Garaffa G, Christopher NA, Ralph DJ. Total phallic reconstruction in female-to-male transsexuals. Eur Urol. 2010;57:715–22.

Management of Urologic Complications Following Metoidioplasty and Phalloplasty

Jessica Schardein, Stephen Blakely, and Dmitriy Nikolavsky

Introduction

Gender affirmation exists on a spectrum. It is entirely dependent on how an individual is affected by their gender dysphoria and what changes they view as necessary to be their true selves. Genital reconstructive surgery may be essential and medically necessary to alleviate gender dysphoria for some, but not all, transgender men [1, 2].

The overall percentage of transgender individuals who pursue gender affirmation surgery ranges from 10–30% [3–5]. According to the American Society of Plastic Surgeons (ASPS) report in 2016, plastic surgeons performed over 1700 transmasculine affirmation surgeries, which represented a 20% increase over the previous year. While the specific number of genital reconstructive surgeries performed by surgeons each year is unknown, there is estimated to be a growing number of patients pursuing genital reconstructive surgery [6, 7].

Transgender patients who pursue gender affirmation surgery may present to a urologist at various stages of their transition for general or specialized urologic care. For those patients who present following genital reconstructive surgery, it is important that the urologist is familiar with the reconstructed anatomy for diagnostic and management purposes. This helps to ensure that some common practices or urological procedures are performed in a safe manner to avoid injury to the reconstructed tissue. An understanding of the reconstructed genitourinary anatomy and of the most common complications can also aide in the most appropriate evaluation. Knowledge regarding surgical techniques to best manage complications can promote better functional and aesthetic outcomes for those pursuing surgical repair. The need for a multidisciplinary approach to patient care through collaboration with other healthcare professionals cannot be overemphasized [8, 9].

Anatomy of Transmasculine Genital Surgery

Broadly, transmasculine genital surgery includes extirpative and reconstructive components. Extirpative procedures include the removal of female reproductive organs (i.e., hysterectomy and vaginectomy) with or without oophorectomy or fertility preservation procedures (Chap. 8). They often follow standard techniques adapted for gender affirming surgery.

Reconstructive procedures include the creation of structures that provide traditionally described

J. Schardein (✉) · S. Blakely
Department of Urology, SUNY Upstate Medical University, Syracuse, NY, USA
e-mail: schardej@upstate.edu

D. Nikolavsky
Urology Department, SUNY Upstate Medical University, Syracuse, NY, USA

© Springer Nature Switzerland AG 2021
D. Nikolavsky, S. A. Blakely (eds.), *Urological Care for the Transgender Patient*,
https://doi.org/10.1007/978-3-030-18533-6_11

masculine functions, such as voiding while standing, and may provide patients with the ability for penetrative intercourse. Metoidioplasty and phalloplasty are grouped into this category along with procedures for implantation of prosthetics. Overall, reconstructive surgery is an innovative area with new developments constantly projecting the field forward and redefining what is possible.

Genital surgery must be tailored to each patient's unique anatomy and goals in order to achieve a successful outcome. In order to manage expectations, it is important to note that an individual's goals may not be able to be met with a single surgery. The number or surgeries necessary may be influenced by patient preference as well as surgeon preference. For example, some surgeons perform hysterectomy, vaginectomy, neophallus construction, and testicular prosthesis in a single surgery [10]. At other institutions, however, these procedures are performed as staged surgeries [11].

Preferences regarding aesthetics, micturition, sexual sensation, and coital ability must all be discussed prior to surgery in order to establish realistic goals and guide the selection of procedures necessary to achieve those goals [12]. Risks of surgery should be discussed up front as part of the informed consent process in order to determine an appropriate surgical plan with an acceptable risk profile.

Minimizing morbidity and complications should always be a goal for both the patient and the surgeon. For greater than 98% of transgender men, voiding from a standing position is another important goal and many will undergo reconstructive surgery with the construction of a neourethra to achieve this goal [13–16]. For patients who prioritize sexual functioning, erogenous sensation and a phallus with sufficient length and girth for penetrative intercourse are important [17]. Upright voiding and sexual functioning can both be achieved with either of the two reconstructive options, metoidioplasty or phalloplasty.

Vaginectomy

Vaginectomy is usually performed prior to or during reconstructive procedures. Generally, vaginectomy involves either resection of the full thickness epithelium of the vagina or de-epithelialization followed by obliteration of the vaginal canal (colpocleisis). These procedures may be performed abdominally or transvaginally. The transvaginal approach is more common when concurrent phalloplasty is planned [18]. The approach involves making an incision at the level of the vaginal introitus, circumferentially dissecting and excising the vaginal epithelium and finally obliterating the space. When there is incomplete removal of vaginal epithelium during vaginectomy and/or distal urinary obstruction diverting urine to fistulize and reopen the cavity, a persistent vaginal cavity may exist between the bladder and the rectum.

Preservation of the vagina until the time of genital reconstruction may be beneficial as vaginal mucosa and full-thickness vaginal flaps can then be used for urethral reconstruction. Specifically, an anterior vaginal wall flap may be salvaged and transposed out of the vagina in order to help lengthen the urethra if needed. A retrospective study by Massie et al. evaluated 224 total phalloplasty patients, 215 who underwent vaginectomy and 9 who underwent vaginal preservation, and found that concurrent vaginectomy and phalloplasty decreased the rate of urethral stricture (OR 0.18) and urethral fistula formation (OR 0.13) [19].

Metoidioplasty

Metoidioplasty is a relatively minimally invasive type of phalloplasty utilizing only local tissue flaps to create a neophallus and a urethra suitable for upright voiding (Chap. 9). This procedure was first described by Durfee and Rowland in 1973 [20]. While there have been several modifications to this procedure over time, it generally involves release of the ventral chordee and lengthening of the native urethra with flaps, similar to proximal hypospadias repairs in pediatric patients [21].

More specifically, the hormonally enlarged clitoris is released from its attachments and elongated to form the glans of the neophallus. The native urethra is extended using local vagi-

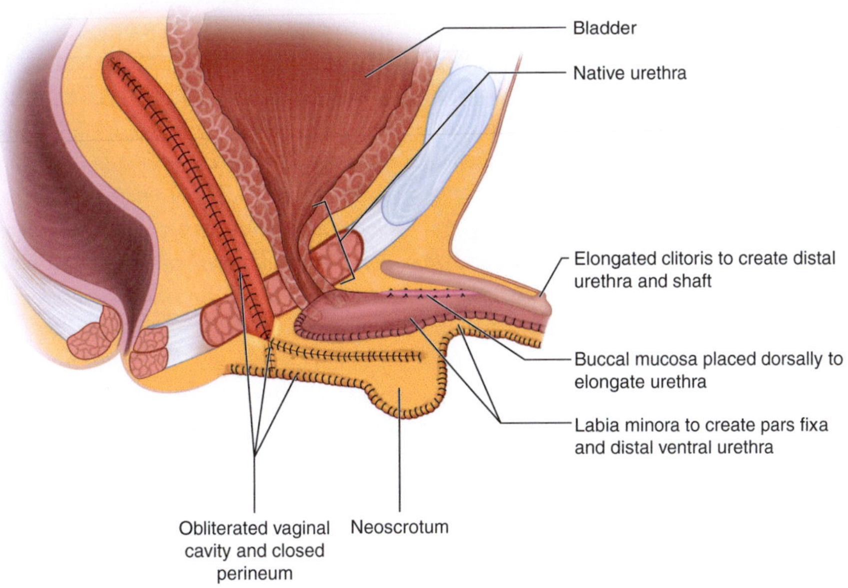

Fig. 11.1 Example of urethral anatomy after metoidioplasty (Belgrade metoidioplasty). In this example urethra from proximal to distal consists of the native portion, tubularized labia minora, dorsally placed buccal mucosa graft (urethral lengthening), distal vestibule, and hypertrophied clitoral glans

nal and labial flaps. *The resulting neourethra consists of the proximal native urethra with its meatus connected to a distal neourethra created from tubularization of the labia minora (Fig. 11.1).* Additional lengthening of the neourethra may be achieved by correction of the chordee and addition of buccal mucosa grafts. Finally, the labia majora is used for the creation of the neoscrotum [18].

Metoidioplasty allows for a sensate neophallus with preserved innervation and allows for upright voiding. Traditionally, this technique was thought to preclude individuals from engaging in penetrative intercourse due to the creation of a microphallus without adequate length or girth. However, for some patients this function is possible. In fact, one systematic review comparing metoidioplasty to radial forearm free flap phalloplasty showed that successful penetration was achieved in 51% vs 43% of patients, respectively [22]. In addition, patient-reported outcomes revealed that 87% vs 70% of patients were satisfied with the aesthetic outcome and 100% vs 69% experienced erogenous sensation, respectively [22]. A newer technique proposed by Cohanzad termed "extensive metoidioplasty" results in a neophallus with an average penile length of 8.7 cm and a range between 6 and 12 cm [23].

Overall, metoidioplasty is less complex compared to phalloplasty. It is, therefore, associated with less morbidity and less frequent urological complications [24]. Moreover, it can be performed in a single procedure within 3–4 hours [18]. Thus, it is an attractive choice for patient who desire a less-invasive option with minimization of scars.

Phalloplasty

Phalloplasty for transmasculine genital reconstructive surgery was first performed by Giles in 1945 as a staged procedure using abdominal pedicle flaps [25]. It is the preferred option for patients interested in a neophallus with increased girth and length. The surgery involves a combination of local and distant tissue transfers to create a neophallus with sufficient dimensions for the desired functions (Chap. 10). Depending on the patient's goals regarding aesthetics, sensation, micturition, and penetrative intercourse, phalloplasty with genital reconstruction can include different combinations of the following: urethroplasty, scrotoplasty, glansplasty, vaginectomy, or colpocleisis, testicular implants and penile prosthesis. The ideal phalloplasty has been described as a single-stage, reproducible procedure that allows for standing urination, tactile and erogenous sensation, sufficient girth to accommodate an erectile prosthesis, and an aesthetically acceptable result [26].

While abdominal pedicle flaps are described as the first flaps used for the creation of a neophallus, several different phalloplasty donor sites now exist for the creation of a neophallus that offer improved sensation and limit the need for additional staged procedures. The type of flaps can be categorized as pedicled flaps or free flaps. Pedicled flaps involve transposition of tissue with an intact blood supply. The most common example of a pedicled flap is the anterior lateral thigh (ALT) flap. Free flaps involve tissue transfer to distant sites with microsurgical vascular anastomoses for detached blood vessels. Examples of free flaps include radial forearm free flaps (RFFF), osteocutenaous flaps, and musculocutaneous latissimus dorsi (MLD) flaps. A combination of a pedicled anteriolateral thigh flap phalloplasty and a radial forearm free flap urethral reconstruction may be a feasible alternative for transgender men who desire a less conspicuous forearm scar [27]. A flap combination phalloplasty involving a combination of either a RFFF and a deep inferior epigastric artery perforator (DIEP) flap, a RFFF and an ALT flap, bilateral superficial circumflex iliac artery perforator (SCIP) flaps, a DIEP flap and an ALT flap, a SCIP flap and an ALT flap, a RFFF with a SCIP flap and an ALT flap and bilateral DIEP flaps has also been utilized in an attempt to reduce the morbidity at each donor site and has similar complication rates to other procedures [28]. The RFFF phalloplasty remains the "gold standard" and is the most commonly employed technique worldwide as it provides the best cosmetic and functional results with an acceptable complication rate [29–32] (Fig. 11.2).

Regardless of the flap, the neophallic urethra is created through a combination of urethral lengthening and urethral formation. The creation of the neourethra can be accomplished with primary urethroplasty or via a staged urethroplasty. *The neourethra can be divided into 5 distinct segments (Fig. 11.3). From proximal to distal, the segments are classified as (1) the native urethra, (2) the fixed perineal urethra (pars fixa), connected by (3) a circular anastomosis to (4) the phallic urethra (pars pendulans) terminating with (5) the meatus (a circular anastomosis to the outer surface of the neophallus)* [14, 33]. The *pars fixa* is the urethral segment that is lengthened by using local vaginal, labial, and/or regional flaps often in conjunction with skin or mucosal grafts [14, 34]. Elongation of this urethral segment is necessary prior to connection to the urinary conduit within the neophallus in order to allow for standing micturition. The *pars pendulans* may be constructed with a variety of techniques, including tube-in-tube techniques and prelamination [14, 16, 33, 34].

Secondary phalloplasty that occurs after metoidioplasty has also been described. A secondary phalloplasty is usually either performed as a planned second stage after metoidioplasty or in patients who are not satisfied with their metoidioplasty [35]. While surgical technique may be varied, the surgery involves a pedicled flap and/or a free flap, similar to a primary phalloplasty. Urethral reconstruction may also proceed in either a one- or two-stage procedure with the urethral anastomosis performed onto the previously lengthened *pars pendulans*, which is the former metoidioplasty meatus, in a spatulated manner [35]. A multi-institutional study by Al-Tamimi et al. retrospectively reviewed 38 patients who underwent secondary phalloplasty and found that urologic complications were comparable [35].

Overall, a typical phalloplasty is more complex than a typical metoidioplasty and may proceed in a staged manner [24, 32, 36]. In general, phalloplasty requires 5 hours with vaginectomy and urethroplasty requiring an additional 3 hours for a total of approximately 8 hours [18].

The placement of testicular implants and/or a penile prosthesis is generally a delayed proce-

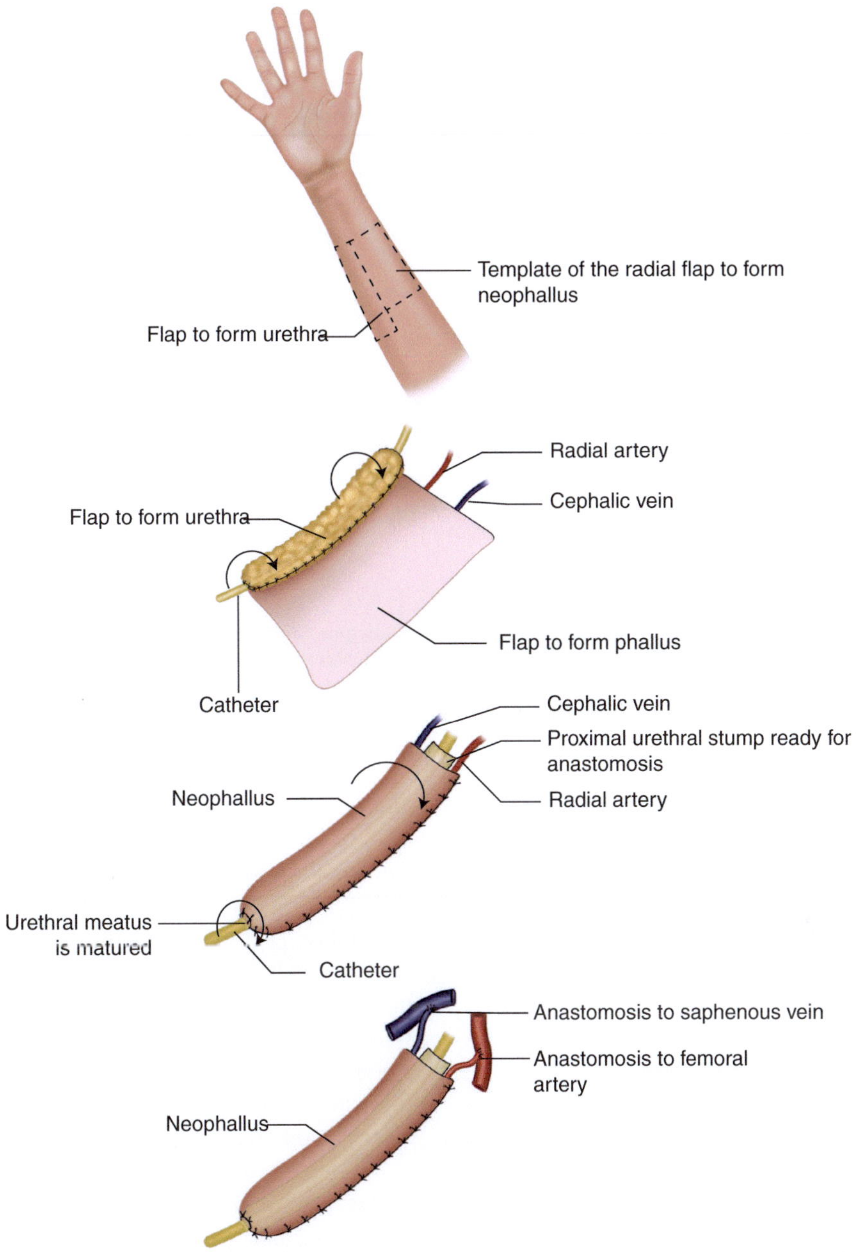

Fig. 11.2 "Tube-within-a-tube" radial forearm flap anatomy. (**a**) A flap template outline on a forearm. (**b**) Tubularization of urethral portion of the flap around a Foley catheter (epithelial surface facing the lumen of the neourethra). (**c**) Rotation of the external neophallic portion of the flap (epithelial surface facing outward). (**d**) Completion of vascular anastomoses, in preparation for urethral anastomoses

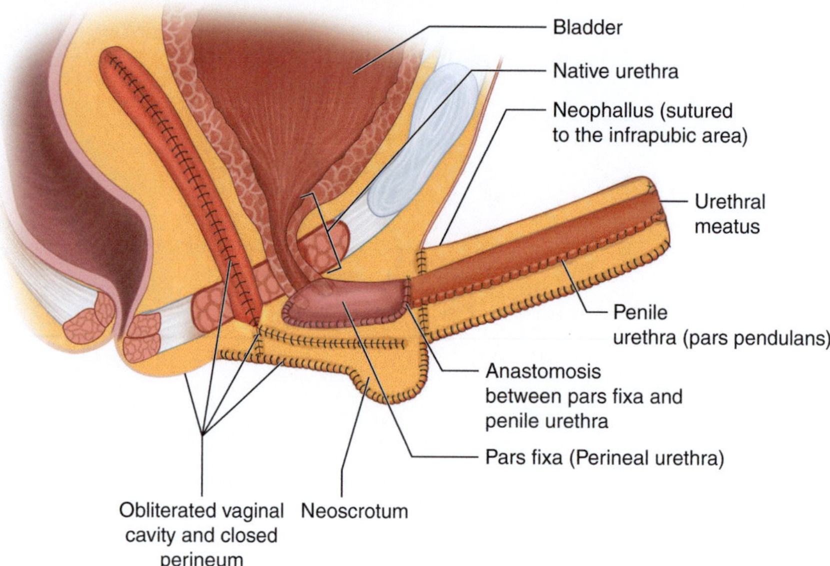

Fig. 11.3 Example of urethral anatomy after phalloplasty. From proximal to distal, the neophallic urethra consists of the native urethra, *pars fixa* (tubularized labia minora), *pars pendulans* (neophallic distal urethra). Numerous suture lines demonstrate anastomotic sites which serve as "vulnerability points" where stricture and fistulae may occur

dure that occurs between 9–12 months, after adequate healing has occurred [9, 17, 37]. The procedure is performed in 2–3 hours. The placement of a penile prosthesis may be deferred if a neophallus is bulky enough on its own for penetrative intercourse [17, 37].

Urologic Complications

Urologic complications are the most common complications following male genital reconstructive procedures [31]. *Urethrocutaneous fistulas, persistent vaginal cavities, and urethral strictures are all examples of urologic complications.* These complications can present within a few weeks up to a few years after surgery [18].

Overall, complications are less common following metoidioplasty compared to phalloplasty due to differences in technique complexity [22, 24, 32]. The rates of urethral strictures or fistulas following metoidioplasty compared to radial forearm phalloplasty are 27% versus 51%, respectively [22]. The overall urethral complication rate among the different phalloplasty techniques was found to be 39%, with even higher rates of complications for staged procedures compared to combined procedures based on a systematic review evaluating 1351 patients across 50 studies [38]. Specifically, rates of urethral complications for phalloplasty techniques utilizing fibula, abdominal, and radial forearm flaps were 22%, 33%, and 41%, respectively [38]. Another study found that compared to the radial forearm free flap phalloplasty, the tube-in-tube anterolateral thigh pedicled flap phalloplasty has a 9% higher urethral complication rate [39]. Based on a multi-institutional retrospective review, secondary phalloplasty has complication rates that are comparable to primary phalloplasty with 30% of patients developing urethral fistulas and 35% of patients developing urethral strictures [35].

Urethrocutaneous Fistulas

A urethrocutaneous fistula is the most common urologic complication following phalloplasty. Multiple studies have found that the rate of fis-

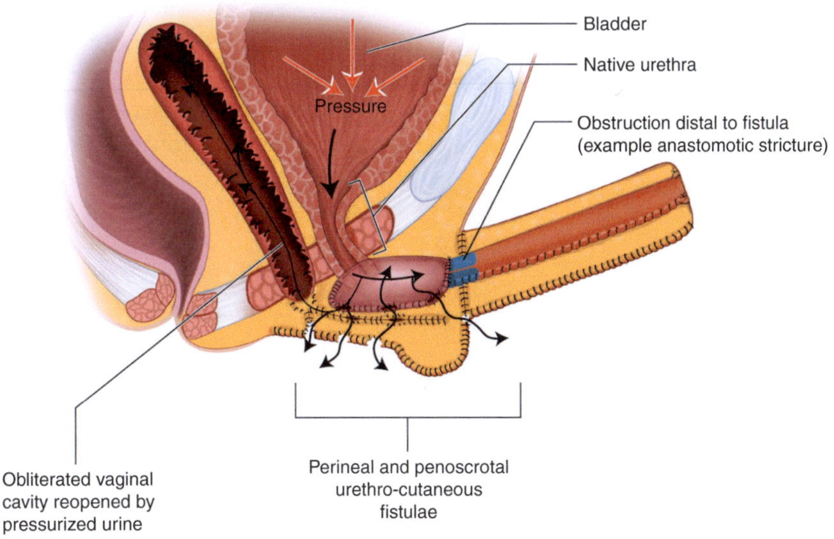

Fig. 11.4 Example of fistulae caused by distal urinary obstruction (i.e., anastomotic stricture). Pressurized urine breaking through proximal suture lines and causing various urethrocutaneous fistulae. Increased urine pressure may also hydrodissect into a previously closed vaginectomy site and produce a persistent (or recurrent) urine-filled vaginal cavity remnant

tula formation associated with radial forearm free flap phalloplasty is between 15% to 75% [31, 40–44].

While fistulas may occur anywhere along the neourethra, anastomotic sites between *pars pendulans* and *pars fixa* and in the ventral suture-line area between *pars fixa* and the native urethra are the most common locations [40, 44] (Fig. 11.4). This is presumably due to decreased vascularity of the flap, poor quality of local tissue in the multilayer closure, as well as the discrepancy between the luminal diameters of the different urethral segments due to primary flap design or secondary to contraction during healing [40, 44]. The size discrepancy in the diameters is unfavorable as it leads to a relative distal obstruction of urinary flow, possibly leading to more proximal fistula formation [44]. This theory also explains how obstruction secondary to urethral strictures can lead to more proximal fistula formation. The reported incidence of fistulas associated with more distal strictures is 40% [44].

Double flap techniques attempt to overcome the issues with blood flow by creating independent vascularized urethral and skin flaps; however, urethral complications still persist [27, 28]. One study by Namba et al. retrospectively reviewed 15 patients who underwent flap combination phalloplasty and found fistulas in 5 (33%) patients [28]. Despite the inability of the double flap to improve outcomes, the use of a well-vascularized flap is considered vital to ensure preservation of the neophallus.

Not surprisingly, fistula formation is also associated with patients who forego vaginectomy and elect vaginal preservation. The higher fistula rate in patients who do not undergo vaginectomy compared to those who do (56% versus 14%) is thought to be related to the lack of available vaginal tissue for flap creation [19].

Spontaneous closure of fistulous tracts may occur in up to 36% of patients within 2 months of diagnosis; however, fistulas that are at multiple sites, large, or persist for greater than 3 months require surgical repair [45, 46] (Fig. 11.5).

Persistent Vaginal Cavity

Communication between the neourethra and a remnant vaginal cavity is another type of fistula and is a commonly encountered urologic complication following phalloplasty. Urologists should have a high index of suspicion for this complication if a patient presents with prolonged post-void dribbling, pelvic pain, or fullness and/or persistent urinary tract infections post phalloplasty.

This complication has been found in approximately half of patients who present for the treatment of a neourethral stricture [24]. *It is suspected that urethral strictures lead to pressurized urine breaking through the ventral suture lines of the fixed urethra into the previously obliterated vaginal cavity* [24] *(Fig. 11.4).* Patients are more susceptible to this complication if there is inadequate vaginal de-epithelialization during colpocleisis or incomplete vaginectomy [18]. In our experience with re-excision and re-obliteration of persistent vaginal cavities, tissue specimens from all 15 patients demonstrate vaginal epithelium on histological examinations (Fig. 11.6).

A persistent vaginal cavity can become quite large and the connection is unlikely to spontaneously close, requiring complete cavity excision and obliteration (Fig. 11.7).

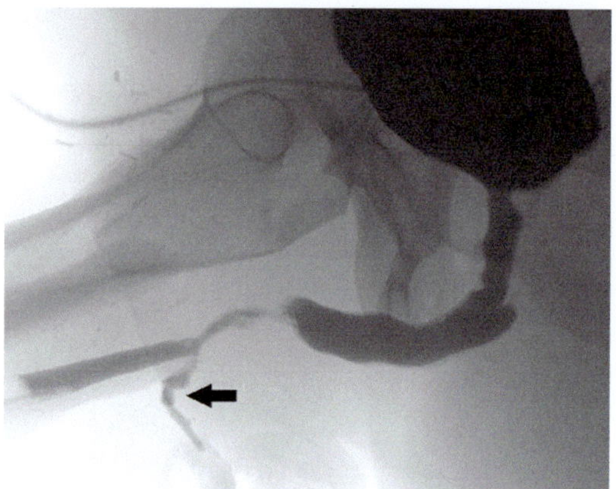

Fig. 11.5 Retrograde urethrogram (RUG) and simultaneous voiding cystourethrogram (VCUG) demonstrating urinary extravasation through a fistulous tract along the neourethra requiring surgical repair

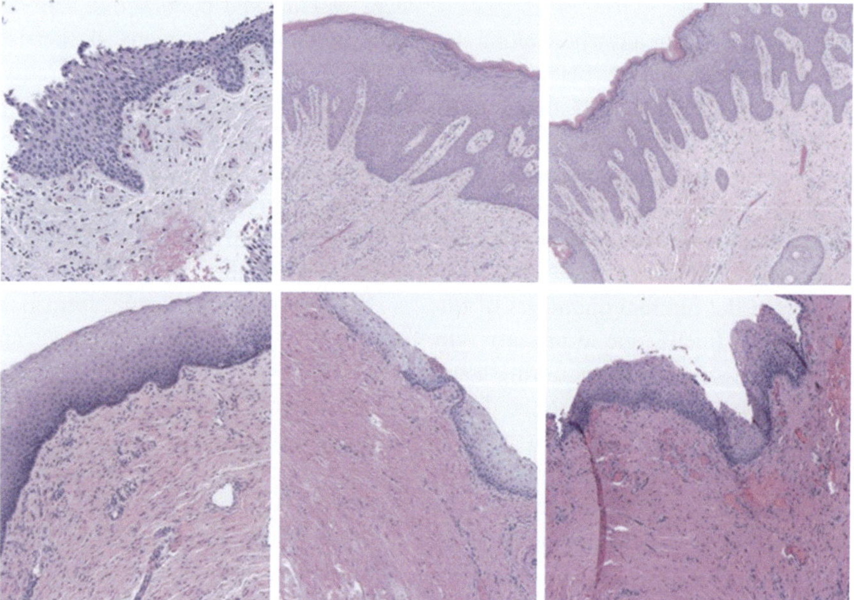

Fig. 11.6 H&E slides of excised remnant vaginal cavity tissue from 6 different patients with the history of prior vaginectomy. The slides demonstrate presence of vaginal epithelium

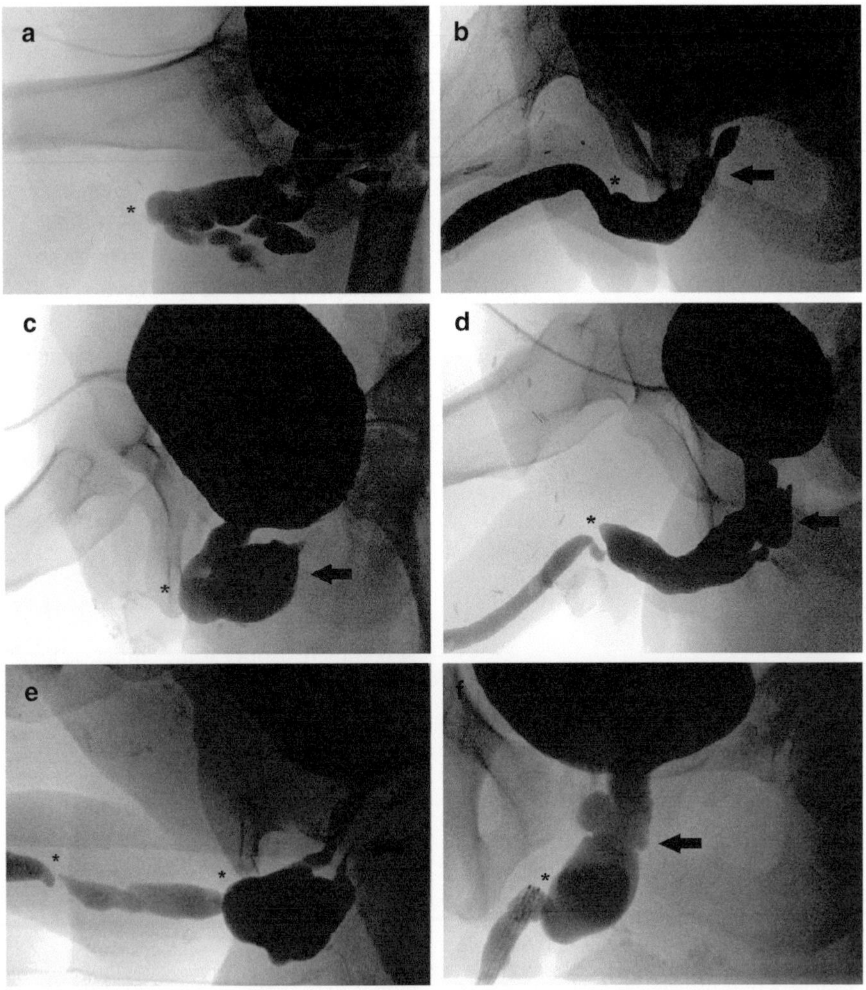

Fig. 11.7 Examples of persistent vaginal cavities detected during preoperative imaging that required surgical repair. The arrow shows the persistent vaginal cavity and the asterisk represents a more distal neourethral stricture

Urethral Strictures

Urethral strictures are a complication with an incidence ranging from 25% to 58% following phalloplasty [44, 47]. Based on a large series, mean stricture length is reported as 3.6 cm with a range of 0.5–15 cm with 41% of strictures in the anastomotic urethra between *pars fixa* and *pars pendulans*, 28% in the phallic urethra, 15% in the meatus, 13% in the fixed urethra, and 8% in multiple urethral segments [33] (Fig. 11.8). *Anastomotic sites are the most common stricture locations likely due to poor vascularization and relative ischemia* [40, 48–50]. During the healing process, contracture may compromise the neo-urethral lumen and potentially lead to complete obliteration that requires surgical repair. Unfortunately, a double flap phalloplasty with an independently vascularized urethra does not appear to improve outcomes [27]. In fact, one retrospective review of 19 transgender men who underwent ALT phalloplasties combined with RFFF urethral reconstruction showed long-term urinary complications occurred in 10 patients (53%), with 9 patients (47%) developing urethral strictures [27].

Urethral strictures can be temporized with catheters until the inflammation surrounding the tissue has abated, but ultimately require surgery in most cases [17] (Fig. 11.9).

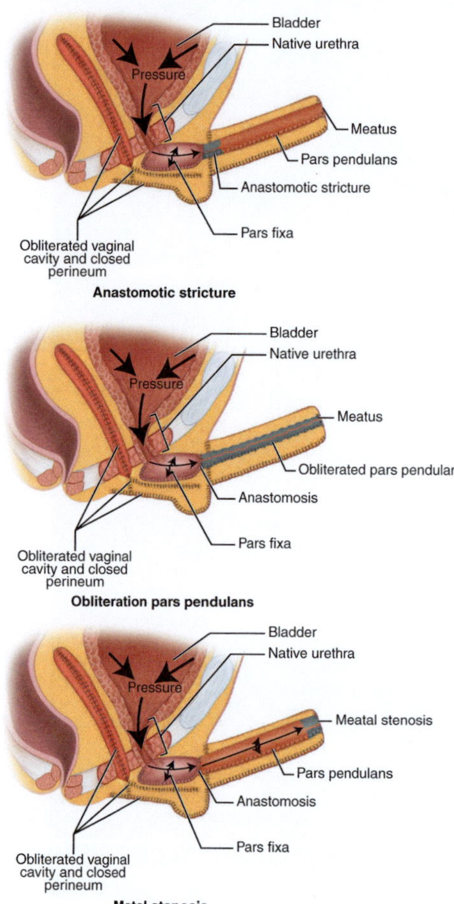

Fig. 11.8 Examples of neophallic urethral strictures. (**a**) Anastomotic stricture between *pars fixa* and *pars pendulans*. (**b**) Panurethral stricture – complete obliteration of *pars pendulans*. (**c**) Meatal stenosis

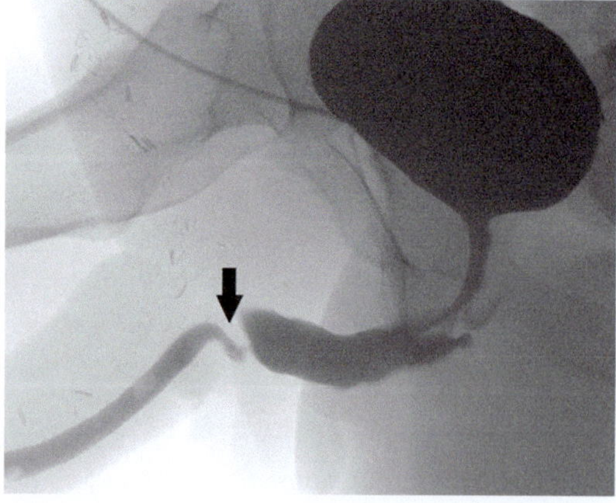

Fig. 11.9 RUG and simultaneous VCUG demonstrating an anastomotic stricture between *pars fixa* and *pars pendulans*

Patient Presentation

Patients may present anytime following transmasculine genital reconstructive surgery for an evaluation of bothersome voiding symptoms. The most common urinary complaints include dysuria, suprapubic pain, weakened urinary stream, post-void dribbling, straining, and feelings of incomplete bladder emptying [24]. There should be a high index of suspicion for a persistent vaginal cavity, urethrocutenous fistula, and/or a urethral stricture when evaluating these patients. Diagnosis and treatment of these complications is important to avoid consequences of chronic infection, sepsis, urinary retention, renal failure, and decreased quality of life.

Evaluation

A complete history is the cornerstone of the evaluation. A well-taken history can elucidate the probable diagnosis and help to determine the next steps. The use of open-ended questions is important to gain a detailed understanding of the clinical picture. More targeted questions can provide information that points to a specific complication. For example, reported passage of urine from a site other than the urethral meatus indicates a urethrocutaneous fistula. In addition, post-void dribbling, which may persist for a long time after each micturition, could indicate a persistent vaginal cavity.

Review of prior operative reports along with corresponding postoperative hospital and clinic notes is necessary for a comprehensive history of presenting illness. These documents provide information regarding exactly what type of genital reconstruction was performed and in how many stages, what type of flaps, if any, were used, how the vascular and urethral anastomoses were completed, what additional procedures were performed, how the patient recovered postoperatively, and what prior attempts were taken to alleviate the bothersome symptoms. Direct communication with the surgeon who performed the earlier operations could be invaluable in obtaining a clear history, and in understanding unique characteristics of each patient's surgical anatomy.

The physical examination should focus on the abdominal, flank, and genital regions. Evaluation of the suprapubic and the flank regions can provide evidence regarding infection or urinary retention. Isolated suprapubic tenderness may indicate cystitis, while costovertebral angle tenderness is concerning for pyelonephritis, especially in a patient with fevers, dysuria, and hematuria. Urinary retention may also be suggested by a palpable bladder.

During the genitourinary examination, the neophallus, neoscrotum, perineum, and surrounding areas should be examined entirely to assess for erythema, induration, fluctuance, fistula formation, or any other abnormality. The urethral meatus should also be examined for its location and patency. *Adequate caliber of the urethra should not be assessed by blind calibration with catheters, dilators, or bougies, but rather under direct vision* via *passage of a flexible cystoscope due to possibility of injury.*

A clean-catch urine sample should be collected for urinalysis and urine culture on any patient with lower urinary tract symptoms or prior to any urologic intervention. Prescription of culture-specific antibiotics is necessary to treat any positive urine cultures. It is important to note that if a urine specimen is collected from an indwelling urinary catheter a positive culture may represent colonization rather than a true infection. Additional laboratory tests including basic metabolic panel (BMP), complete blood count (CBC), and blood cultures should be obtained based on clinical judgement.

A uroflow and post-void residual (PVR) are noninvasive ways to measure the maximal urine flow rate and evaluate for urinary retention. Immediate bladder drainage is important if urinary retention is identified to avoid potential urinary tract infections and/or damage to the upper urinary tracts. In an effort to avoid blind and potentially traumatic urethral catheterizations, especially given the high likelihood of a urethral stricture, suprapubic catheterization by a urologist in a procedure room or in the operating room or by an interventional radiologist in a radiology suite is the preferred method of drainage. It is important to place at least a 16 French catheter 2–3 cm above the pubis, in the midline. A large bore catheter ensures adequate drainage in addition to offering a reliable channel for the

evaluation of the bladder and proximal urethra via antegrade cystourethroscopy.

Imaging combined with endoscopy is essential to delineate stricture and/or fistula location as well as the presence of a persistent vaginal cavity. While feasible to perform in an office setting, the complex anatomy may warrant an examination under anesthesia. Initial imaging should include a retrograde urethrogram (RUG), in which contrast is injected retrograde through the urethra, and a voiding cystourethrogram (VCUG), in which contrast is instilled in the bladder and voided [49]. Additional imaging is dictated by the initial evaluation and may include ultrasound, computed tomography (CT) scan, or pelvic magnetic resonance imaging (MRI). It is important to personally review imaging as not all radiologists are aware of the wide variety of anatomic and pathologic changes unique to patients who undergo gender affirmation surgery [49]. Any sequestered fluid collection or abscess seen on imaging should be drained, and urine and cavity cultures should be sent to determine appropriate antibiotic treatment prior to urologic intervention.

Endoscopy can be performed with a 16 French flexible cystoscope for direct visualization of the urethra as previously mentioned. When the urethral lumen is unable to accommodate a flexible cystoscope, an 8 French flexible pediatric cystoscope or a ureteroscope may be used for evaluation. When the neourethra is tortuous, a guidewire ensures safe gradual advancement of a flexible scope. A simultaneous retrograde urethrogram can be performed by injecting contrast through the working channel of the scope. Flexible cystourethroscopy through a suprapubic tract may be performed if the distal urethra is completely obliterated. The presence of a persistent vaginal cavity, the location of any fistula as well as the location, length, and caliber of any strictures should be noted.

Preoperative Planning

After completing the comprehensive preoperative assessment, the patient should be counseled regarding the clinical findings, implications of those findings and treatment options, including alternatives to surgery. *In order to make an informed decision regarding treatment, patients should be educated regarding the individual risks and benefits of the 3 possible approaches: (1) conservative management, (2) further reconstruction, and (3) urinary diversion (i.e., perineal urethrostomy).* Proper patient counseling involves establishing realistic preoperative expectations as well as providing detailed information about the surgical risks, the possibility of multistage procedures, and the risk of partial or total loss of the neophallus or loss of previously placed penile or testicular prosthetics [35]. *Management options depend on the severity of the problem, availability of healthy tissue for reconstruction, and the patient's personal preferences.* Patients with poor health or tissue quality may not be candidates for heroic reconstructive measures despite their preference to pursue further reconstruction.

Once the decision to pursue surgery is made, medical clearance should be obtained, and the patient should be optimized for surgery. Optimization may include tobacco cessation, discontinuation of recreational drugs, nutritional support, diabetic control, and treatment of ongoing infections. Pre-anesthesia clearance and planning can help to ensure that surgery is safe from an anesthesia and pain control perspective as well.

The placement of a suprapubic catheter should be considered for preoperative urinary diversion to circumvent the passage of pressurized urine across damaged neourethral structures and avoid further injury to the underlying tissues. A suprapubic catheter may also benefit patients postoperatively by allowing adequate drainage of urine.

Given that further reconstruction is a unique surgical challenge, prior operative reports should be re-reviewed prior to surgery to ensure the specific details regarding each prior reconstructive effort are known. *The location of a vascular pedicle is of utmost importance in order to avoid compromising the blood supply of the neophallus during surgery.*

After adequate anesthesia and intubation, the patient should be placed in lithotomy position. It is important to remember to avoid positioning the patient in a high-lithotomy position as this position can possibly compress and obstruct blood supply to the neophallus.

If the surgical plan includes intraoperative harvesting of buccal mucosa graft, prior harvest site and endotracheal tube placement should be considered preoperatively. The tube should be placed on the side opposite of the intended harvest site.

Fistula Repair Techniques

Successful repair of urinary fistula involves several key principles. These include complete excision of the fistula tract, the use of absorbable sutures, a tension-free closure, a multilayer closure with well-vascularized tissue, nonoverlapping suture lines, and low-pressure healing, which means elimination of distal obstruction (i.e., stricture repair), maximal urinary drainage through a catheter (urethral and/or suprapubic), and prevention of detrusor overactivity [18].

The surgery begins with cystourethroscopy in order to gain an understanding of the lower urinary tract anatomy. This may be performed in a retrograde or antegrade manner depending on the clinical scenario. External probing of the fistula tract with a guidewire or lacrimal duct probe during endoscopy can assist in the identification of the fistula within a tortuous neourethra in the absence of other anatomic landmarks [24]. External probing is also useful for delineating the fistula tract trajectory and for measuring the distance of the cutaneous opening to the neourethra. Once the fistula is properly identified, the placement of concentric retraction sutures at the edges of the fistula tract can be used to facilitate excision. Although not necessary, sharp excision of the tract may be performed in a "cut to the light" procedure in the presence of an intraluminal cystoscope [24]. Following excision, the resultant opening of the neourethra may be closed in multiple nonoverlapping layers using absorbable sutures to bring well-vascularized tissue across the repair. Coverage of the fistula repair site with a fasciocutaneous groin flap, a labial fat pad flap, or a musculofascial gracilis flap should be considered to decrease the risk of fistula recurrence [45]. Repair of any communicating persistent vaginal cavity or distal neourethral stricture should also be pursued in the same setting to decrease the risk of fistula recurrence [51]. Maintaining a suprapubic or urethral catheter for 3–4 weeks postoperatively achieves low-pressure healing through maximal urinary drainage. Anticholinergics can prevent bladder spasms during this time period as well.

When patients present for postoperative catheter removal, a RUG or a VCUG can be used to assess the effectiveness of fistula repair. Any evidence of contrast extravasation on imaging requires maintenance or replacement of the catheter for an additional 2–3 weeks to allow for further drainage and healing. Repeat imaging at follow-up ensures the resolution of the fistula prior to catheter removal.

Techniques for Obliteration of a Persistent Vaginal Cavity

Although a persistent vaginal cavity may not be apparent during the preoperative evaluation, a high index of suspicion should remain for this potential complication until its absence is proven intraoperatively. If a remnant cavity is identified preoperatively or intraoperatively, it should be completely excised and obliterated. This can be accomplished through a transabdominal robotic-assisted laparoscopic approach or an open perineal approach, similar to colpocleisis [51] (Fig. 11.10). In our experience, subepithelial injection of lidocaine with epinephrine into the lining of the cavity is helpful in tissue hydrodissection and in reducing intraoperative bleeding [45]. The placement of bilateral ureteral stents and a urethral catheter prior to the dissection may help with the identification and avoidance of injury to the ureters, or at the least may aid in early intraoperative detection of an injury [18].

Endoscopic Stricture Management

Endoscopic management of urethral strictures may be a non-invasive first-line treatment option for short, single strictures. The two endoscopic options include dilation and direct visualization internal urethrotomy (DVIU). These approaches must be performed under direct endoscopic or radiographic guidance to ensure the proper location is dilated or incised. The placement of a catheter for at least 2 weeks postoperatively allows for urinary drainage to promote healing [52]. In an effort to maintain long-term urethral patency, self-catheterization or self-calibration of the anterior urethral segment can be used following catheter removal [18].

Unfortunately, endoscopic procedures are unlikely to result in durable success, with the rate of recurrence as high as 88% likely due to the lack of a corpus spongiosum and poor blood supply in a neophallus [6, 24, 47]. It is therefore our preference to perform reconstruction in this setting. Lumen et al., however, describe DVIU as a reasonable first-line approach when the neophallic stricture is less than 3 cm in length and no prior DVIU has been performed based on their retrospective review that showed success rate of first-time DVIU to be 43.8% at a mean of 51 months [52]. A shorter time to stricture formation following neophallus construction was identified as a significant risk factor for failure of endoscopic intervention [52].

Urethroplasty Techniques

For definitive treatment of long, multifocal, or recurrent urethral strictures, urethral reconstruction via urethroplasty is the best option. Urethroplasty can be very challenging due to the poor blood supply of the neourethra as previously described [50]. The type of urethroplasty depends upon the location and length of the stricture as well as the availability and quality of the local tissue surrounding the stricture. Examples of various urethroplasty techniques following neophallus construction include meatal reconstruction,

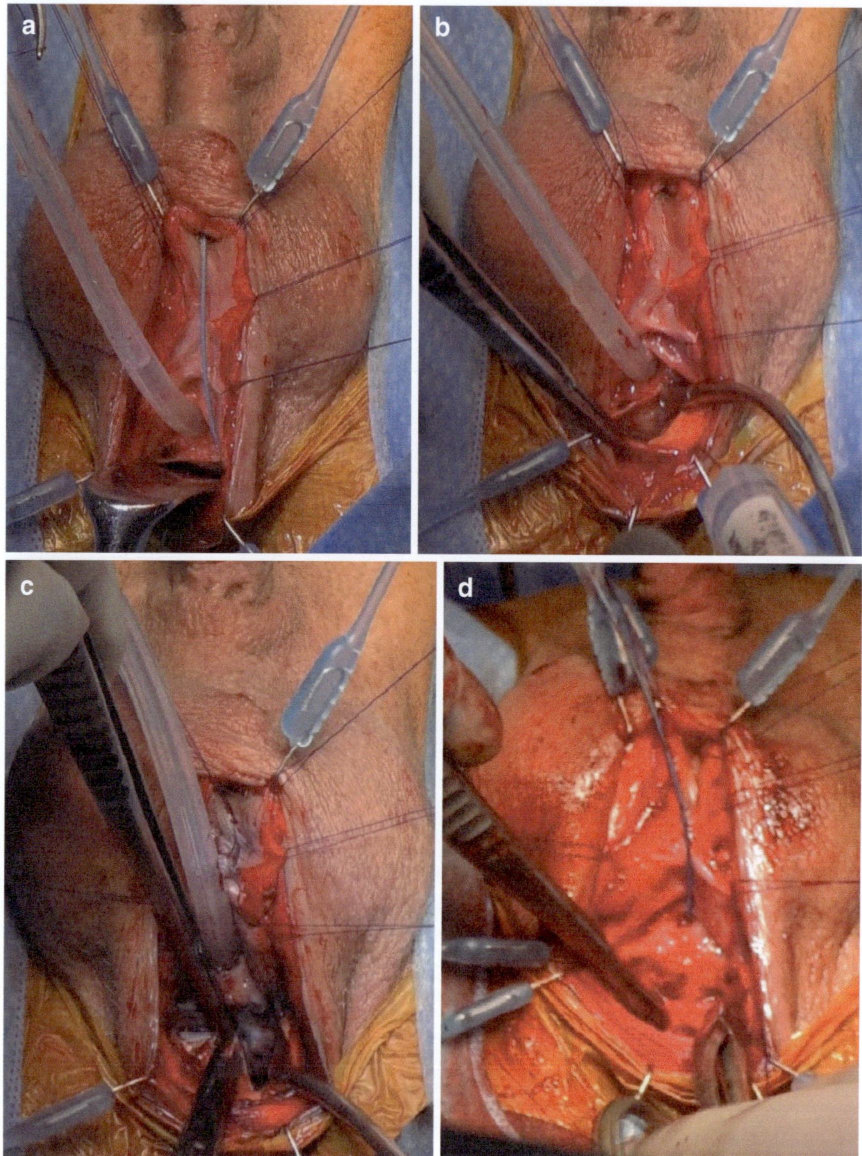

Fig. 11.10 Persistent vaginal cavity re-excision. (**a**) Intraoperative view: persistent vaginal cavity seen posterior to the neourethra. (**b**) Epinephrine-lidocaine solution injected into epithelium of persistent vaginal cavity to facilitate re-excision of the vaginal tissue. (**c**) Sharp dissection to ensure meticulous cavity de-epithelialization (**d**) and obliteration of persistent vaginal cavity

excision and primary anastomosis (EPA), free graft urethroplasty, pedicled flap urethroplasty, and two-stage urethroplasty [17, 33, 45].

In general, meatal reconstruction is achieved by (1) meatotomy, (2) advancement meatoplasty, or (3) single or staged buccal mucosa graft augmentation (i.e., dorsal or ventral inlay techniques). Panurethral or long pendulous urethral strictures/obliteration always requires a staged approach with urethral plate augmentation via buccal mucosa or other substitution materials. Anastomotic strictures or obliteration can be approached in various ways. In these scenarios, it is not uncommon to consent the patient for several different possibilities and make the final surgical plan intraoperatively based on intraoperative findings related to surrounding tissue quality (i.e., vascularity, degree of scarring) and presence of infection (i.e., abscess cavities). In our practice, staged procedures are offered to all patients with previous single-stage procedure failures. Perineal urethrostomy is performed for patients with multiple failed reconstructive attempts or those who choose to avoid extensive reconstruction.

Meatal Reconstruction

Extended meatotomy is the standard approach for surgical correction of short stenotic segments at the meatus [53]. This technique involves incising the meatus with a simple ventral incision followed by reapproximating the inner urethral mucosa and glanular tissue with sutures. This can result in a hypospadic-appearing meatus with an unpredictable urinary flow direction (Fig. 11.11a).

Meatoplasty is usually reserved for more complex patients with recurrent or longer meatal strictures. Numerous techniques can be employed that may incorporate flaps or grafts and be performed in single or staged procedures similar to more proximal urethral reconstruction [53]. While various techniques for distal urethral reconstruction in cisgender males have been proposed, most utilizing genital skin flaps with a dartos pedicle, these techniques cannot be applied in patients with neophallus due to unique vascular anatomy (i.e., absence of dartos tissue) and lack of quality local skin available for reconstruction [54–58]. In contrast, graft augmentation techniques have become highly versatile options for the treatment of distal urethral strictures in cis-gender males and could be applied for the treatment of distal neophallic strictures.

The Asopa urethroplasty is a one-stage technique that involves ventral sagittal urethrotomy and dorsal graft placement without mobilization of the urethra [59] (Fig. 11.11). Another distal urethroplasty technique developed by Chowdhury et al. is a single-stage ventral onlay repair with buccal mucosal graft [60]. Alternatively, a double-face buccal mucosal graft technique is described by Goel et al. [61]. Briefly, this technique involves opening the stenosed segment ventrally and raising glanular wings for the placement of a ventral graft followed by a dorsal urethrotomy incision for the placement of a dorsal graft [61]. We have previously developed a novel transurethral approach for fossa navicularis strictures that involves a ventral transurethral wedge resection of the stenosed segment and transurethral delivery and spread fixation of appropriate buccal mucosal graft inlay into the resultant urethrotomy [62]. This technique, originally described for use in cis-gender males, was subsequently applied to 5 transgender males with distal urethral strictures and resulted in 80% (4/5) recurrence-free success at intermediate-term follow-up.

For patients with completely obliterated meatus, those with prior failures or patients seeking to reverse extended meatotomy due to poor aesthetics or urine flow deviation, augmented staged urethroplaty techniques are available. These techniques, similar to staged repairs for failed hypospadias, begin with ventral urethral spatulation and creation of dorsal urethral plate with use or grafts as a first stage. Four to six months later, patients return for the tubularization stage. Graft contractures between the stages are common and may require additional graft placement at the time of tubularization or further intermediate stages to create adequate urethral plate. Patients seeking distal urethral reconstruction should be educated on the possible need for numerous operations, risks of urethrocutaneous fistula, glans dehiscence, suboptimal cosmetic outcomes, and likelihood of persistent or worsened urinary stream deviation or spraying.

Single-Stage Anastomotic Techniques for Anastomotic Strictures

For a primary short urethral anastomotic stricture, a single-stage anastomotic technique without the use of additional flaps or grafts is possible. Excision and primary anastomosis (EPA) or a

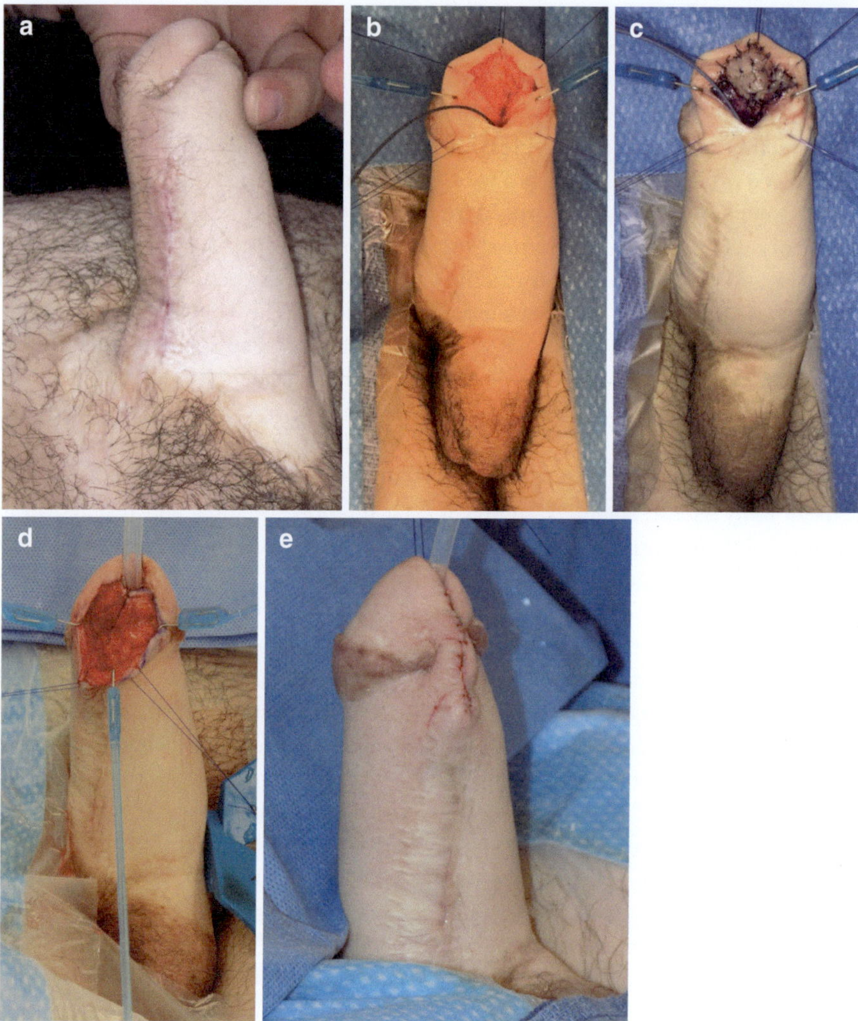

Fig. 11.11 Example of a single-stage meatal reconstruction (**a**) Preoperative image of patient with prior failed extended meatotomy. (**b**) Stenosed segment incised dorsally. (**c**) Dorsal placement of buccal mucosal graft inlay. (**d**) Tubularization of neourethra over a catheter. (**e**) Postoperative image immediately after tubularization and ventral skin closure

non-transecting anastomotic urethroplasty may be performed when there is a short anastomotic stricture with the presence of reliable well-vascularized local tissue. This technique involves excising the stenosed urethral segment, spatulating the proximal and distal stumps in opposite, complementary directions, and then reapproximating the edges over an indwelling catheter [24]. While this is considered a "gold standard" approach for short strictures in cis-gender male urethras, decreased tissue mobility, absence of corpus spongiosum, and reduced blood supply limit its success in transgender men with neourethras [16, 47]. The overall success rate for this technique is cited as 57% [33]. This poor success rate is one of the reasons we argue against using primary anastomosis techniques in any patient with a stricture in the neophallus. In addition, it is our reconstructive philosophy to avoid subjecting patients to repeated techniques they have previously failed and, conceptually, we treat an anastomotic stricture between *pars fixa* and *pars pendulans* as a previously failed anastomotic urethroplasty. Thus, we prefer to utilize other reconstructive techniques for all anastomotic strictures in patients with a neophallus.

Single-Stage Substitution Techniques for Anastomotic Strictures

Single-stage substitution techniques rely on flaps or grafts and are typically used for repairs of longer or more complex strictures. One of the most commonly performed techniques is a dorsal inlay approach with buccal mucosal graft [59]. Buccal mucosal grafts have become the tissue of choice for urethral reconstruction due to the pan-laminar vascular plexus that is ideal for engraftment and the thick, non-keratinized epithelium that is compatible with a wet environment [47]. Skin, vaginal epithelium, enteric, and bladder mucosa have also been described as possible graft options [47, 59, 63–66]. It is important to note that circumferential mobilization of the neourethra is not performed as it is in cis-urethras since it could compromise the vascular supply to the neophallus [18]. The surgery typically begins with a ventral urethrotomy followed by a vertical dorsal incision through the stenosed segment of the urethra and advances 1–2 cm into the patent lumen proximally and distally. The graft is placed as a dorsal inlay (Asopa-type technique) that increases the size of the lumen and ensures patency prior to closure [59]. Although dorsal placement may avoid the frequently unreliable vascularity and coverage of the ventral tissue, ventral repairs have also been described [47, 67].

It is our preference to perform simultaneous dorsal inlay and ventral onlay buccal mucosa urethroplasty whenever possible (Fig. 11.12). This technique sometimes called "double-face" repair, now adapted for repairs of neophallic strictures, was first described by Palminteri et al. for the treatment of strictures in cis-gender males with bulbar urethral strictures [68]. Each graft is quilted on an independent vascular bed. During a neourethral stricture repair, we typically utilize neo-scrotal fat (similar to a Martious flap) for the

ventral graft. However, a gracilis flap may also be present in the perineum from the original neophallus construction [24]. If available, gracilis can be carefully recycled for use as a vascular bed for the ventral buccal mucosa graft [24] (Fig. 11.13). A fasciocutaneous flap may also be used to support a ventral onlay graft and improve its blood supply [69].

Staged Techniques

A staged urethroplasty is the preferred method of choice for long penile or recurrent anastomotic neophallic strictures (Figs. 11.14, 11.15 and 11.16). This technique begins with a ventral urethrotomy through the stenosed segment, or a complete ventral spatulation of the anterior urethral segment in cases of panurethral strictures. The urethral plate can either be augmented with a graft or a new neourethral plate can be created with a graft. As previously mentioned, there are several types of grafts available, with buccal mucosal graft being the most common. The lateral edges of the urethral plate are then sutured to the borders of the skin incision. The distal urethral plate remains exposed during healing and the patient voids through a temporary more proximal urethrostomy. The urethral plate matures over the next 3–6 months. During the second stage, tubularization of the neourethra occurs over a catheter following lateral mobilization of the urethral plate. Overall, this technique has been reported to have a success rate of up to 70%, which is the highest success rate among all types of neophallic urethroplasties [33].

Perineal Urethrostomy

Unfortunately, when considering all the different reconstructive options, overall stricture recurrence rates are typically greater than 40% and many patients require several additional interventions [33, 44]. Perineal urethrostomy is an alternate option for patients who are not interested in reconstructive surgery or who have failed multiple reconstructive efforts. In other situations, it

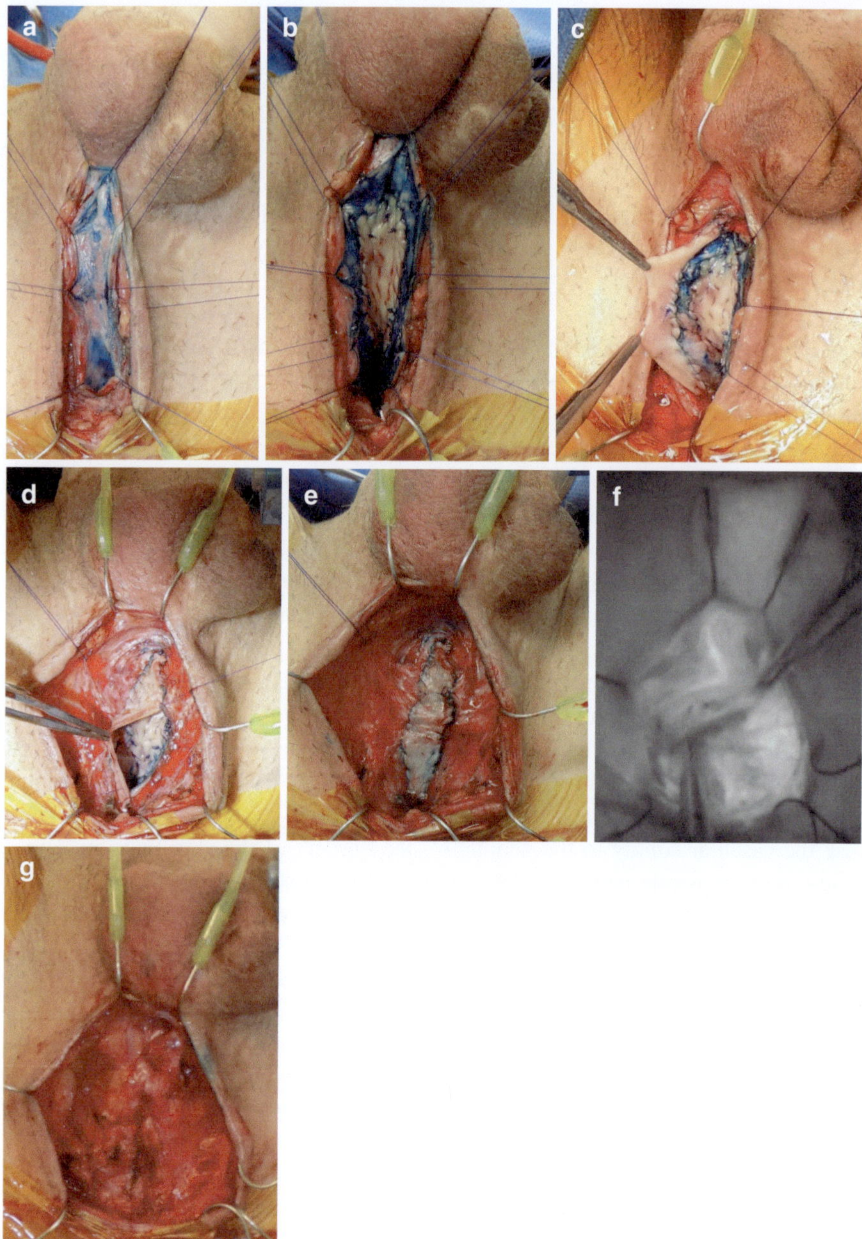

Fig. 11.12 Single-stage double-face buccal mucosal graft for repair of anastomotic stricture (**a**) Neourethral stricture with narrow urethral plate prior to repair. (**b**) Dorsal inlay of buccal mucosal graft after sagittal dorsal incision of stenosed segment. (**c**) Ventral onlay of buccal mucosal graft. (**d**) Double-face buccal mucosal graft for the creation of larger caliber urethral lumen. (**e**) Exposed ventral onlay graft. (**f**) Indocyanine green (ICG) perfusion study demonstrating local tissue perfusion prior to its rotation over the ventral graft. (**g**) Closure in multiple layers

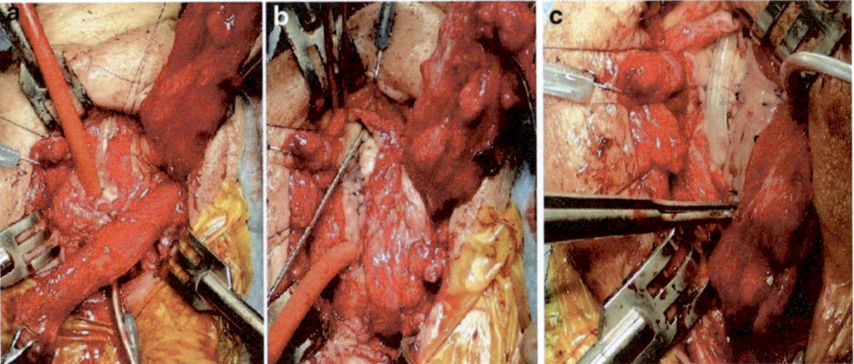

Fig. 11.13 Recycled gracilis: an alternate approach to a single-stage double-face repair in a patient with a gracilis flap previously placed in the perineum at the time of phalloplasty. (**a**) Dissected and preserved gracilis is divided into two tails – one for vaginal cavity obliteration and another as graft bed for a ventral buccal mucosal graft. (**b**) Dorsal inlay of buccal mucosal graft. (**c**) Ventral onlay of buccal mucosal graft on gracilis prior to tubularization of neourethra over catheter and closure

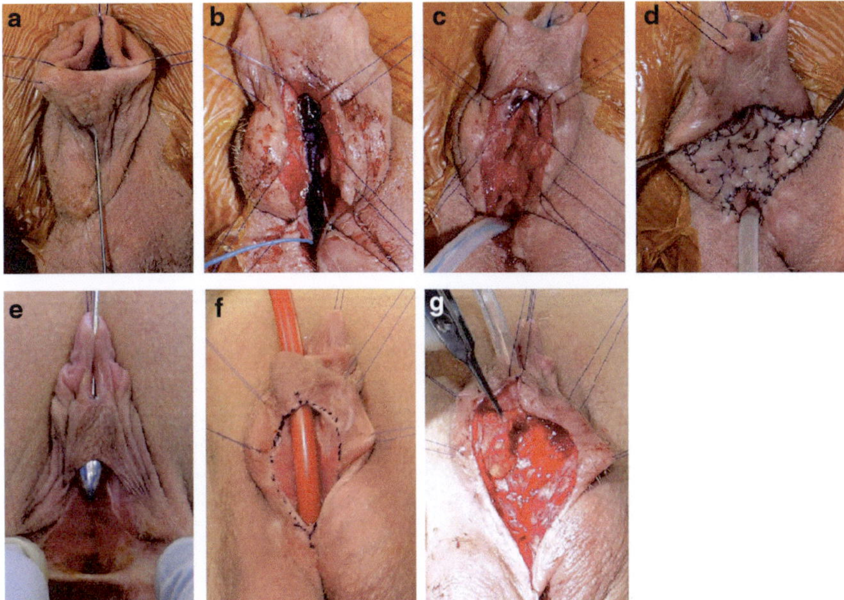

Fig. 11.14 Staged repair of a urethrocutaneous fistula and neourethral stricture in a patient with a prior metoidioplasty. (**a**) A bougie is placed to demonstrate urethrocutaneous fistula. (**b**) Neourethral stricture with a narrowed urethral plate is highlighted with methylene blue dye. (**c**) Healthy tissue is exposed for the placement of buccal mucosal graft following excision of the stenosed avascular segment. (**d**) A buccal mucosal graft inlay is tailored and quilted into the dorsal incision. (**e**) Second stage: preoperative image of viable buccal mucosal graft at 6 months' follow-up. (**f**) Wide caliber urethral plate prior to tubularization of neourethra and (**g**) closure in multiple layers over catheter

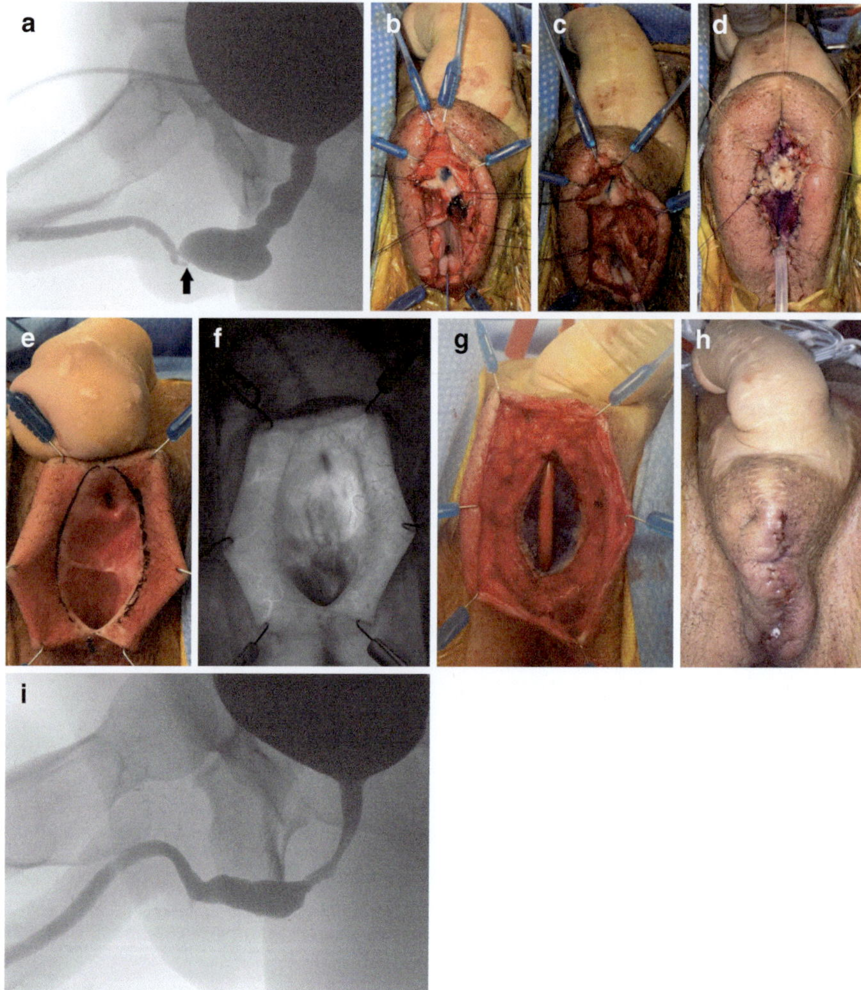

Fig. 11.15 Staged repair of anastomotic stricture in a patient with a prior phalloplasty. (**a**) Preoperative RUG and VCUG. (**b**) Anastomotic stricture between *pars pendulans* and *pars fixa*. (**c**) Dorsal incision of stenosed anastomotic segment. (**d**) Completion of stage one repair with dorsal placement of buccal mucosal graft to serve as a temporary augmented perineal urethrostomy. (**d**) Second stage: preoperative image showing wide urethral plate at 6 months postoperatively. (**e**) Indocyanine green (ICG) perfusion study demonstrating well-perfused buccal graft tissue. (**f**) Urethral tubularization over a urethral catheter and skin closure. (**g**) Postoperative VCUG showing a wide caliber urethral lumen without evidence of fistula or stricture

may be used as a temporary treatment until definitive reconstruction is pursued. This surgery results in the creation of a perineal urethral meatus under the neoscrotum by opening the fixed urethra and approximating the lateral edges of the urethra to the perineum (Fig. 11.17). It allows for unobstructed urine flow from the newly created urethra. It is important to note that patients are able to retain their continence since the native urethra and the bladder neck are not manipulated during this procedure.

Challenges of Reconstructive Surgery

Reconstructive surgery in this patient population is challenging due to the nature of the neo-anatomy. There is a lack of spongiosum, pedicle blood supply, and multiple anastomoses between structures of varying tissue types with differing physical properties [44]. Additionally, surgical options may be impacted by the limited availability of local flaps and distant grafts [47]. No long-term results for any types of revision urethroplasty after

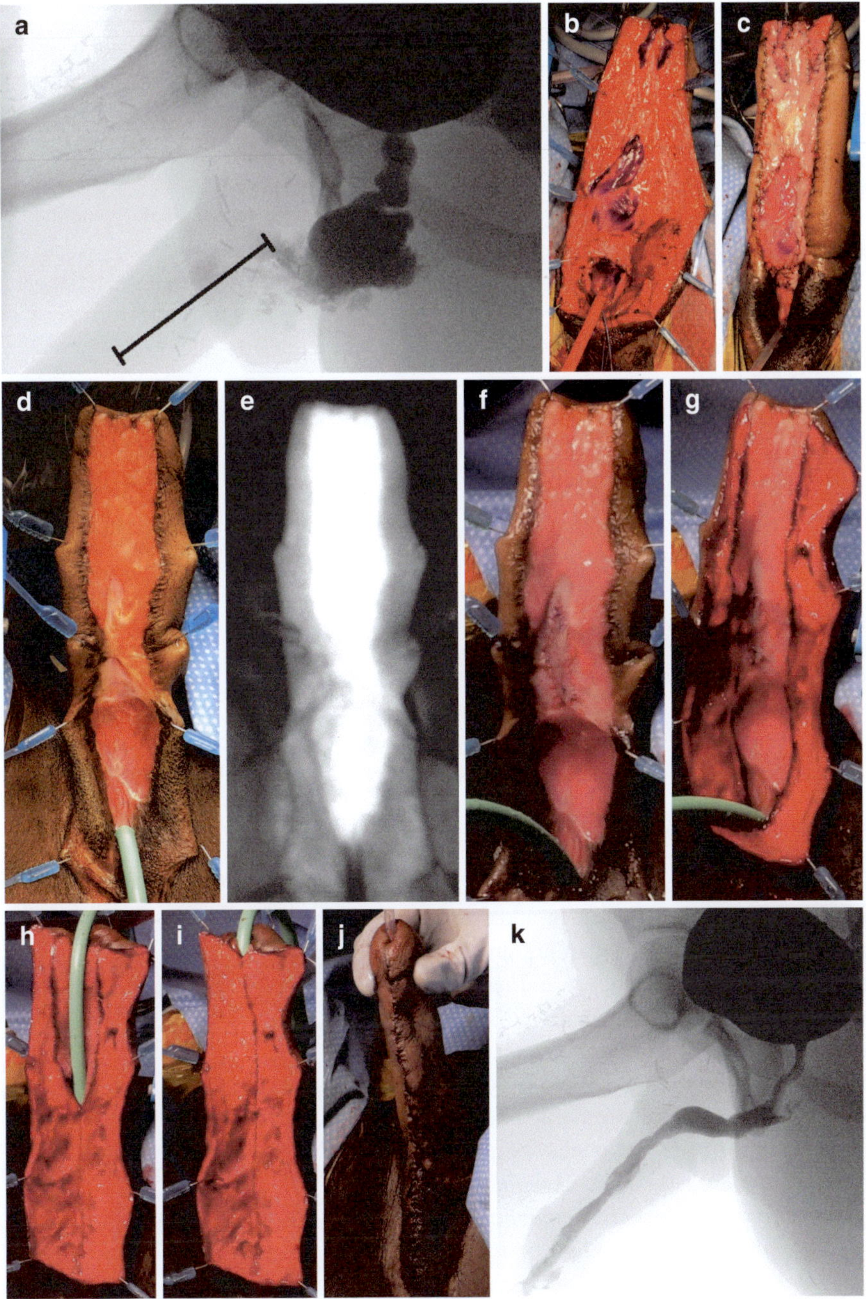

Fig. 11.16 Staged panurethral stricture repair in a patient with a history of prior radial forearm phalloplasty with a prelaminated urethra. (**a**) Preoperative RUG and VCUG showing a completely obliterated neophallic urethra. (**b**) Intraoperative image showing largely absent neourethral plate. (**c**) Fixation of re-harvested buccal mucosal graft in multiple "mosaic" pieces. (**d**) Second stage: intraoperative image of matured neourethral plate at 6 months' follow-up. (**e**) Indocyanine green (ICG) perfusion study showing well-perfused buccal mucosal tissue. (**f**) Placement of additional dorsal buccal mucosal graft inlay within narrowed portion of neo-urethral plate. (**g**) Lateral mobilization of the urethral plate. (**h** and **i**) Tubularization of neourethra over catheter prior to closure. (**j**) Final postoperative image. (**k**) Postoperative VCUG demonstrating a widely patent neophallic urethra

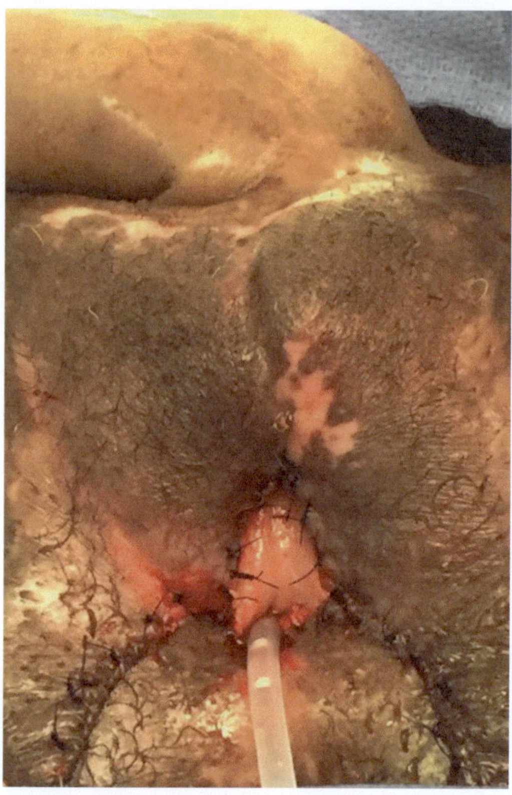

Fig. 11.17 Perineal urethrostomy posterior to the scrotum

metoidioplasty or phalloplasty exist. In addition, there is a lack of understanding regarding urodynamic changes after the initial surgery and reconstructive efforts. Urinary complaints despite successful reconstruction are not uncommon. For example, perceived urinary incontinence (postvoid dribble) may occur after reconstruction due to trapping of urine in the fixed and phallic portions of the urethra [70]. *Given the high likelihood of urinary complaints or recurrent complications, lifelong urologic follow-up is essential for transgender men who have undergone genital reconstructive surgery* [45, 48].

> **Take Home Points**
> 1. Metoidioplasty and phalloplasty are the two options for genital reconstructive surgery.
> 2. Urologic complications of metoidioplasty and phalloplasty include urethro-

cutaneous fistulas, persistent vaginal cavities, and urethral strictures.
3. Unique anatomical considerations and patient preferences dictate surgical planning.
4. Surgical repair of urethrocutaneous fistulas and persistent vaginal cavities may be performed in a single-stage procedure while surgical repair of urethral strictures may require staged procedures.
5. Urologic follow-up is necessary to manage postoperative expectations and any additional or recurrent urologic complications.

References

1. Wernick JA, Busa S, Matouck K, et al. A systematic review of the psychological benefits of gender-affirming surgery. Urol Clin N Am. 2019;46:475–86.
2. Hage JJ, Karim RB. Ought GIDNOS get nought? Treatment options for nontranssexual gender dysphoria. Plast Reconstr Surg. 2000;105(3):1222–7.
3. Giami A, Beaubatie E. Gender identification and sex reassignment surgery in the trans population: a survey study in France. Arch Sex Behav. 2014;43:1491–501.
4. James SE, Herman JL, Rankin S, et al. The report of the 2015 U.S. transgender survey. Washington, DC: National Center for Transgender Equality; 2016.
5. Kailas M, Lu H, Rothman E, et al. Prevalence and types of gender-affirming surgery among a sample of transgender endocrinology patients prior to state expansion of insurance coverage. Endocr Pract. 2017;23(7):780–6.
6. Dy GW, Sun J, Granieri MA, et al. Reconstructive management pearls for the transgender patient. Curr Urol Rep. 2018;19:36.
7. Nolan IT, Dy GW, Levitt N. Considerations in gender-affirming surgery. Urol Clin N Am. 2019;46:459–65.
8. Coleman E, Bockting W, Botzer M, et al. Standards of care for the health of transsexual, transgender, and gender-nonconforming people: version 7. Int J Transgend. 2012;13(4):165–232.
9. Pan S, Honig SC. Gender-affirming surgeferrry: current concepts. Andrology and infertility. Curr Urol Rep. 2018;19:62.
10. Stojanovic B, Bizic M, Bencic M, et al. One-stage gender-confirmation surgery as a viable surgical procedure for female-to-male transsexuals. J Sex Med. 2017;14:741.
11. Garcia MM, Christopher NA, De Luca F, et al. Overall satisfaction, sexual function, and the durability of

neophallus dimensions following staged female to male genital gender confirming surgery: the Institute of Urology, London U.K. experience. Transl Androl Urol. 2014;3:156.

12. World Professional Association for Transgender Health (WPATH). Standards of care for the health of transsexual, transgender, and gender nonconforming people. Version 7. 2011. www.wpath.org/publications/soc. Accessed 5 Dec 2019.

13. Hage JJ, Bout CA, Bloem JJ, et al. Phalloplasty in female-to-male transsexuals: what do our patients ask for? Ann Plast Surg. 1993;30(4):323–6.

14. Hage JJ, Bloem JJ. Review of the literature on construction of a neourethra in female-to-male transsexuals. Ann Plast Surg. 1993;30(3):278–86.

15. Dubin BJ, Sato RM, Laub DR. Results of phalloplasty. Plast Reconstr Surg. 1979;64(2):163–70.

16. Puckett CL, Montie JE. Construction of male genitalia in the transsexual, using a tubed groin flap for the penis and a hydraulic inflation device. Plast Reconstr Surg. 1978;61(4):523–30.

17. Morrison SD, Chen ML, Crane CN. An overview of female-to-male gender-confirming surgery. Nat Rev Urol. 2017;14(8):486–500.

18. Ferrando C, Zhao LC, Nikolavsky D. Transgender surgery: female to male. In: Eckler K, editor. UpToDate. Waltham, MA: UpToDate; 2019. www.uptodate.com. Accessed February 9, 2019.

19. Massie JP, Morrison SD, Wilson SC, et al. Phalloplasty with urethral lengthening: addition of a vascularized bulbospongiosus flap from vaginectomy reduces postoperative urethral complications. Plast Reconstr Surg. 2017;140(4):551.

20. Durfee R, Rowland W. Penile substitution with clitoral enlargement and urethral transfer. In: Laub DR, Gandy P, editors. Proceedings of the second interdisciplinary symposium on gender dysphoria syndrome. Standford: Stanford University Press; 1973.

21. Perovic SV, Djordjevic ML. Metoidioplasty: a variant of phalloplasty in female transsexuals. BJU Int. 2003;92(9):981–5.

22. Frey JD, Poudrier G, Chiodo MV, Hazen A. A systematic review of metoidioplasty and radial forearm flap Phalloplasty in female-to-male transgender genital reconstruction: is the "ideal" neophallus an achievable goal? Plast Reconstr Surg Glob Open. 2016;4:1131.

23. Cohanzad S. Extensive metoidioplasty as a technique capable of creating a compatible analogue to a natural penis in female transsexuals. Aesthet Plast Surg. 2016;40:130.

24. Nikolavsky D, Yamaguchi Y, Levine JP, et al. Urologic sequelae following phalloplasty in transgendered patients. Urol Clin N Am. 2017;44:113–25.

25. Giles H. Congenital absence of the penis. Br J Plast Surg. 1948;1:8.

26. Gilbert DA, Horton CE, Terzis JK, et al. New concepts in phallic reconstruction. Ann Plast Surg. 1987;18:128–36.

27. van der Sluis WB, Smit JM, Pigot GLS, et al. Double flap phalloplasty in transgender men: surgical technique and outcome of pedicled anteriolateral thigh flap phalloplasty combined with radial forearm free flap urethral reconstruction. Microsurgery. 2017;37:917–23.

28. Namba Y, Watanabe T, Kimata Y. Flap combination phalloplasty in female-to-male transsexuals. J Sex Med. 2019;16:934–41.

29. Chang TS, Hwang WY. Forearm flap in one-stage reconstruction of the penis. Plast Reconstr Surg. 1984;74:251–8.

30. Song R, Gao Y, Song Y, Yu Y, Song Y. The forearm flap. Cin Plast Surg. 1982;9:21–6.

31. Monstrey S, Hoebeke P, Selvaggi G, et al. Penile reconstruction: is the forearm flap really the standard technique? Plast Reconstr Surg. 2009;124:510–8.

32. Garaffa G, Ralph DJ, Christoper N. Total urethral construction with the radial artery-based forearm free flap in the transsexual. BJU Int. 2010;106:1206–10.

33. Lumen N, Monstrey S, Goessaert AS, et al. Urethroplasty for strictures after phallic reconstruction: a single-institution experience. Eur Urol. 2011;60(1):150–8.

34. Rashid M, Tamimy MS. Phalloplasty: the dream and the reality. Indian J Plast Surg. 2013;46(2):283–93.

35. Al-Tamimi M, Pigot GL, van der Sluis WB, et al. The surgical techniques and outcomes of secondary phalloplasty after metoidioplasty in transgender men: an international, multi-center case series. J Sex Med. 2019;16:1–11.

36. Schechter LS, Safa B. Introduction to Phalloplasty. Clin Plast Surg. 2018;45:387.

37. Neuville P, Morel-Journel N, Maucourt-Boulch D, et al. Surgical outcomes of erectile implants after phalloplasty: retrospective analysis of 95 procedures. J Sex Med. 2016;13:1758–64.

38. Remington AC, Morrison SD, Massie JP, et al. Outcomes after phalloplasty: do transgender patients and multiple urethral procedures carry a higher rate of complication? Plast Reconstr Surg. 2018;141:220.

39. Ascha M, et al. Outcomes of single stage phalloplasty by pedicled anterolateral thigh flap versus radial forearm free flap in gender confirming surgery. J Urol. 2018;199(1):206–13.

40. Blaschke E, et al. Postoperative imaging of phalloplasties and their complications. Am J Roentgenol. 2014;203:323–8.

41. Kim SK, Moon JB, Heo J, Kwon YS, Lee KC. A new method of urethroplasty for prevention of fistula in female-to-male gender reassignment surgery. Ann Plast Surg. 2010;64(6):759–64.

42. Leriche A, Timsit MO, Morel-Journel N, Bouillot A, Dembele D, Ruffion A. Long-term outcome of forearm flee-flap phalloplasty in the treatment of transsexualism. BJU Int. 2008;101(10):1297–300.

43. Rashid M, Sarwar SR. Avulsion injuries of the male external genitalia: classification and reconstruction with the customised radial forearm free flap. Br J Plast Surg. 2005;58(5):585–92.

44. Rohrmann D, Jakse G. Urethroplasty in female-to-male transsexuals. Eur Urol. 2003;44(5):611–4.

45. Schardein JN, Zhao LC, Nikolavsky D. Management of vaginoplasty and phalloplasty complications. Urol Clin N Am. 2019;46:605–18.

46. Fang RH, Kao YS, Ma S, Lin JT. Phalloplasty in female-to-male transsexuals using free radial osteocutaneous flap: a series of 22 cases. Br J Plast Surg. 1999;52(3):217–22.

47. Levine LA, Elterman L. Urethroplasty following total phallic reconstruction. J Urol. 1998;160(2):378–82.

48. Monstrey SJ, Ceulemans P, Hoebeke P. Sex reassignment surgery in the female-to-male transsexual. Semin Plast Surg. 2011;25(3):229–44.

49. Stowell JT, Grimstad FW, Kirkpatrick DL, et al. Imaging Findings in Transgender Patients after Gender-affirming surgery. Radiographics. 2019;39(5):1368–92.

50. Santucci RA. Urethral complications after transgender phalloplasty: strategies to treat them and minimize their occurrence. Clin Anat. 2018;31(2):187–90.

51. Groenman F, et al. Robot-assisted laparoscopic colpectomy in female-to-male transgender patients; technique and outcomes of a prospective cohort study. Surg Endosc. 2017;31(8):3363–9.

52. Lumen N, Oosterlinck W, Decaestecker K, et al. Endoscopic incision of short (<3 cm) urethral strictures after phallic reconstruction. J Endourol. 2009;23(8):1329–32.

53. Daneshvar M, Hughes M, Nikolavsky D. Surgical management of fossa navicularis and distal urethral strictures. Curr Urol Rep. 2018;19(6):43.

54. Coney BC. A penile flap procedure for the relief of meatal stricture. Br J Urol. 1963;35:182–3.

55. Blandy JP, Tresidder GC. Meatoplasty. Br J Urol. 1967;39(5):633–4.

56. Jordan GH. Reconstruction of the fossa navicularis. J Urol. 1987;138(1):102–4.

57. De Sy WA, Oosterlinck W, Verbaeys A. European experience with 1-stage urethroplasty with free full thickness skin graft. J Urol. 1981;125(4):502–3.

58. Gelman J, Sohn W. 1-stage repair of obliterative distal urethral strictures with buccal graft urethral plate reconstruction and simultaneous onlay penile skin flap. J Urol. 2011;186(3):935–8.

59. Asopa HS, Garg M, Singhal GG, et al. Dorsal free graft urethroplasty for urethral stricture by ventral sagittal urethrotomy approach. Urology. 2001;58(5):657–9.

60. Chowdhury PS, Nayak P, Mallick S, et al. A single stage ventral onlay buccal mucosal graft urethroplasty for navicular fossa strictures. Indian J Urol. 2014;30(1):17–22.

61. Goel A, Goel A, Dalela D, Sankhwar SN. Meatoplasty using double buccal mucosal graft technique. Int Utol Nephrol. 2009;41(4):885–7.

62. Nikolavsky D, Abouelleil M, Daneshvar M. Transurethral ventral buccal mucosa graft inlay urethroplasty for reconstruction of fossa navicularis and distal urethral strictures: surgical technique and preliminary results. In Urol Nephrol. 2016;48(11):1823–9.

63. Zhang Y, Liu C, Qu C, et al. Is vaginal mucosa graft the excellent substitute material for urethral reconstruction in female-to-male transsexuals? World J Urol. 2015;33:2115–23.

64. Mundy AR, Andrich DE. Entero-urethroplasty for the salvage of bulb-membranous stricture disease or trauma. BJU Int. 2010;105:1716–20.

65. Xu YM, Qiao Y, Sa YL, et al. Urethral reconstruction using colonic mucosa graft for complex strictures. J Urol. 2009;182:1040–3.

66. Vanni AJ. New frontiers in urethral reconstruction: injectables and alternative grafts. Trawl Androl Urol. 2015;4(1):84–91.

67. Pariser JJ, et al. Buccal mucosal graft urethroplasty for the treatment of urethral stricture in the neophallus. Urology. 2015;85(4):927–31.

68. Palminteri E, Manzoni G, Berdondini E, et al. Combined dorsal plus ventral double buccal mucosa graft in bulbar urethral reconstruction. Eur Urol. 2008;53(1):81–90.

69. Wilson, et al. Fasciocutaneous flap reinforcement of ventral onlay buccal mucosa grafts enables neophallus revision urethroplasty. Ther Adv Urol. 2016;8(6):331–7.

70. Hoebeke P, Selvaggi G, Ceulemans P, et al. Impact of sex reassignment surgery on lower urinary tract function. Eur Urol. 2005;47(3):398–402.

Geolani W. Dy, Ian T. Nolan, Nabeel A. Shakir, and Lee C. Zhao

Introduction

Indications for Phalloplasty

Phalloplasty is one option for genital-related gender-affirming surgery (GAS) in transgender men. For the purpose of this chapter, the term "transgender man" will encompass all patients assigned female at birth who identify as a gender other than female. Many transgender patients may seek GAS in order to relieve gender dysphoria or to better align their body with their gender identity. Transgender and gender nonbinary patients are a growing demographic, estimated to comprise up to 0.6% of the US population [1]. While relatively few transgender men (about 3%) have had any type of genital GAS [2], rates are increasing. Gender dysphoria is emerging as one of the most common indications for phalloplasty, alongside other indications such as exstrophy-epispadias complex, differences of sexual development, micropenis, traumatic penile amputation, and post-penectomy reconstruction [3–10].

Considerations in Neophallus Creation

Several studies have elucidated transgender men's goals while considering phalloplasty and suggest that erectile function is important to many. In a Dutch questionnaire, 86% of patients desired a neophallus with erectile function [11]. Another questionnaire from Sweden reported a slightly lower but still sizable proportion (49%) seeking erectile capacity [12]. Other historic goals of phalloplasty include a single-stage, reproducible procedure; ability for standing micturition with urinary continence; tactile (protective) and erogenous sensation; sufficient girth to accommodate a prosthesis; and aesthetic acceptability [13].

Overview of Phalloplasty Technique
(Table 12.1)

A number of flaps are available for neophallus creation. The flaps used for transgender men are similar to those used for cisgender men who undergo phalloplasty for other indications [5, 6, 8–10, 14]. Each approach has benefits and

G. W. Dy · L. C. Zhao (✉)
Department of Urology, New York University, New York, NY, USA
e-mail: Geolani.dy@nyumc.org; lee.zhao@nyumc.org

I. T. Nolan
New York University School of Medicine, New York, NY, USA
e-mail: Ian.nolan@nyulangone.org

N. A. Shakir
Department of Urology, University of Texas Southwestern Medical Center, Dallas, TX, USA
e-mail: Nabeel.shakir@phhs.org

© Springer Nature Switzerland AG 2021
D. Nikolavsky, S. A. Blakely (eds.), *Urological Care for the Transgender Patient*,
https://doi.org/10.1007/978-3-030-18533-6_12

Table 12.1 Prosthesis placement techniques and perioperative care in large series of neophallus prostheses

Study	Study type	No. pts	Phalloplasty technique	Population	Prosthesis type	Preoperative antibiotics	Prosthesis placement delay	Dissection technique	Fixation technique	Protective sheath	Postoperative care
Hoebeke [45]	Retrospective review	35	RFFF	Trans	AMS one-piece Dynaflex [10];AMS three-piece hydraulic CX or CXM [25]	Pre: cefazolin 2 × 2 gm; post: ciprofloxacin 500 mg/d × 5d	>12 months	Blunt dissection with Hegar dilators to 0.5 cm below tip of phallus. Choice of single or double implant based on ease of dilation	Two polyester fiber 1 sutures from pubic periosteum to proximal end of polyester sock, around smallest part of prosthesis	Polyester vascular prosthesis in all but three-piece implants	Erection maintained 4 days. Bed rest 4 days
Leriche [30]	Retrospective review	38[a]	RFFF	Trans	Special prototype (no longer available) or Ambicor, AMS 600 and AMS 700S	n/a	3–9 months	Basal lateral incision of phalloplasty	n/a	n/a	n/a
Hoebeke [51]	Case review	129	RFFF	Trans	AMS CX or CXM [50];Ambicor [47];AMS CX InhibiZone [17]; Dynaflex single-cylinder inflatable [9];Coloplast/ Mentor [6].	Cefazolin 3 x1g	23 months (9–127 months)	Blunt dissection with Hegar dilators to 0.5 cm below tip of phallus. Choice of single or double implant based on ease of dilation	Base of cylinder, covered by a rear tip extender, is fixed to pubic bone via nonresorbable suture	Dacron vascular prosthesis used until February 2006	n/a
Zuckerman [49]	Retrospective review	31	RFFF [30]; pedicled groin flap [1]	Trans [15]; trauma [7]; DSD or micropenis [7]; cancer [2]	Duraphase malleable [21];AMS CX/ CXR or Coloplast Titan [10]	Vancomycin; gentamycin	56.3 months	Bilateral incisions at ischial tuberosities. Blunt dissection with Hegar dilators, leaving tissue below tip of phallus	Anchored to inferior pubic rami	Gore-Tex	n/a

Neuville [46]	Retrospective review	69	40 RFFF [40]; suprapubic [23]; other/ unknown [6]	Trans [63]; malformation [4]; trauma [3]	AMS Ambicor two-piece (71);Ambicor with vascular graft [19];AMS CXR, CX, 600–650 [5]	Cefazolin 2 g	19 months (8–84)	Lateral incision to neoscrotum. Blunt dissection with Hegar dilators. Choice of single or double implant based on ease of dilation	Polyester graft slit at base of pipe and sutured to pubis	Vascular graft prosthesis occasionally used. Polyester (Hemashield Gold)	n/a
Cohen [47]	Retrospective review	10	RFFF	Trans	AMS 700 LGX [5]; AMS 700 CX [5]	n/a	Median 206 days, at least 6 months	Infrapubic incision. Dissection to pubic symphysis with electrocautery. Corticotomy created in pubic symphysis via Stryker TPS bone drill	Anchoring sutures connect corticotomy defect to rear tip and proximal cylinder of implant	Gore-Tex	n/a
Falcone (2018)	Retrospective review	247	RFFF (157); infraumbilical (90)	Trans	AMS 700 CX, CXM/R, or AMS Ambicor	Gentamicin 80 mg; amoxicillin/ clavulanic acid 2 g/200 mg	12–37 months	2-stages: (1) reservoir insertion at time of glans sculpture and testicular prosthesis; (2) groin incision ipsilateral to reservoir, dilation to 18 Hegar	Sock at rear anchored to pubic symphysis and at tip via Ethibond suture	Polyethylene terephthalate sock	Cylinders left semi-inflated for 1 week

[a]38 of 56 total patients received a penile prosthesis

drawbacks regarding donor site morbidity, potential for long-term urologic complications following urethral construction, sensory capacity, and the need for erectile prostheses [14, 15]. Most common are the radial forearm free flap (RFFF) [6, 16, 17] and pedicled locoregional flap from the anterolateral thigh (ALT) [18–20], although inferiorly based abdominal flaps [21], the latissimus dorsi, and fibular flaps [15] have been reported as well. We will describe basic principles of RFFF and ALT techniques below.

Of all phalloplasty techniques, the RFFF has the most extensive literature base [3, 14, 16, 17, 22]. In RFFF phalloplasty, donor site dissection preserves the circulating radial artery and vein as well as local nerves. Common recipient structures include arteries, common femoral, lateral, circumflex femoral, circumflex iliac, or inferior epigastric artery and venae comitantes; veins, deep inferior epigastric or greater saphenous veins; and nerves, ilioinguinal and branches of the internal pudendal nerves (the dorsal penile nerves in cisgender men or clitoral nerves in transgender men).

The flap is tubularized and the urethral tube constructed (so-called tube within a tube). The donor flap is then delivered to the pubic region, and its pedicle and nerves are anastomosed to the corresponding recipient vessels. The recipient site is typically prepared concurrently or at a separate stage with vaginectomy and scrotoplasty, as well as mobilization and lengthening of the native urethra for anastomosis. Urethral anastomosis to the recipient site may be performed in a single stage or at a later time.

Benefits of RFFF include capacity for standing micturition, tactile and erogenous sensation, and potential for erectile prosthesis placement [3]. Rates of flap loss are generally low. The primary drawback is donor site morbidity, often requiring a skin graft and resulting in highly visible scarring, with conflicting reports regarding risk of functional loss [17, 23–25]. Urethral complications such as stricture and fistulae are common, with rates ranging from 25% to 75% [14, 17, 26–30].

The ALT rotational pedicled flap is a popular alternative to RFFF. This flap is dissected, tubularized, and passed beneath an inguinal tunnel [18]. Benefits of ALT relative to RFFF include a discreet donor site without the need for microvascular anastomosis and capacity to use the femoral cutaneous nerves for reinnervation. However, the greater thickness of thigh skin and subcutaneous fat often lead to excess girth. Excess flap girth can make neourethral tubularization more technically challenging and can also impair perceived rigidity after penile prosthesis placement.

Alternatives to Prostheses

Erectile prosthesis placement is the most common technique currently used to afford neophallic rigidity and is the main focus of this chapter. However, other options such as autologous grafts (cartilage or the bone) or implantable splints may also afford some erectile rigidity [31].

Cartilage grafts were first described in 1936 by Borgoras [32] but are not commonly used. Osteocutaneous grafts in RFFF have been reported since 1988 [33]. They are most commonly taken from either the fibula or radius. If taken from the radius, they are incorporated into the RFFF with fixation of the bone segment to the pubic symphysis using permanent suture [34]. However, after the first year postoperatively, neophallus rigidity and skin elasticity decline due to the thin, unicortical nature of the radius [34–36]. The fibula is another potential donor site with greater durability. In this approach, the fibula is fixed to the periosteum of the pubic symphysis with nonabsorbable nylon suture to allow for an oscillating motion in all directions during intercourse [36, 37].

A more recent development is the external prosthetic penis, or penile epithesis, described by Selvaggi [38, 39]. The epithesis is installed in a staged approach: first, osteointegrated titanium implants are drilled into the pubic bone, and then, epithesis is placed 6 months later.

Penile Prosthesis

Penile prosthesis placement is now the most widely utilized approach for achieving erectile neophallus rigidity. The penile prosthesis was introduced for cisgender men in 1973 before adaptation for use in transgender individuals in 1977 [40, 41]. Several challenges exist in the placement of erectile prostheses, which largely stem from the use of implants designed for cisgender penile anatomy in the neophallus.

Prosthesis Types

Two main categories of implantable erectile devices are in current use: semirigid (malleable) and inflatable prostheses. Inflatable prostheses are more widely used, as they allow for a depressurized, deflated state that improves concealability and may decrease the risk of extrusion from chronic pressure [41–44]. Multicomponent prostheses (AMS 700 from Ambicor, American Medical Systems, Minnetonka, MN, USA, and Coloplast/Mentor Mentor Corporation, Santa Barbara, CA, USA) have been increasingly common since single-component Dynaflex (American Medical Systems, Minnetonka, MN, USA) was removed from the market in 1997 [45].

However, multicomponent inflatable prostheses are subject to mechanical failure. There is limited data regarding longevity of inflatable penile prostheses in the phalloplasty population, with one study of 247 patients reporting an implant 5-year survival rate of 78% and another study of 95 patients reporting median implant life expectancy of 4.2 years, with no reported difference between AMS Ambicor or AMS CXR prostheses [22, 46]. As transgender men tend to undergo erectile prosthesis placement at younger ages (mean age 23.6–41.7 years) compared with cisgender men with erectile dysfunction, they may require more revisions throughout their lifetime [44, 46–49].

Semirigid prostheses are less common. However, they do carry the advantage of fewer components, as they require no scrotal pump or reservoir, which may make them more appropriate in patients with limited scrotal space or prior abdominal surgery. Comparative studies are sparse, although a single study of 31 erectile prostheses patients demonstrated a trend for higher overall complications with the malleable devices (28% vs 10%, inflatable devices), although the study was not powered to reach statistical significance [49].

Surgical Technique

Surgical Preparation and Approach

In order to decrease the risk of pressure necrosis, a phallus should ideally be sensate prior to implant placement. Most modern series describe waiting 6–9 months between creation of the neophallus and implant placement in order to allow time for nerve coaptation and return of protective sensation [22, 30, 42, 45, 47–51].

Preoperative considerations include antibiotic prophylaxis and urinary drainage. Preoperative antibiotic prophylaxis has been reported by several studies. The exact regimen is institution dependent and often includes cephalosporins and aminoglycosides prior to incision, although there is no specific dosing protocol that has clearly demonstrated superiority. Preoperative urinary drainage by having the patient void or via small urethral catheter placement is generally recommended, to limit risks of urethral or bladder injury. Standard surgical field prep and sterilization are routine.

Erectile prostheses may be placed via a number of approaches, including infrapubic (penopubic), penoscrotal, parascrotal, and perineal approaches. The authors prefer a parascrotal approach (Fig. 12.1). Avoidance of the neourethra and neurovascular supply of the flap is critical and requires careful consideration of the initial approach used for neophallus creation [45]. Intraoperative Doppler ultrasound has been used to localize and avoid the phallus' vascular supply [44]. Dissection to the pubic symphysis for prosthesis anchoring must be carried out carefully. Hegar or Brooks dilators may be used to develop infrapubic or distal subcutaneous spaces.

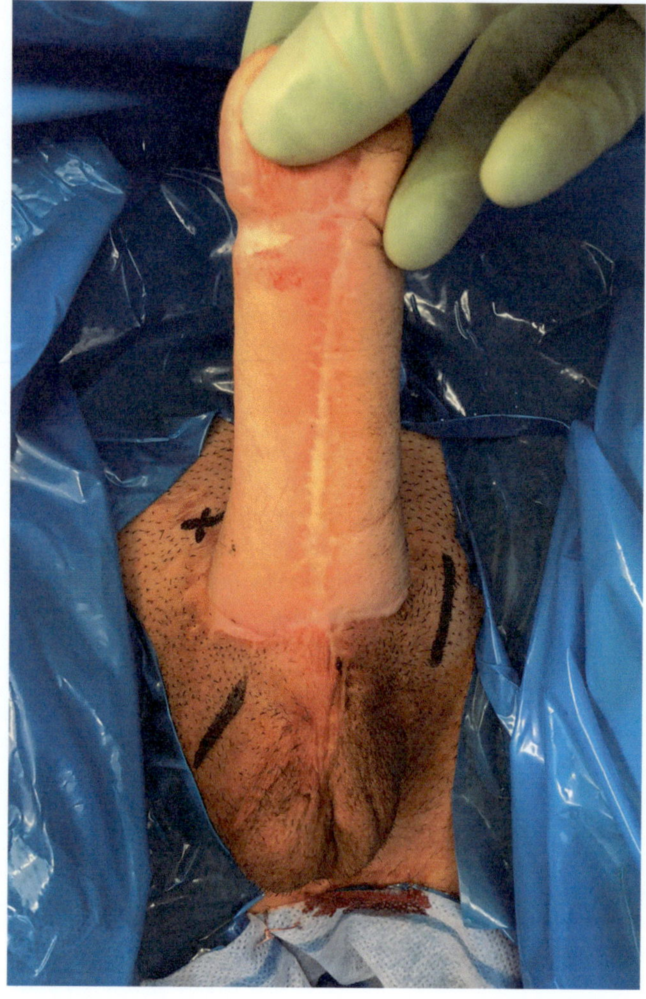

Fig. 12.1 Preoperative markings for erectile device and testicular prosthesis placement. The erectile device is placed through an incision contralateral to the vascular pedicle and the testicular device through a scrotal incision opposite the inflatable erectile device pump

Distal dilation of the neophallus should also be undertaken carefully to avoid compromising distal prosthesis cushioning. After dissection and prior to prosthesis placement, intraoperative measurements should be taken to determine the optimal size of erectile implant to be placed.

Single vs Dual Cylinders

Choice of single- or dual-cylinder implants is highly patient-specific and typically depends on factors such as girth of neophallus and difficulty of dilation [44, 47, 51]. Hoebeke et al. conclude that single-cylinder devices may be aesthetically superior to dual-cylinder devices [45]. Insufficient distal cushioning may lead to a poor cosmetic result if dual cylinders are placed (Fig. 12.2).

Vascular Grafts for Neotunical Reconstruction and Proximal Anchoring

Many institutions have described the use of neo-tunical sheaths or "socks" (Gore-Tex or Dacron vascular grafts) to provide distal cushioning and scaffolding for proximal attachment in the absence of distal corporal bodies [44–46, 48–51].

Transgender individuals with neophallus, unlike cisgender men who have had phallic recon-

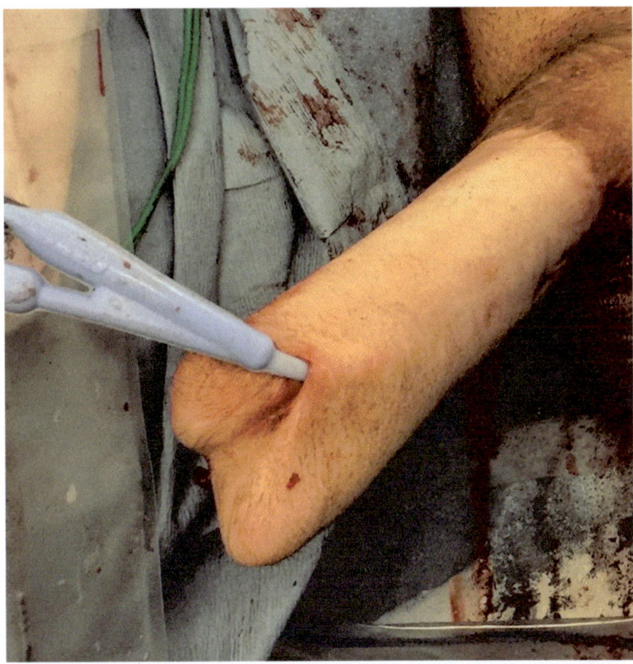

Fig. 12.2 Dual cylinders with poor aesthetic result due to lack of distal cushioning

struction after penectomy, do not have the residual proximal corporal tissue that is typically used to anchor erectile prostheses [3, 9, 44, 46]. In cisgender men, the proximal aspect of the cylinder is inserted into the dilated crura of the corpora, and the cuff of the PTFE sheath may then be sutured to the residual tunica albuginea. In transgender patients or cisgender patients without proximal corpora remnants, the proximal PTFE sheath is instead closed along the length of the implant cylinder, leaving an open slit as an exit site for tubing if an inflatable prosthesis is used.

If native corpora are not present, as in transgender male patients, then bone anchoring must be used to achieve proximal fixation of the prosthetic cylinders. Anchor sites include the pubic symphysis or less commonly the ischial tuberosity [49]. In either case, the implant is secured to the bone via proximal Gore-Tex or Dacron grafts or via rear tip extenders fixed to the inferior aspect of the pubic symphyseal periosteum via nonresorbable sutures [22].

Alternatively, the proximal portion of the implant may be directly inserted into the pubic ramus [47, 52]. In this anchoring technique, a 1cm^2 corticotomy is created in the inferior aspect of the pubic ramus using an electric drill. A bone anchor is drilled and impacted on either side of the corticotomy. The bone anchor is preloaded with permanent double-armed suture, which is then guided through the rear tip extender, seating the proximal aspect of the device into the corticotomy.

The authors prefer a proximal anchoring approach which includes insertion of Smith & Nephew TwinFix bone anchors directly into the pubic ramus, securing the preloaded permanent suture into the rear tip extender of the prosthesis (Fig. 12.3). The potential advantage of this approach is the ease of bone anchor explantation, given the known high rates of revision prosthesis in the neophallus population.

For distal fixation, the Furlow tool and Keith needle are used to seat the cylinders, with care to avoid the urethra in those who have undergone urethral lengthening. The authors prefer use of an acellular matrix "cap" sewn onto the distal tip of the prosthesis with permanent suture, to provide additional cushioning and to augment distal fixation through scarring (Fig. 12.4).

For multicomponent prostheses, the reservoir is placed in the space of Retzius or a subrectus

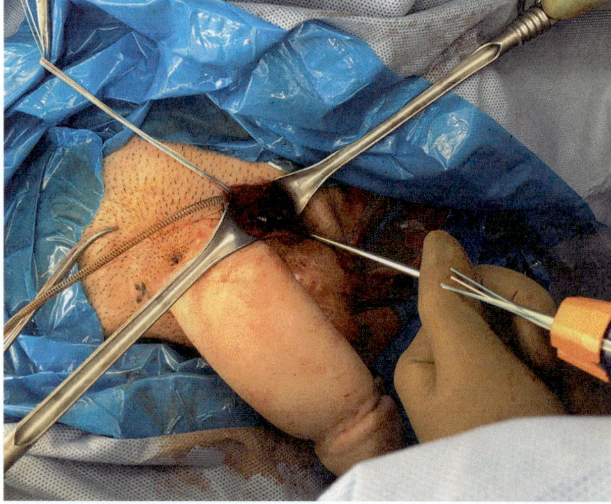

Fig. 12.3 Bone anchors are inserted into the pubic ramus

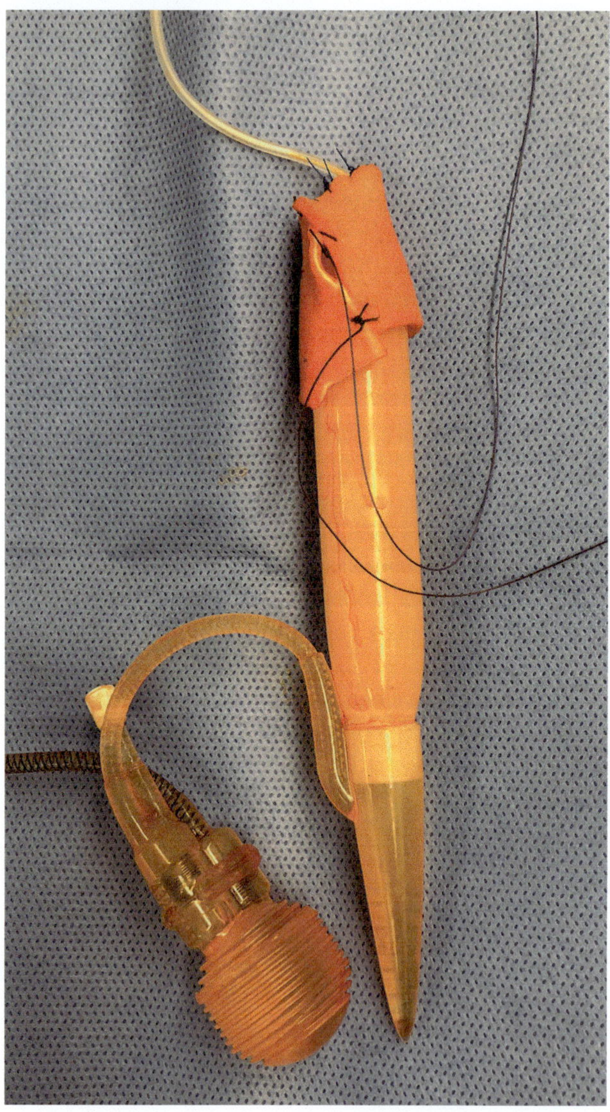

Fig. 12.4 Adapted inflatable erectile implant with single cylinder and acellular matrix cap secured to distal tip

Fig. 12.5 Inflated prosthesis 6 weeks after implantation

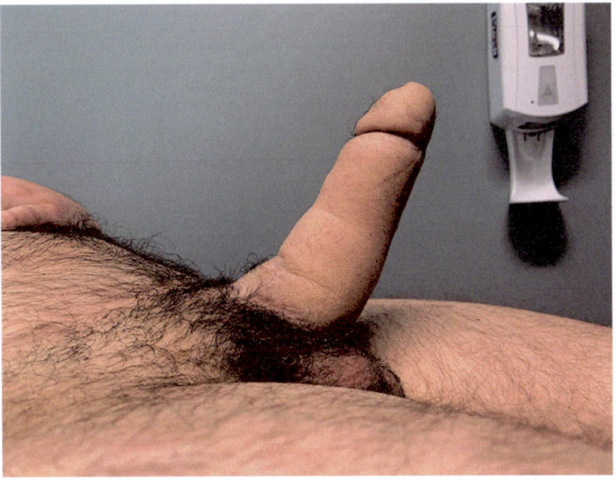

pouch. The pump is placed in the neoscrotum and the incisions closed in multiple layers.

Postoperative Care

Postoperative care is highly institution dependent; however, some trends emerge in the literature. Patients are typically admitted for postoperative observation, with mean lengths of stay reported between 1.3 and 3.7 days in recent series [46, 47], though the authors tend to discharge patients home postoperatively after uncomplicated procedures. Any closed-suction drain systems and urinary catheters are typically removed prior to discharge [9]. If urinary drainage is required long term, suprapubic tube placement may be the best option for infection control. Implanted devices are often left partially inflated for 7–10 days [3, 9] with initial cycling of the prosthesis at 6 weeks (Fig. 12.5) [46].

Complications (Table 12.2)

Rates of complication and revision following erectile prosthesis placement in phalloplasty range from 20% to 80% [22, 30, 48, 49, 51, 53, 54]. Potential complications include infection, extrusion or erosion, injury to the neurovascular supply of the neophallus, device migration, inadequate rigidity, poor aesthetic result, pain, and device failure. Typically, these complications are managed by implant revision or removal and replacement. Complications such as infection and erosion are more prevalent in transgender men, likely due to absence of protective corporal tissue in the neophallus and the preexisting surgical burden on the site of implantation from neophallus creation. However, long-term survival of implants is relatively good. One study reported that in patients whose devices remained intact through the early postoperative period, the majority retained their original prostheses at nearly 5 years [49].

Infection

Prosthesis infection risk is considerably higher in neophallus than in cisgender men with impotence (approximately 10% vs 1.1%, respectively) [55]. Several factors may contribute to the elevated infection rates: lack of corporal bodies and minimal barrier from the urethra and skin and limited vascular supply in the setting of a flap-based phallus, thereby leading to poorer wound healing. The most recent and largest study of 247 transgender men after RFFF and IPP reported an infection rate of 8.5%, which was not clearly associated with any predictive factors including number of cylinders or protective measures such as silver Dacron sleeve or InhibiZone [22]. Another relatively large study of 129 patients reported an 11.9% infection rate, which also was not associated with type of prosthesis or number or size of cylinders [51]. Other recent series including transgender and cisgen-

Table 12.2 Postoperative outcomes in large series of neophallus prosthesis

Study	No. pts	Phalloplasty technique	Population	Mean F/u (range)	Mean age, yr (range)	Prosthesis type	Surgical outcomes[a]	Sexual outcomes[a]	QoL and satisfaction outcomes	Complications
Hoebeke [45]	35	RFFF	Trans	2.3 years	n/a	AMS one-piece Dynaflex [10]; AMS three-piece hydraulic CX or CXM [25]	Uneventful prosthesis placement (80%). Original prosthesis at follow-up (92%)	Sexually active (90.6% of 32)	"91.5% success rate"	Overall (20%): infection and partial necrosis (3%); infection (9%); perforation (3%); technical failure (9%)
Leriche [30]	38[b]	RFFF	Trans	110 months[c]	30 (20–44)[c]	Special prototype (no longer available) or Ambicor, AMS 600 and AMS 700S	Functional prosthesis (51%)	Satisfied with penetrative sexual intercourse (51%)	n/a	Replacement due to infection or mechanical failure (29%); explantation (8%)
Hoebeke [51]	129	RFFF	Trans	30.2 months (0–132)	31.9 (15–52)	AMS CX or CXM [50]; Ambicor [47]; AMS CX InhibiZone [17]; Dynaflex single-cylinder inflatable [9];Coloplast/ Mentor [6]	Original implant in place (58.9%)	n/a	n/a	Replacement (32%). Explantation or revision (41%). Malposition (15%); dysfunction (13%); infection (12%); prosthesis leak (9%); protrusion (8%). Dysfunction highest in Dynaflex group (53.3%, other implants <25%).
Zuckerman [49]	31	RFFF [30], pedicled groin flap [1]	Trans [15]; trauma [7]; DSD or micropenis [7]; cancer [2]	59.7 months	35.6	Duraphase malleable [21]; AMS CX/CXR or Coloplast Titan [10]	Five-year survival rate 65%–70%	Sexually active (81%)		Explantation (19%). Intraoperative (6%): bladder injury (3%); flap arterial injury (3%). Postoperative (23%): infection (10%); erosion (6%); mobility (3%); malleable fracture (3%). Trend toward higher rate of complications with malleable device (28% vs 10%, $p = 0.10$)

Neuville [46]	69	40 RFFF [40]; 23 suprapubic [23]; other/ unknown [6]	Trans [63]; malformation [4]; trauma [3]	4 years (0.5–6.1)	40.3	AMS Ambicor two-piece (71);Ambicor with vascular graft [19]; AMS CXR, CX, 600–650 [5]	Original prosthesis in place (62.3%). Mean life expectancy 4.2 years	n/a	n/a	Replacement (37%). Explantation (7%). Early (6.3%): infection (4.3%). Late (31.6%): malpositioning (12.6%); dysfunction (10.5%); erosion (4.2%); infection (4.2%).No difference in malpositioning and dysfunction with or without vascular graft
Cohen [47]	10	RFFF	Trans	49 months	41.7	AMS 700 LGX [5]; AMS 700 CX [5]	Functional prosthesis (81%)	n/a	n/a	Perioperative complications (20%). Reoperation (70%): infection (50%); migration (30%); mechanical failure (20%)
Falcone (2018)	247	RFFF (157); infraumbilical (90)	Trans	20 months	38 (21–69)	AMS 700 CX, CXM/R, or AMS Ambicor	Five-year survival rate 78%, no device superior. Original prosthesis in place (56.6%). Satisfactory sensation (83%); ability to cycle device (100%)	Using for penetration (77%). Achieving orgasm (61%)	Overall satisfaction (88%); dissatisfaction (19%); partner dissatisfaction (60%)	Revision (43%). Infection (8.5%). Mechanical failure (15.4%), due to cylinder rupture (11%); cylinder aneurysm (3%); connecting tube rupture (2%). Revision higher in suprapubic than RFFF (HR 0.74, $p = 0.013$)

[a]At latest follow-up
[b]38 of 56 total patients received a penile prosthesis
[c]Data only reported for 56 total patients, of whom only 38 received penile prosthesis

der male patients with neophallus report infection rates from 8.4% in a series of 95 procedures [46] to 50% in a cohort of ten patients who underwent bone anchoring with corticotomy [47]. Of note, infections were largely attributable to the implant and not to corticotomy-induced osteomyelitis [47].

Infection is typically managed with immediate explantation and washout of the wound with delayed reimplantation. Some may choose to perform immediate reimplantation based on the clinical severity of the infection.

Extrusion and Erosion

Extrusion of an implant may occur at various sites, including cylinder erosion through the glans or neourethra and scrotal pump erosion through the neoscrotum (Fig. 12.6). These are indications for immediate explantation. Rates are higher in patients without corpora (typically 4–8% and as high as 33%) [44, 46, 51] than in cisgender men (1.3%) [56].

Migration

Migration of erectile prostheses is another concern that may lead to revision surgery to the device or anchoring mechanism or device replacement. Rates range from 3.2% in one study of 31 cisgender and transgender men who underwent proximal fixation at the inferior pubic rami [49] to 14.6% in one study of transgender patients with RFFF and suture fixation to the pubic bone [51].

Vascular grafts around the prosthesis may be protective against migration through adherence to adjacent flap tissue. Consequently, removal of devices with vascular grafts may be especially challenging due to the same principle of graft

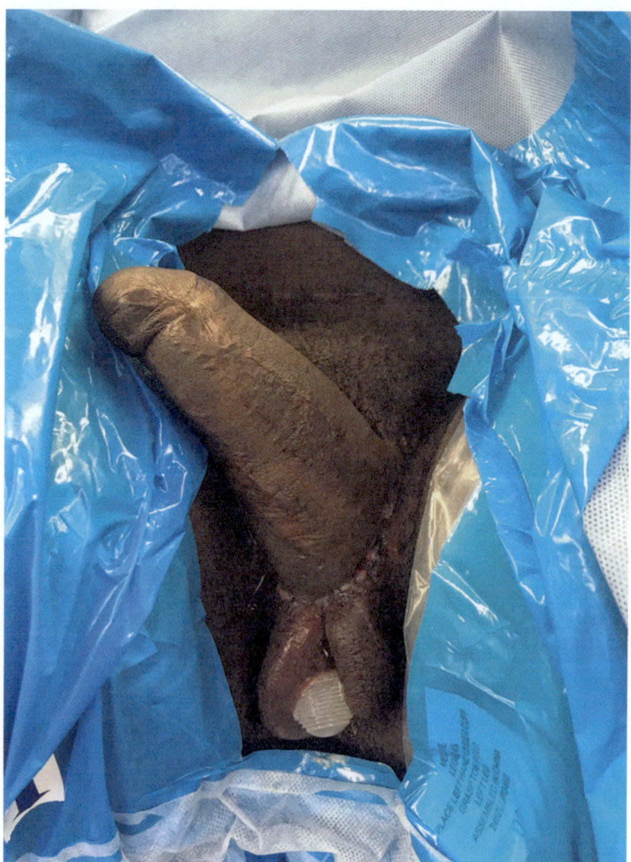

Fig. 12.6 Erosion of a prosthetic pump through neoscrotum

Fig. 12.7 Removal of a vascular graft and prosthesis in a neophallus at risk of distal prosthesis extrusion

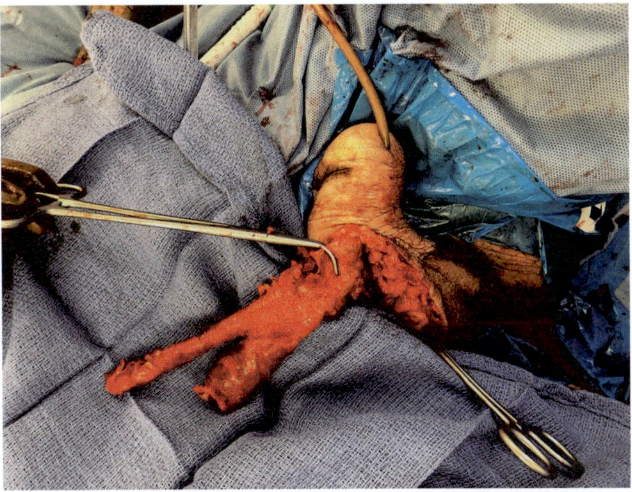

adherence (Fig. 12.7). One study showed that vascular grafts were potentially associated with lower rates of malpositioning (OR 0.86) in patients with AMS Ambicor implants, though this did not reach statistical significance [46]. In one small study of ten patients who had bone anchoring via cortical drilling, three (30%) had inadequate fixation requiring revision [47]. Of note, these cases were linked with self-reported vigorous sexual activity.

Device Leak and Failure

Early mechanical failure is also more common in neophallus patients. Falcone and colleagues reported a mechanical failure rate of 15.4% in a large series of transgender men who underwent RFFF with IPP [22]. The most common causes were cylinder rupture (69%), cylinder aneurysm (19%), or rupture of the tubing connecting the pump to the cylinder (12%). Hoebeke [51] reported that rates of dysfunction and leakage were higher in transgender men than in cisgender men with impotence: 14.5% vs 4.3% for dysfunction and 17.4% vs 10.8% vs for leakage in three-piece prostheses [56]. Repeated friction against vascular grafts during intercourse may contribute to mechanical dysfunction [57]. While vascular grafts are generally regarded as protective, one study comparing outcomes with or without vascular grafts was unable to find a significant difference between dysfunction rates between the groups [46].

Vascular Compromise

Injury to the vascular supply of the neophallus is rare but severe complication requiring emergent microvascular repair and likely implant removal. This complication was only reported by a single patient from a single study [49].

Device-Specific Adaptations

Currently, patients within the USA are limited to devices that are designed for cisgender male anatomy. Ideally, erectile prostheses for transgender men should have a number of modifications optimizing them for use in phalluses without preexisting corpora. These include a rear tip amenable to bony fixation; a wider distal tip to decrease pressure at the distal tissue and decrease erosion risk; and a single, wider cylinder implant capable of providing rigidity and girth. One such device is the ZSI 475 FTM hydraulic implant (Zephyr Surgical Implants, Switzerland) specifically for patients with neophallus, which features a broad base for proximal fixation and a realistically rigid glans. However, it is not FDA approved for use in the USA and has only very limited data with few patients and follow-up of less than 1 year [54, 55].

Patient-Reported Outcomes

While several studies reveal generally high satisfaction following gender-affirming phalloplasty [3, 5, 8, 9, 22, 30, 53, 58], few report on degree of satisfaction with the erectile prostheses specifically. Falcone reported that in a large cohort of 247 patients, 88% reported high overall satisfaction, 83% were satisfied with sensation, 77% were able to penetrate a partner during intercourse, 61% achieved orgasm, and 60% reported high partner satisfaction [22]. Leriche et al. reported that 51% of a cohort of 35 transgender phalloplasty patients had satisfactory penetrative sexual intercourse [30]. Eighty-one percent of Zuckerman's cohort of 31 cisgender and transgender male patients were sexually active following phalloplasty and prosthesis placement. In a cohort of 20 transgender men with the transgender-specific ZSI implant, Neuville reports 92.8% satisfaction, with 85.7% regularly engaging in penetrative intercourse [54, 55]. In a series of six cisgender men who underwent RFFF and prosthesis placement following traumatic penile amputation, all were sexually active [3]. Patients with congenital penile insufficiency due to exstrophy or micropenis appear to report lower rates of regular sexual activity, between 17% and 58% [6, 44].

Patient-reported outcome data are significantly limited by the lack of a standardized measurement tool to assess satisfaction and subjective outcomes after erectile prosthesis placement, phalloplasty, or gender-affirming surgery generally.

Testicular Prostheses

Criteria for Placement

For patients who desire testicular prostheses, placement should be considered once the scrotoplasty has healed completely [59]. However, a one-stage insertion at the time of gender-affirming surgery has been described, with a reported rate of testicular implant loss of 3/473 patients (0.6%) [60].

While there is little data on ideal surgical approaches in this setting, we recommend using a low groin or high scrotal incision where feasible and avoiding skin penetration when fixing the prosthetics' positions. Concomitant insertion of an inflatable penile prosthesis is feasible, and if this is pursued, a single testicular implant can be placed through a separate incision opposite the prosthesis pump [51].

Types of Testicular Prostheses

Currently, only silicone-coated, saline-filled prostheses are FDA approved for use in the USA, on the basis of a large multicenter study establishing their safety [61]. Prostheses filled with silicone-based gel or elastomer were withdrawn from the market due to concerns for silicone migration but are available outside the USA [62]. The Coloplast Torosa® (Coloplast, Minneapolis, MN, USA) is the principal device available in the USA at the time of writing and comes in four sizes: extra small, small, medium, and large, corresponding to increasing saline volumes. The injection port on the prosthetic can be accessed up to five times for filling or withdrawing saline.

Silicone-gel- or elastomer-filled implants are available in the European and Asian markets and include devices manufactured by Polytech (Polytech, Dieburg, Germany) and the Promedon N&S® prosthesis (Promedon, Cordoba, Argentina). These implants cannot be filled additionally intraoperatively. Common to all devices are variety in size of implants (ranging from 5 to 36 mL) and a tab allowing for suture anchoring of the prosthetic.

Postoperative Care for Testicular Implants

Patients are discharged with a course of empiric antibiotics and followed up within 2–4 weeks for evaluation of the wound. Afterward, patients are counseled to observe for device-associated malposition, extrusion, concern for infection, or pain.

Complications of Testicular Implants

From the cisgender literature, the most common complications following testicular prosthesis placement include infection (0.6%–4%), hematoma (0.3%–3%), and extrusion (3%–8%) [63]. As with penile prostheses, ensuring sterile urine, perioperative antibiotics, and antimicrobial irrigation of the incision are advocated, ensuring broad-spectrum coverage. Additional suggestions for preventing device-associated infections, described in the cisgender prosthetic literature, include preoperative chlorhexidine bath, clipping of pubic hair, double gloving, and avoiding hematomas [64]. The labial fat pads, left in situ after scrotoplasty with labia majora skin flaps, may offer protection against device extrusion [65].

The rate of dissatisfaction with prosthetic location has been reported as 30% for cisgender men undergoing orchiectomy for testicular cancer [66]. The incidence of testicular prosthetic migration for transgender men is unclear. However, implantation of testicular prosthesis is relatively simple. Studies of improvement in body image and self-esteem, as well as outcomes of device placement in the trans men population, are warranted.

> **Key Points**
> 1. Neophallus prosthesis implantation requires avoidance of critical vascular and urinary tract structures, proximal prosthesis anchoring, and distal cushioning.
> 2. Erectile prostheses are associated with increased risk of infection, extrusion, erosion, and device migration relative to prosthesis placement in cisgender men, with a high revision rate.
> 3. Surgeons performing neophallus prosthesis placement should have a thorough understanding of neophallic reconstructive technique prior to proceeding with device placement.
> 4. Testicular prosthesis placement techniques, complications, and satisfaction rates have not been well-described in the transgender population. Position and size of testicular prostheses depend on neoscrotal anatomy.
> 5. Validated assessment tools for neophallus and testicular prosthesis are needed to inform provider counseling and patient expectations.

Conclusions

Literature reporting outcomes of erectile prosthesis placement is limited to retrospective reviews with varying techniques, follow-up, and outcome measures, with even fewer studies describing outcomes of testicular prosthesis. Unique to transgender patients or others without preexisting corpora, successful implantation requires (a) protective sensation, achieved through nerve coaptation and a 6–9 month waiting period after initial phalloplasty; (b) proximal bony fixation to mitigate the risk of migration and malpositioning; and (c) distal cushioning, with assistance of prosthetic graft "socks" or acellular dermis caps to further solidify placement. Complication and reoperation rates for prosthesis placement remain high, likely due to unique anatomy in transgender male patients. Therefore, these procedures should only be undertaken with the assistance of experienced surgeons who are able to manage microvascular complications as they arise. Modification of the existing prostheses to accommodate unique aspects of neophallus anatomy may be beneficial. As with all gender-affirming surgery, erectile and testicular prosthesis placement would benefit from a standardized patient-reported outcome measure to enable assessment and comparison of techniques.

References

1. Flores AR, Herman JL, Gates GJ, Brown TNT. How many adults identify as transgender in the United States? The Williams Institute: Los Angeles; 2016.

2. Grant JMML, Tanis J, Herman JL, Harrison J, Keisling M. National transgender discrimination survey report on health and health care. Washington, DC: National Center for Transgender Equality and the National Gay and Lesbian Task Force; 2010.

3. Falcone M, Garaffa G, Raheem A, Christopher NA, Ralph DJ. Total phallic reconstruction using the radial artery based forearm free flap after traumatic penile amputation. J Sex Med. 2016;13(7):1119–24.

4. Amukele SA, Lee GW, Stock JA, Hanna MK. 20-year experience with iatrogenic penile injury. J Urol. 2003;170(4 Pt 2):1691–4.

5. Callens N, Hoebeke P. Phalloplasty: a panacea for 46, XY disorder of sex development conditions with penile deficiency? Endocr Dev. 2014;27:222–33.

6. Garaffa G, Spilotros M, Christopher NA, Ralph DJ. Total phallic reconstruction using radial artery based forearm free flap phalloplasty in patients with epispadias-exstrophy complex. J Urol. 2014;192(3):814–20.

7. Kayes O, Shabbir M, Ralph D, Minhas S. Therapeutic strategies for patients with micropenis or penile dysmorphic disorder. Nat Rev Urol. 2012;9(9):499–507.

8. Lumen N, Monstrey S, Selvaggi G, Ceulemans P, De Cuypere G, Van Laecke E, et al. Phalloplasty: a valuable treatment for males with penile insufficiency. Urology. 2008;71(2):272–6. discussion 6-7

9. Garaffa G, Raheem AA, Christopher NA, Ralph DJ. Total phallic reconstruction after penile amputation for carcinoma. BJU Int. 2009;104(6):852–6.

10. Bluebond-Langner R, Redett RJ. Phalloplasty in complete aphallia and ambiguous genitalia. Semin Plast Surg. 2011;25(3):196–205.

11. Hage JJ, Bout CA, Bloem JJ, Megens JA. Phalloplasty in female-to-male transsexuals: what do our patients ask for? Ann Plast Surg. 1993;30(4):323–6.

12. Jacobsson J, Andreasson M, Kolby L, Elander A, Selvaggi G. Patients' priorities regarding female-to-male gender affirmation surgery of the genitalia – a pilot study of 47 patients in Sweden. J Sex Med. 2017;14(6):857–64.

13. Gilbert DA, Horton CE, Terzis JK, Devine CJ Jr, Winslow BH, Devine PC. New concepts in phallic reconstruction. Ann Plast Surg. 1987;18(2):128–36.

14. Frey JD, Poudrier G, Chiodo MV, Hazen A. An update on genital reconstruction options for the female-to-male transgender patient: a review of the literature. Plast Reconstr Surg. 2017;139(3):728–37.

15. Selvaggi G, Bellringer J. Gender reassignment surgery: an overview. Nat Rev Urol. 2011;8(5):274–82.

16. Chang TS, Hwang WY. Forearm flap in one-stage reconstruction of the penis. Plast Reconstr Surg. 1984;74(2):251–8.

17. Monstrey S, Hoebeke P, Selvaggi G, Ceulemans P, Van Landuyt K, Blondeel P, et al. Penile reconstruction: is the radial forearm flap really the standard technique? Plast Reconstr Surg. 2009;124(2):510–8.

18. Lee GK, Lim AF, Bird ET. A novel single-flap technique for total penile reconstruction: the pedicled anterolateral thigh flap. Plast Reconstr Surg. 2009;124(1):163–6.

19. Rubino C, Figus A, Dessy LA, Alei G, Mazzocchi M, Trignano E, et al. Innervated island pedicled anterolateral thigh flap for neo-phallic reconstruction in female-to-male transsexuals. J Plast Reconstr Aesthet Surg. 2009;62(3):e45–9.

20. Morrison SD, Son J, Song J, Berger A, Kirby J, Ahdoot M, et al. Modification of the tube-in-tube pedicled anterolateral thigh flap for total phalloplasty: the mushroom flap. Ann Plast Surg. 2014;72(Suppl 1):S22–6.

21. Bettocchi C, Ralph DJ, Pryor JP. Pedicled pubic phalloplasty in females with gender dysphoria. BJU Int. 2005;95(1):120–4.

22. Falcone M, Garaffa G, Gillo A, Dente D, Christopher AN, Ralph DJ. Outcomes of inflatable penile prosthesis insertion in 247 patients completing female to male gender reassignment surgery. BJU Int. 2018;121(1):139–44. https://doi.org/10.1111/bju.14027. Epub 2017 Oct 20. PMID: 28940910.

23. Selvaggi G, Monstrey S, Ceulemans P, T'Sjoen G, De Cuypere G, Hoebeke P. Genital sensitivity after sex reassignment surgery in transsexual patients. Ann Plast Surg. 2007;58(4):427–33.

24. Hoebeke P, Selvaggi G, Ceulemans P, De Cuypere G, T'Sjoen G, Weyers S, et al. Impact of sex reassignment surgery on lower urinary tract function. Eur Urol. 2005;47(3):398–402.

25. Van Caenegem E, Verhaeghe E, Taes Y, Wierckx K, Toye K, Goemaere S, et al. Long-term evaluation of donor-site morbidity after radial forearm flap phalloplasty for transsexual men. J Sex Med. 2013;10(6):1644–51.

26. Rohrmann D, Jakse G. Urethroplasty in female-to-male transsexuals. Eur Urol. 2003;44(5):611–4.

27. Ascha M, Massie JP, Morrison SD, Crane CN, Chen ML. Outcomes of single stage phalloplasty by pedicled anterolateral thigh flap versus radial forearm free flap in gender confirming surgery. J Urol. 2018;199(1):206–14. https://doi.org/10.1016/j.juro.2017.07.084. Epub 2017 Jul 29. PMID: 28765066.

28. Lumen N, Monstrey S, Goessaert AS, Oosterlinck W, Hoebeke P. Urethroplasty for strictures after phallic reconstruction: a single-institution experience. Eur Urol. 2011;60(1):150–8.

29. Levine LA, Elterman L. Urethroplasty following total phallic reconstruction. J Urol. 1998;160(2):378–82.

30. Leriche A, Timsit MO, Morel-Journel N, Bouillot A, Dembele D, Ruffion A. Long-term outcome of forearm flee-flap phalloplasty in the treatment of transsexualism. BJU Int. 2008;101(10):1297–300.

31. Noe JM, Birdsell D, Laub DR. The surgical construction of male genitalia for the female-to-male transsexual. Plast Reconstr Surg. 1974;53(5):511–6.

32. Borgoras N. Uber die volle plastische wiederhersteuung eines zum koitus fahigen penis (peniplastica totalis). Zentralbl Chirurg. 1936;63:1271–6.

33. Biemer E. Penile construction by the radial arm flap. Clin Plast Surg. 1988;15(3):425–30.

34. Kim SK, Lee KC, Kwon YS, Cha BH. Phalloplasty using radial forearm osteocutaneous free flaps in

female-to-male transsexuals. J Plast Reconstr Aesthet Surg. 2009;62(3):309–17.

35. Kim SK, Kim TH, Yang JI, Kim MH, Kim MS, Lee KC. The etiology and treatment of the softened phallus after the radial forearm osteocutaneous free flap phalloplasty. Arch Plast Surg. 2012;39(4):390–6.

36. Schaff J, Papadopulos NA. A new protocol for complete phalloplasty with free sensate and prelaminated osteofasciocutaneous flaps: experience in 37 patients. Microsurgery. 2009;29(5):413–9.

37. Papadopulos NA, Schaff J, Biemer E. The use of free prelaminated and sensate osteofasciocutaneous fibular flap in phalloplasty. Injury. 2008;39(Suppl 3):S62–7.

38. Selvaggi G, Elander A, Branemark R. Penile epithesis: preliminary study. Plast Reconstr Surg. 2010;126(5):265e–6e.

39. Selvaggi G, Branemark R, Elander A, Liden M, Stalfors J. Titanium-bone-anchored penile epithesis: preoperative planning and immediate postoperative results. J Plast Surg Hand Surg. 2015;49(1):40–4.

40. Scott FB, Bradley WE, Timm GW. Management of erectile impotence. Use of implantable inflatable prosthesis. Urology. 1973;2(1):80–2.

41. Puckett CL, Montie JE. Construction of male genitalia in the transsexual, using a tubed groin flap for the penis and a hydraulic inflation device. Plast Reconstr Surg. 1978;61(4):523–30.

42. Levine LA, Zachary LS, Gottlieb LJ. Prosthesis placement after total phallic reconstruction. J Urol. 1993;149(3):593–8.

43. Hage JJ, Bloem JJ, Bouman FG. Obtaining rigidity in the neophallus of female-to-male transsexuals: a review of the literature. Ann Plast Surg. 1993;30(4):327–33.

44. Segal RL, Massanyi EZ, Gupta AD, Gearhart JP, Redett RJ, Bivalacqua TJ, et al. Inflatable penile prosthesis technique and outcomes after radial forearm free flap neophalloplasty. Int J Impot Res. 2015;27(2):49–53.

45. Hoebeke P, de Cuypere G, Ceulemans P, Monstrey S. Obtaining rigidity in total phalloplasty: experience with 35 patients. J Urol. 2003;169(1):221–3.

46. Neuville P, Morel-Journel N, Maucourt-Boulch D, Ruffion A, Paparel P, Terrier JE. Surgical outcomes of erectile implants after Phalloplasty: retrospective analysis of 95 procedures. J Sex Med. 2016;13(11):1758–64.

47. Cohen AJ, Bhanvadia RR, Pariser JJ, Hatcher DM, Gottlieb LJ, Bales GT. Novel technique for proximal bone anchoring of penile prosthesis after radial forearm free flap neophallus. Urology. 2017;105:2–5.

48. Hage JJ. Dynaflex prosthesis in total phalloplasty. Plast Reconstr Surg. 1997;99(2):479–85.

49. Zuckerman JM, Smentkowski K, Gilbert D, Storme O, Jordan G, Virasoro R, et al. Penile prosthesis implantation in patients with a history of Total phallic construction. J Sex Med. 2015;12(12):2485–91.

50. Jordan GH, Alter GJ, Gilbert DA, Horton CE, Devine CJ Jr. Penile prosthesis implantation in total phalloplasty. J Urol. 1994;152(2 Pt 1):410–4.

51. Hoebeke PB, Decaestecker K, Beysens M, Opdenakker Y, Lumen N, Monstrey SM. Erectile implants in female-to-male transsexuals: our experience in 129 patients. Eur Urol. 2010;57(2):334–40.

52. Large MC, Gottlieb LJ, Wille MA, DeWolfe M, Bales GT. Novel technique for proximal anchoring of penile prostheses in female-to-male transsexual. Urology. 2009;74(2):419–21.

53. Callens N, De Cuypere G, T'Sjoen G, Monstrey S, Lumen N, Van Laecke E, et al. Sexual quality of life after total phalloplasty in men with penile deficiency: an exploratory study. World J Urol. 2015;33(1):137–43.

54. Neuville P, Morel-Journel N, Cabelguenne D, Ruffion A, Paparel P, Terrier JE. First outcomes of the ZSI 475 FtM, a specific prosthesis designed for Phalloplasty. J Sex Med. 2019;16(2):316–22. https://doi.org/10.1016/j.jsxm.2018.11.013. Epub 2019 Jan 9.

55. Carson CC III, Mulcahy JJ, Harsch MR. Long-term infection outcomes after original antibiotic impregnated inflatable penile prosthesis implants: up to 7.7 years of followup. J Urol. 185(2):614–8.

56. Carson CC, Mulcahy JJ, Govier FE. Efficacy, safety and patient satisfaction outcomes of the AMS 700CX inflatable penile prosthesis: results of a long-term multicenter study. AMS 700CX study group. J Urol. 2000;164(2):376–80.

57. Perovic SV. Editorial comment on: erectile implants in female-to-male transsexuals: our experience in 129 patients. Eur Urol. 57(2):340.

58. De Cuypere G, T'Sjoen G, Beerten R, Selvaggi G, De Sutter P, Hoebeke P, et al. Sexual and physical health after sex reassignment surgery. Arch Sex Behav. 2005;34(6):679–90.

59. Selvaggi G, Hoebeke P, Ceulemans P, Hamdi M, Van Landuyt K, Blondeel P, et al. Scrotal reconstruction in female-to-male transsexuals: a novel scrotoplasty. Plast Reconstr Surg. 2009;123(6):1710–8.

60. Stojanovic B, Bizic M, Bencic M, Kojovic V, Majstorovic M, Jeftovic M, et al. One-stage gender-confirmation surgery as a viable surgical procedure for female-to-male transsexuals. J Sex Med. 2017;14(5):741–6.

61. Turek PJ, Master VA. Testicular prosthesis study G. safety and effectiveness of a new saline filled testicular prosthesis. J Urol. 2004;172(4 Pt 1):1427–30.

62. Kogan S. The clinical utility of testicular prosthesis placement in children with genital and testicular disorders. Transl Androl Urol. 2014;3(4):391–7.

63. Lucas JW, Lester KM, Chen A, Simhan J. Scrotal reconstruction and testicular prosthetics. Transl Androl Urol. 2017;6(4):710–21.

64. Bodiwala D, Summerton DJ, Terry TR. Testicular prostheses: development and modern usage. Ann R Coll Surg Engl. 2007;89(4):349–53.

65. Dy GW, Sun J, Granieri MA, Zhao LC. Reconstructive management pearls for the transgender patient. Curr Urol Rep. 2018;19(6):36.

66. Dieckmann KP, Anheuser P, Schmidt S, Soyka-Hundt B, Pichlmeier U, Schriefer P, et al. Testicular prostheses in patients with testicular cancer – acceptance rate and patient satisfaction. BMC Urol. 2015;15:16.

Perioperative Care and Follow Up

Nim Christopher

Introduction

Transgender patients have specific considerations when assessing the neo-urethra. Broadly, there are 2 categories, namely, transgender female urethras for patients who have had any kind of vaginoplasty and transgender male urethras for patients who have had phalloplasty or metoidioplasty. For those who have not had their urethra altered surgically in the context of genital gender-affirming surgery (GGAS), the care is exactly the same as for cisgender males and cisgender females. There is also a heterogeneous group of transgender patients who identify as non-binary who have some aspects of both male and female identity. These individuals should have urologic care appropriate to the type of neo-urethra constructed, or if no urethral surgery has been performed, then appropriate to the born gender.

Anatomy of Transgender Female Urethras

Essentially, these patients are dealt with in exactly the same way as any cisgender female. The neo-urethra is fairly short and the meatus is in the perineum. There are some specific anatomical issues that must be considered. Firstly, there may be quite a lot of corpora spongiosum remaining after reconstruction around the well-vascularised urethra. Secondly, the prostate is typically left in situ and is encircling the proximal urethra between the membranous urethra and the bladder neck. Finally, the seminal vesicles are also left in situ at the time of vaginoplasty. The prostate and seminal vesicles are usually small and atrophic but this may not always be the case.

Catheters

Catheterisation should be performed as usual for cisgender females either with short female urethral catheters or the longer male catheters. Occasionally these patients will have meatal stenosis, which can be treated exactly as in a female urethra, i.e., using curved Cluttons urethral sounds or straight meatal dilators. In difficult cases specialised dilators may have to be used, such as S-Curve™ urethral dilators (Cook Medical®, USA) over a Nitinol coated hydrophilic guide wire (Terumo®, Japan). There should be no issue with performing clean intermittent self-catheterisation (CISC) if required as the meatus should be in an anatomically correct female position.

N. Christopher (✉)
University College London Hospital, London, UK

St Peters Andrology Centre, London, UK
e-mail: nim@andrology.co.uk

© Springer Nature Switzerland AG 2021
D. Nikolavsky, S. A. Blakely (eds.), *Urological Care for the Transgender Patient*,
https://doi.org/10.1007/978-3-030-18533-6_13

Cystourethroscopy

The perineal urethra is analogous to that of a cisgender male bulbar urethra with the same calibre; therefore, standard endoscopic equipment including a 21/22F cystoscope with a terminal lip, or a resectoscope, could be used without a problem. In cases of meatal stenosis or a stricture, it would be useful to place a safety guidewire and utilize a flexible or paediatric cystoscope.

Haematuria

Visible haematuria should be assessed and investigated in the normal fashion as for cisgender females. There are some extra potential causes which should be considered. These are bleeding from the prostate and/or seminal vesicles. These male structures would normally be shrunken and atrophic due to loss of testosterone after bilateral orchidectomy, if the patient has already had GGAS or due to Gonadotrophin Releasing Hormone (GnRH) agonists or Androgen receptor blockade if they have not had GGAS yet. However, if the patient has transitioned late in life, then there may already be significant natural benign prostatic enlargement. These patients may also suffer from orgasmic bleeding. They should be investigated as per the normal protocol for male haemospermia, i.e. seminal or urine culture, Prostatic Specific Antigen (PSA) blood test and transvaginal or transrectal ultrasound to assess prostate and seminal vesicles. It would be sensible to also perform digital transvaginal examination of the prostate if there is an accessible full-depth vaginoplasty in much the same way as a digital rectal examination (DRE) of prostate for cisgender males. Obviously in zero-depth vaginoplasty, a standard DRE of prostate is indicated.

Urinary Tract Infections

Lower urinary tract infections (UTIs) are relatively common in cisgender females because of the short native urethra [1]. The same will apply for transgender female urethras and will be treated in exactly the same way [2]. Transgender females may also develop bladder outflow obstruction secondary to benign prostatic obstruction (BPO) which can also present with UTIs. Standard investigations include digital transvaginal/transrectal examination of the prostate, urinary flow rate and post-void bladder residual volume scan. If there is poor bladder emptying secondary to BPO, then standard urological treatment protocols apply, i.e. alpha-blockers such as Alfuzosin, Tamsulosin and/or 5-alpha reductase inhibitors such as Finasteride and Dutasteride. In some patients, the symptoms may be severe enough to warrant ablative prostate surgery to reduce obstruction [3, 4]. This could be in the form of a standard transurethral resection of prostate, bladder neck incision, newer technologies such as laser prostatectomy with different laser wavelengths and/or the latest technologies such as hydro-jet ablation prostatectomy and so on [5]. The patient should be clinically assessed in exactly the same way as for a cisgender male.

Stones

The transgender female urethra is made from the normal male bulbar urethra with transitional cell epithelium so is unlikely to suffer from stone formation unless keratinised or hair-bearing squamous epithelium has been used for urethral repair. All reconstructed urethras, particularly those made from keratinised skin with potential hair follicles, have a risk of urinary stone formation. Bladder stones would be rare except in cases of chronic urinary retention. The risk of upper urinary tract stone formation should not be influenced by the oestrogen therapy in the under 50y age group. If anything, the incidence of upper urinary tract stone formation should be reduced for the younger transgender females when compared to cisgender males due to the protective effect of oestrogen [6]. In the over 50y age group, the data is mixed in that postmenopausal cisgender females on oestrogen replacement therapy may have a higher incidence of renal stone formation than those not on hormone replacement therapy [7, 8]. There is no published data on older transgender females regarding renal stone formation. The neo-urethra is wide and there is easy access for all the normal endoscopic stone clearing equipment.

Surgical Positioning

If a transgender female needed endoscopic urological intervention, the standard lithotomy position for rigid cystoscopy under general anaesthesia or supine with hips/knees flexed and abducted for flexible cystoscopy under local anaesthesia is perfectly adequate. For open/reconstructive surgery for urethral stenosis, a low or extended lithotomy could be required for surgical access. Neovaginal stenosis is one of the most common problems in transgender females after vaginoplasty and is usually due to lack of regular self-vaginal dilation. Again, depending on surgeon preference, either a low or extended lithotomy position would give good access for surgical repair

Transgender Male Urethras

Transgender male patients after a phalloplasty are expected to have a thinner-walled bladder analogous to a cisgender female bladder as opposed to the bladder of a cisgender male. The bladder then empties through a native urethra into a perineal urethra (*pars fixa*) which is anastomosed to an extended skin-tube neo-urethra (*pars pendulans*). The longer neo-urethra increases the resistance to flow, following Poiseuille's Law, which may conceivably cause bladder muscular hypertrophy [9–11].

For patients with metoidioplasty who void from the tip of the micro-penis, the proximal part of the urethra (*pars fixa*) is constructed from native meatal skin or an anterior vaginal mucosal flap [12, 13]. Native meatal skin is non-secretory and is not keratinised. Vaginal mucosa does contain a significant secretory component and because of the multiple skin folds can stretch considerably. The middle and distal part of the neo-urethra is typically formed from thin inner labial skin and/or buccal mucosa graft embedded onto the corpora cavernosa of the clitoris. The labial skin portion of the neourethra is expandable under hydrostatic voiding pressure whereas the buccal graft portion does not expand much.

For phalloplasty, there are various methods of urethral reconstruction. The proximal part is exactly the same as the metoidioplasty urethra. The middle or scrotal part of the neo-urethra is made from thin inner labial skin like for metoidioplasty. The phallic portion of the neo-urethra can be made in many different ways. Commonest is a vascularised free/pedicled flap of keratinised skin, e.g. radial artery phalloplasty or anterolateral thigh phalloplasty [14–21]. Other methods include the use of long non-hair bearing inner labial/clitoral hood skin flaps and buccal grafts on to the phallus [22, 23]. In our experience, if skin grafts are placed onto the fat of the phallus at the time of single-stage phalloplasty, the graft take is not so good because of the lesser blood supply in fat at the time of flap transfer. If the skin grafts are placed on a well-perfused muscle, as in the muscular latissimus dorsi flap, the graft take is expected to be better [22]. A third method is to use a prelaminated urethra [24]. This is performed by wrapping a 40F stent with split thickness skin graft with the raw surface on the outside and tunnelling it into the phallus donor site. The stent is left in for 3 months for the skin graft to 'take' and then the phallus is transferred with the urethra embedded inside. A caution must be taken with this approach as circular grafts are known to be unreliable and are strongly discouraged in urologic literature [AUA Urethral Stricture Guidelines statement 21] [25]. The survivability of the phallic neo-urethra is dependent on the blood supply, so free/pedicled flaps would be better than long local skin flaps which would then be better than a prelaminated skin graft neo-urethra. This is particularly important if a penile erectile prosthesis is inserted as this will disturb the underlying blood supply and patients are then more likely to develop an ischaemic urethral stricture. It is also extremely important to avoid using hair-bearing skin for the neo-urethra as this would make complications more likely.

Catheters

The neo-urethra in transgender males is usually very difficult to catheterise. First, because the urethral calibre at the level of pendulous urethra is normally expected to be 14–16 French. Second, the connection of the often tortuous perineal urethra (*pars fixa*) to the native urethra is usually at almost a 90-degree angle. Lastly, almost 40 percent of patients after phalloplasty present with small residual or recurrent vaginal cavity under the native urethra, and a blindly placed catheter may preferentially pass into such a cavity [26]. Still, a careful attempt could be made with a generously lubricated 14F silicone catheter. For metoidioplasty, a smaller 12F or 10F catheter may be needed. The regular latex catheters are usually too soft.

The phallus should be firmly pulled away from the body and slightly downwards to straighten out the curve of the scrotal urethra and make the 90-degree bend at the native meatus less to help with catheter passage. This is usually very difficult to negotiate just with a catheter. An experienced practitioner could carefully try a 12–14 French Coude tip catheter which has a slightly angled and stiffer pointy tip which might be safely negotiated through. Care must be taken to never try and force the catheter through as this will lead to false passages and urethral damage and lots of bleeding.

The other relatively safe approach would be an attempt to pass a guide wire blindly into the phallus neo-urethra until almost no wire is left outside the phallus. If the other end of the guidewire has not come back out of the phallus, then it is very likely in the bladder. An open-ended catheter can then be passed over the guidewire to prove passage into the bladder. The demonstration of the urine drip from the open-ended catheter, however, may not prove placement into the bladder – a large vaginal remnant filled with urine may produce the same urine drip [26]. Therefore, the safest approach to urethral catheterisation is with a use of a flexible cystoscope to insert a guidewire over which a catheter can be passed. If available, a flexible pediatric cystoscope or an 8-french ureteroscope could be used

and could help navigating even through some non-obliterated strictures. Obviously if there is a very narrow stricture causing urinary retention, the safest and most sensible thing to do is to place a suprapubic catheter. With the suprapubic tube in place, the patient can have a retrograde and voiding urethrogram to assess the stricture and plan future management.

Cystourethroscopy

Because the neo-urethras are typically narrow and tortuous, standard 21/22 French rigid cystoscopes or 24–26 French resectoscopes are not suitable for use in patients after phalloplasty or metoidioplasty. In general, the use of rigid endoscopic instruments should be avoided in patients with neo-urethra. However, if no other alternative is present, we recommend using the most narrow instrument available, ideally ≤17 French calibre. Again, it is preferable to use a smaller flexible 16 French cystoscope or better yet 7–8 French paediatric cystoscopes in patients with a neourethra. The practitioner should be aware that the scrotal neo-urethra has a 90-degree or greater acute bend in the transition to the native urethra so the entrance to the bladder may not be immediately obvious. There is often a posterior pouch just before the native urethra which represents the distended vaginal/urethral flap used in the original urethroplasty, and it is easy to miss the native urethral opening which is high up at the 12 o'clock position. With these considerations, it is more appropriate to use a flexible cystoscope.

Haematuria

Transgender male patients will have all the usual potential causes for haematuria in addition to several that are specific to phalloplasty. Bleeding from granulation tissue on the neo-urethral suture line is common and is often seen soon after the neo-urethra has been made. We suspect the acidic urine causes the granulation tissue to subside naturally. If granulation tissue persists, it could be easily treated with diathermy applied through a flexible cystoscope. Because the neo-urethra swells from the heat artefact, it is recommended to always leave a catheter afterwards for a few days. Of note, in some cisgender patients after undergoing phalloplasty, such as those with urinary diversion for bladder exstrophy complex, only seminal fluid is expected to be passing through the neo-urethra. The alkaline nature of the seminal discharge seems to promote excessive granulation tissue in the neo-urethra in this author's experience

Urinary Tract Infections

The rate of urinary tract infections in transgender males is unknown at this point. In our experience, in the absence of urinary obstruction, it is exceedingly rare for transgender males to present with urinary tract infections. Although random urine culture frequently shows presence of bacteria, due to skin-tube urethra colonisation by bacteria, these are usually asymptomatic bacteriuria.

Transgender male patients with symptomatic urinary tract infections should be investigated as any cisgender male with a UTI: upper urinary tract ultrasound, urinary flow rate and post-void bladder volume scan and cystoscopy. Unless the patient is immunocompromised, they should only receive antibiotic treatment for microbiologically proven UTI with symptoms. Asymptomatic patients can just be monitored as long as the rest of the urinary tract is normal. If the urine cultures are persistently positive, it is worth investigating for strictures, stones and remnant vaginal cavities which could serve as reservoirs of infected urine. The only other exception is for patients having a penile prosthesis inserted where any UTI should be treated prior to surgery. In the author's experience, about 5% of transgender male patients with a neo-phallus will have very severe recurrent UTIs. If full investigations reveal no treatable abnormality, then rotating low-dose prophylactic antibiotic therapy can be tried for 3–6 months to allow the bladder lining to recover. If this fails, then a temporary defunctioning perineal urethrostomy can be made to give the bladder mucosa a rest for 6 months and to recover. The neo-urethra can be reconnected at a later date if the patient is UTI free.

In this era of increasing antibiotic resistance, there is much interest in non-antibiotic therapies such as D-Mannose, Probiotics, Cranberry supplements, Methenamine Hippurate, Oestrogens, Intravesical Glycosaminoglycans, Immunostimulants, Novel Vaccines and other agents in cisgender females with recurrent UTIs [27]. The evidence is mixed and there is no high-level data supporting any single treatment, and it is suggested that a multimodal approach is more likely to be successful. Unfortunately, there is no data for transgender male patients. The author has also empirically tried both transurethral and bladder instillations of hyaluronic acid in selected patients who did not respond to prophylactic antibiotics with some success. Hyaluronic acid bladder instillations have been used for cisgender females with chronic UTIs to reduce the number of UTIs by about 50% [28]. In the transgender male patient, the problem is bacterial colonisation in the skin tube urethra. Because the neo-urethra is difficult to catheterise, the patient would need a flexible cystoscopy to insert the 40 mg/40 ml of hyaluronic acid into the bladder. The patient retains it for at least 1 hour before voiding. Treatments are weekly for 6 weeks and then monthly for 1 year if there is a good response. Concomitant prophylactic antibiotics can be gradually weaned off over the year. Alternatively, the patient can inject about 20 mg/20 ml of hyaluronic acid into the urethra with a syringe and then use a penile clamp or finger compression to keep it in the neo-urethra for about 1 hour before voiding. The treatment protocol frequency is the same as for bladder instillations. Most patients will not be keen on a perineal urethrostomy even if it is temporary. Intravesical antibiotic therapy has also been tried in the short term for cisgender females with recurrent UTIs using gentamicin, neomycin/polymyxin, neomycin or colistin [29]. Treatment was well tolerated with 78% seeing a reduction in UTIs. As with other therapies, there are no data on transgender individuals.

Stones

Keratinised skin will be constantly rejuvenated with the old keratin falling off as the epithelium replaces itself. In normal skin, this becomes house dust. In the neo-urethra, this keratin reacts with the urine to form a white sticky sediment that attaches to the neo-urethra and any hairs present. A good flow of urine usually washes most of this out, but because the neo-urethra is not a perfectly smooth cylindrical tube, eddies and currents from turbulent flow occur. This means that particles can be trapped in parts of the neo-urethra. This will lead to urethral stone formation. Patients may have almost no symptoms because the proximal or scrotal neo-urethra just expands to accommodate the stones and urine can flow round the outside. In the phallic portion of the urethra, they are usually more symptomatic because this neo-urethra is much less expandable. Hence, patients are more likely to present with obstructive urinary symptoms or UTIs or passing lots of debris in the urine. Sometimes, the problem is only discovered when it proves impossible to pass a catheter during other surgery.

A urethrogram is recommended to check for strictures and also if the bladder end of the neo-urethra is normal. These urethral stones can be dealt with endoscopically with a narrow rigid or flexible cystoscope and Holmium laser fibre. Unfortunately, urethral stones are often in association with a stricture and/or hairy skin, so it is usually easier to perform an open urethro-lithotomy to extract all the stones and lay open the stricture and expose the hairy area. Once the inflammation has settled down, the neo-urethra can be reassessed to determine how to repair it.

Bladder stones are unusual and present a problem in urethral access. Because the neo-urethra is relatively narrow and has a 90-degree bend in the perineum, and is therefore much less flexible than a native urethra, it is usually impossible to get a standard rigid cystoscope in to use a Pneumatic, Electrohydraulic, Laser or Ultrasonic lithoclast. Also, even if the bladder stone can be broken up, there is still the problem of how to get the fragments out. A percutaneous transpubic bladder puncture is one alternative using the same equipment as for Percutaneous Nephro-lithotomy. This allows good visualisation and access to the bladder stone and fragments can be easily removed with grasper forceps. A suprapubic catheter would be left in the suprapubic tract for 10–14 days. If the surgeon is experienced in transgender male neo-urethral reconstruction or has access to a colleague that does, then a temporary perineal urethrostomy can be made to allow access for the standard cystoscopic equipment. Subsequently, a routine bladder stone destruction with the various lithoclasts can be performed and fragments washed out in the usual fashion. The neo-urethra would have to be reformed afterwards and a catheter left in for 2–3 weeks until healed.

Ureteric stones are treated in exactly the same way as for cisgender males with one difference. It would not be possible to perform a rigid ureteroscopy because of the difficulties of access via the neo-urethra so flexible ureteroscopy and a laser lithotripter would be the replacement option.

Surgical Positioning

If a transgender male patient needs urethral surgery, a lithotomy would be the best position to achieve access to the entire urethra. In cases where the problem is only at the meatus or phallic urethra, a supine position would be adequate.

For penile erectile prosthesis and testis prosthesis, there are 2 positions depending on surgeon preference and patient body habitus. For average size patients, a supine position with the legs 45–60° apart gives access to both sides of the neo-scrotum for testes prosthesis insertion and also penile prosthesis insertion. Penile prosthesis insertion could be either via an infrapubic-type approach at the phallus base or an infero-lateral approach via the side of the neo-scrotum over the adductor tendon. There is good access for pubic bone fixation for both single- and double-cylinder penile prosthesis. For overweight patients needing a double cylinder penile prosthesis via the infero-lateral approach, the lithotomy position would give easier access. For non-transgender phalloplasty patients with a native scrotum and existing crura of corpora cavernosa, a scrotal approach in the supine position with legs together is appropriate. If there are no native crura, the approach is the same as for transgender males.

Take Home Points

- External phenotype and urologic anatomy do not always match, so be vigilant.
- If no history of urethral reconstruction, then transgender urologic surgery is exactly the same as for patient's native gender.
- For transgender female urethroplasty urologic surgical access is exactly as for cisgender females.
    - Remember there is still a prostate and a much thicker and vascular bulbo-spongiosum.
    - Standard urological instrumentation can be used.
- For transgender male urethroplasty the urethra is narrower, tortuous and less forgiving.
    - Insert catheters over a guide wire or via flexible cystoscopy.
    - Use smaller calibre instruments.
    - Open urethral stone removal is usually quicker and safer than endoscopic as you can deal with the cause at the same time.
    - Bladder stones can be accessed via suprapubic puncture or open cystolitholopaxy.
    - Ureteric stones can be accessed with the flexible ureteroscope or in antegrade fashion via renal puncture.
    - Urinary tract infections can be difficult to clear because of bacterial colonisation of the skin tube urethra.

References

1. Minardi D, d'Anzeo G, Cantoro D, Conti A, Muzzonigro G. Urinary tract infections in women: etiology and treatment options. Int J Gen Med. 2011;4:333–43.

2. Middleton I, Holden FA. Urological issues following gender reassignment surgery. Br J Nurs. 2017;26(18):S28–33.

3. Miksad RA, Bubley G, Church P, Sanda M, Rofsky N, Kaplan I, et al. Prostate cancer in a transgender woman 41 years after initiation of feminization. JAMA. 2006;296(19):2316–7.

4. Molokwu CN, Appelbaum JS, Miksad RA. Detection of prostate cancer following gender reassignment. BJU Int. 2008;101(2):259; author reply -60.

5. Srinivasan A, Wang R. An update on minimally invasive surgery for benign prostatic hyperplasia: techniques, risks, and efficacy. World J Mens Health. 2019

6. Heller HJ, Sakhaee K, Moe OW, Pak CY. Etiological role of estrogen status in renal stone formation. J Urol. 2002;168(5):1923–7.

7. Maalouf NM, Sato AH, Welch BJ, Howard BV, Cochrane BB, Sakhaee K, et al. Postmenopausal hormone use and the risk of nephrolithiasis: results from the women's health initiative hormone therapy trials. Arch Intern Med. 2010;170(18):1678–85.

8. Zhao Z, Mai Z, Ou L, Duan X, Zeng G. Serum estradiol and testosterone levels in kidney stones disease with and without calcium oxalate components in naturally postmenopausal women. PLoS One. 2013;8(9):e75513.

9. Sutera SP, Skalak R. The history of Poiseuille's law. Annu Rev Fluid Mech. 1993;25(1):1–20.

10. Kuhn A, Hiltebrand R, Birkhauser M. Do transsexuals have micturition disorders? Eur J Obstet Gynecol Reprod Biol. 2007;131(2):226–30.

11. Hoebeke P, Selvaggi G, Ceulemans P, De Cuypere G, T'Sjoen G, Weyers S, et al. Impact of sex reassignment surgery on lower urinary tract function. Eur Urol. 2005;47(3):398–402.

12. Djordjevic ML, Bizic M, Stanojevic D, Bumbasirevic M, Kojovic V, Majstorovic M, et al. Urethral lengthening in metoidioplasty (female-to-male sex reassignment surgery) by combined buccal mucosa graft and labia minora flap. Urology. 2009;74(2):349–53.

13. Djordjevic ML, Stojanovic B, Bizic M. Metoidioplasty: techniques and outcomes. Transl Androl Urol. 2019;8(3):248–53.

14. Garaffa G, Christopher NA, Ralph DJ. Total phallic reconstruction in female-to-male transsexuals. Eur Urol. 2010;57(4):715–22.

15. Garaffa G, Ralph DJ, Christopher N. Total urethral construction with the radial artery-based forearm free flap in the transsexual. BJU Int. 2010;106(8):1206–10.

16. Baumeister S, Sohn M, Domke C, Exner K. [Phalloplasty in female-to-male transsexuals: experience from 259 cases]. Handchir Mikrochir Plast Chir. 2011;43(4):215–21.

17. Monstrey S, Hoebeke P, Dhont M, Selvaggi G, Hamdi M, Van Landuyt K, et al. Radial forearm phalloplasty: a review of 81 cases. Eur J Plast Surg. 2005;28(3):206–12.

18. Chang TS, Hwang WY. Forearm flap in one-stage reconstruction of the penis. Plast Reconstr Surg. 1984;74(2):251–8.

19. Felici N, Felici A. A new phalloplasty technique: the free anterolateral thigh flap phalloplasty. J Plast Reconstr Aesthet Surg. 2006;59(2):153–7.
20. Ascha M, Massie JP, Morrison SD, Crane CN, Chen ML. Outcomes of single stage phalloplasty by pedicled anterolateral thigh flap versus radial forearm free flap in gender confirming surgery. J Urol. 2018;199(1):206–14.
21. van der Sluis WB, Smit JM, Pigot GLS, Buncamper ME, Winters HAH, Mullender MG, et al. Double flap phalloplasty in transgender men: surgical technique and outcome of pedicled anterolateral thigh flap phalloplasty combined with radial forearm free flap urethral reconstruction. Microsurgery. 2017;37(8):917–23.
22. Perovic SV, Djinovic R, Bumbasirevic M, Djordjevic M, Vukovic P. Total phalloplasty using a musculocutaneous latissimus dorsi flap. BJU Int. 2007;100(4):899–905; discussion.
23. Djordjevic ML. Novel surgical techniques in female to male gender confirming surgery. Transl Androl Urol. 2018;7(4):628–38.
24. Salgado CJ, Fein LA, Chim J, Medina CA, Demaso S, Gomez C. Prelamination of neourethra with uterine mucosa in radial forearm osteocutaneous free flap phalloplasty in the female-to-male transgender patient. Case Rep Urol. 2016;2016:8742531.
25. Wessells H, Angermeier KW, Elliott S, Gonzalez CM, Kodama R, Peterson AC, et al. Male urethral stricture: American Urological Association guideline. J Urol. 2017;197(1):182–90.
26. Dy GW, Granieri MA, Fu BC, Vanni AJ, Voelzke B, Rourke KF, et al. Presenting complications to a reconstructive urologist after masculinizing genital reconstructive surgery. Urology. 2019;132:202–6.
27. Sihra N, Goodman A, Zakri R, Sahai A, Malde S. Nonantibiotic prevention and management of recurrent urinary tract infection. Nat Rev Urol. 2018;15(12):750–76.
28. Goddard JC, Janssen DAW. Intravesical hyaluronic acid and chondroitin sulfate for recurrent urinary tract infections: systematic review and meta-analysis. Int Urogynecol J. 2018;29(7):933–42.
29. Pietropaolo A, Jones P, Moors M, Birch B, Somani BK. Use and effectiveness of antimicrobial intravesical treatment for prophylaxis and treatment of recurrent urinary tract infections (UTIs): a systematic review. Curr Urol Rep. 2018;19(10):78.

Care of Transgender Patients: Oncological Concerns

Kathryn Scott, Gennady Bratslavsky, and Elizabeth Ferry

Introduction

Oncologic concerns in the transgender population are an area of medicine set to become more prominent in everyday practice as the rate of transgender surgery continues to rise. Cancer remains the second leading cause of death among all persons in the United States and the transgender population is not exempt from baseline oncologic risk. This population however is often under-screened [1]. With the increasing number of patients receiving gender affirmation surgery, it is important to consider and evaluate for baseline and other additional risks in these patients.

Current research focuses on the medical transition undergone by transgender individuals and its potential oncologic effects. However, this remains an under-researched topic due to the relatively small cohorts of patients. Literature reviews of the transgender population often produce studies of low-quality evidence that thus far lack enough data to cite cancer rates in this population or determine precise oncologic risks [2].

Currently, we do not know the effects medical treatment for gender affirmation has on cancer development in these individuals [3]. What we do know is the transgender population has a higher prevalence of other risk factors for malignancy. Examples include high rates of HIV and higher smoking rates [4, 5]. The U.S. Transgender Survey released by the National Center for Transgender Equality found transgender persons to be five times more likely to have HIV [6]. This places them at a higher risk for AIDS-defining cancers, as well as other malignancies. Higher rates of smoking place these patients at heightened risk for multiple malignancies.

With these and other risk factors, it is highly important that transgender patients are screened appropriately. However, there are often barriers to the transgender population receiving care that not only limit their access to oncologic screening and treatment, but also their inclusion in epidemiological data and research that allows for better characterization of these issues. One of the largest of these barriers is a fear of discrimination. Twenty-eight percent of transgender patients reported delaying their care due to fear of discrimination [7]. Additionally, a quarter of patients experience insurance-related issues that are specific to being transgender [6]. This may be denial of coverage for either care or medications related to their transition process and in some instances denied coverage for being transgender [6]. These issues lead to a lack of preventative care.

K. Scott
Department of Urology, SUNY Upstate Medical Center, Syracuse, NY, USA
e-mail: scottkath@upstate.edu

G. Bratslavsky · E. Ferry (✉)
Department of Urology, Upstate University Hospital, SUNY Upstate Medical University, Syracuse, NY, USA
e-mail: bratslag@upstate.edu; ferrye@upstate.edu

© Springer Nature Switzerland AG 2021
D. Nikolavsky, S. A. Blakely (eds.), *Urological Care for the Transgender Patient*,
https://doi.org/10.1007/978-3-030-18533-6_14

However, even when care is sought, it has been shown that the transgender population received cancer screening at lower rates than the cisgender population [8]. This is in part due to lack of standardized screening recommendations for those who have undergone gender affirmation surgery.

Screening in the transgender population may be further complicated by implicit bias or potential transgender-specific knowledge deficits. The fact that a majority of physicians receive no training with regard to the care of a transgender patient can inhibit the delivery of high-quality care to these patients [9]. A potential area of confusion for providers is the various ways in which a patient may undergo gender affirmation. Patients may undergo medical transitioning in which they take hormones to induce secondary sex characteristics consistent with the self-identified gender. In addition to this, they may also undergo surgical procedures to remove or create gender-specific anatomy. This is referred to as gender affirmation surgery. For patients undergoing surgery, they may undergo "top" surgery, "bottom" surgery, or both. Top surgery refers to surgery performed to remove breast tissue or place implants. Bottom surgery encompasses the spectrum of procedures performed on the genitalia and organs of reproduction, as discussed in other chapters.

Given the numerous issues detailed above, it is easy to see how the transgender community is one at high risk of mismanagement, especially regarding potential malignancies. This chapter focuses on the care of the transgender patient regarding oncologic concerns.

Standard Screening

It is well demonstrated that the transgender population faces many barriers to care. A very important barrier this group faces is that of screening. Regarding cancer screening, multiple studies have demonstrated that the transgender population is screened at lower rates than the cisgender population [6, 8]. For example, transgender men are less likely to be up to date on their Pap smear testing. In a study of transgender males, 8% had

undergone hysterectomy. Of the remaining 92%, only 27% of those studied had a Pap smear test within the last year compared to 43% of cisgender women [6].

One reason for this discrepancy is the lack of national guidelines regarding cancer screening in the transgender population. Various societies offer system-based recommendations and many researchers have also offered recommendations based on their work. The World Professional Association for Transgender Health (WPATH) notes that organ systems which are not affected by hormone use may be monitored by guidelines developed for the general population. In regard to post-transition care, no screening recommendations are provided.

As there is a lack of standardized guidelines or recommendations, we provide our own expert opinion here. For those areas not covered, standard screening should be applied.

Prostate Cancer Screening

In hypogonadal men, especially African American and Afro-Caribbean males, particularly aggressive forms of prostate cancer are known to develop [10]. As of yet, the behavior of the prostate gland in the hypogonadal environment is unknown. Until larger prospective trials of the transgender population are conducted, we recommend annual PSA screening is commenced at age 40.

Testicular Cancer

Considering the fact the testicles are removed, we do not believe that patients require continued screening unless they have a history of testicular cancer prior to procedure.

Penile Cancer

No additional screening is required for penile cancer. Any remaining penile skin should be viewed as skin on any other part of the body and treated accordingly. As of 2019 there are no reports of penile cancer in transgender women. Nevertheless, the incidence of penile cancer is approximately 2080 in the United States, likely making the probability for penile cancer in the transgender population exceedingly low [11]. Patients should be informed to consult with their gynecologist or urologist as this would be part of a typical genital or pelvic examination.

Endometrial Cancer

Considering the known increase risk of endometrial cancer with estrogen use, we would recommend periodic surveillance using ultrasound or biopsy as determined by patients' physician [12]. The authors acknowledge the low incidence of uterine cancer (approximately 62,000 per year) in the United States; however, it has been shown that several factors increase risk, including hormone use, by two to ten-fold [11, 13]. While no epidemiological studies have shown a decrease in mortality with screening, transgender men should be informed and offered, if requested, the opportunity for periodic (biennial) ultrasound-based screening. Additionally they should be promptly referred for any concerning signs of gynecological malignancy. The lack of vagina precludes adequate examination of pelvic viscera, but in this case transrectal ultrasound could provide reasonable ultrasound assessment.

Patient History

The beginnings of oncologic care in the transgender patient start with a thorough history. It is important to ascertain not only the patient's medical affirmation process, but also the surgical procedures performed to both create and remove gender-specific organs. While cancers that may occur in the retained organs of the patient's birth gender are of concern, there are reports of malignancy in neo-organs that also must be considered.

A thorough general history should be obtained for the overall health of the patient, including prior screening history, and the presence of onco-logic risk factors should be determined. Family history should assess for conditions that may be affected by the use of hormones as well as malignancies. A sexual history is important to help determine sexually transmitted infection screening needs. Finally, a social history provides a look at the patient's support structure and is a chance to uncover any non-medical areas in which the patient may need assistance but be hesitant to bring to the attention of the medical provider.

It is critical to obtain information specific to the transgender process, including prior and current hormonal and surgical interventions. The care provider should review hormone use for types and duration. If this cannot be obtained from the patient, records from other providers should be requested. It is important to remember that many patients may obtain their hormones outside of medical practice. These are especially important to confirm that the patient is on appropriate and safely dosed medications.

Of utmost importance is the patient's surgical history. Prior surgical procedures should be discussed with attention paid to which gender-specific organs have been removed and which remain following any gender-affirming procedures. As the specifics may be unknown to the patient, it is important to communicate with the patient's surgeon and obtain operative reports for a complete surgical history. Since gender affirmation surgeries are not standardized among surgeons, it is important to specifically confirm what procedures were performed with respect to which organs are removed and which are preserved in order to provide the best oncologic screening and care.

Transgender Surgery: Surgical Extirpation Specifics

One of the most important aspects of caring for a transgender patient who has undergone gender affirmation surgery is to understand their new anatomy. This entails knowledge of organs removed, organs retained, and neo-organs consistent with their preferred gender.

Table 14.1 Structures removed and retained following gender affirmation surgery

Transgender female	
Removed	**Remains**
Testicles	Penile skin, foreskin, and scrotal skin as neovagina and labia minora/majora
Corpora spongiosa[a], cavernosa[a] (penis)	Glans as the neoclitoris
	Prostate, seminal vesicles
Transgender male	
Removed	**Remains**
Vagina[bc] (colpectomy)	Labia majora[b,c]
Uterus	Clitoris
Breast tissue	Ovaries, fallopian tubes[b]
	Cervix[b]

[a]Indicates partial removal
[b]Removal is variable depending on the patient and surgeon discussion
[c]Portions of the vagina and labia majora may remain as flaps or as components of the pars fixa. In other cases, they may remain due to incomplete excision or regeneration of the cavity due to presence of distal obstruction. Finally, patients may request to preserve this tissue on purpose

Table 14.1 demonstrates the typical structures that are removed or remain after gender-affirming surgery.

Genital Surgery for a Transgender Female

Transfeminine genital affirmation surgery consists of removal of the external male organs of reproduction with the creation of female genitalia. Additionally, patients may undergo breast augmentation independent of the above procedures.

Removal

The testicles and penis are typically removed as part of the complete gender affirmation surgery. Removal of the testicles (orchiectomy) may be done as a solitary procedure, as staged or "early" orchiectomy or at the time of vaginoplasty in conjunction with penectomy. Orchiectomy not only aids in the visual transformation of these patients, but also allows for the cessation of anti-androgen therapy and reduction in estrogen dose by 20–50% [14]. It is important to remember that the entire prostate and seminal vesicles will remain in place after complete genital affirmation surgery. Additionally, proximal portions of corpora cavernosa, corpus spongiosum, and parts or spermatic cord are typically left in place.

Reconstruction

The most common method of neovagina creation is the penile inversion technique with or without scrotal graft [15]. This is an important point due to the risks of having skin incorporated in the genital tract. The newly formed vagina is made of penile shaft skin. Risk factors for penile cancer, such as HPV, may place patients at risk of forming cancers of the neovagina. Finally, the glans is used as part of the neoclitoris and the penile and scrotal skin are used for labioplasty. While penile cancer generally occurs at a low rate, it is important to recognize that this vulnerable tissue would be found in a new location in a transgender female. Additionally, some patients undergo vaginoplasty using bowel segments. These tissues remain at risk for the development of cancer and other intestinal pathologies that may develop in this new location. A single case report describes a cis-female with a history of vaginal agenesis who underwent sigmoid colon neovagina creation. On the work-up of vaginal bleeding 53 years later, a large mass was found; pathology revealed a well-differentiated adeno-carcinoma which was eventually managed with total pelvic exenteration [16]. The same issues may occur in transgender females who have undergone bowel segment vaginoplasty. Other intestinal pathologies have also been described, including the development of simultaneous colonic and neovaginal ulcerative colitis in a previously constructed neovagina using sigmoid colon. This patient ultimately required subtotal colectomy and neovaginectomy [17].

Genital Surgery for the Transgender Male

The cis-gender female reproductive organs including uterus, cervix, ovaries, fallopian tubes, and vagina are not readily visible if totally or partially left in place. Additionally, gender affirmation surgery in transgender males is often more variable as far as which organs are spared and which are removed. Furthermore, the reconstructive options differ based on the desires of the patient. Therefore, patients may undergo some or all of the following described procedures, once again emphasizing the importance of taking thorough surgical history.

Removal

Patients undergo vaginectomy or removal of the vagina. This is done with the closure of the perineum and typically performed at the time of metoidioplasty or phalloplasty. At the discretion of the patient and surgical team, hysterectomy (with or without removal of the cervix) and concurrent salpingo-oophorectomy may also be performed, removing the internal female organs of reproduction. These procedures make up what is typically referred to as "bottom" surgery. An additional component of affirmation surgery that may be completed is mastectomy, or "top" surgery. It is important to note that the mastectomy performed in transgender male patients is not an oncologic procedure and some residual breast tissue remains [18, 19].

Reconstruction

The options are variable depending on the desire and expectations of the patient. A scrotoplasty is performed to create a scrotum from the labia majora. In terms of phallus creation, patients may undergo metoidioplasty or phalloplasty. A metoidioplasty uses local tissues while phalloplasty is accomplished through the use of reconstructive flaps, typically from the leg or forearm.

Organ-Specific Cancer Concerns

The literature regarding cancer cases in the transgender population is limited to small series and case studies. The specific concerns are different for transgender males and transgender females.

Transgender Females

In the transgender female population, clinicians must be cognizant of 3 primary oncologic concerns: prostate cancer, testicular cancer, and penile cancer. Additionally, transgender females may be at risk of both breast and neovaginal cancer.

Prostate Cancer

While prostate cancer is one of the most common cancers in men, the incidence of prostate cancer in the transgender population is low, cited at 0.04% in one large cohort review [20]. With just 9 total cases reported in the literature, our knowledge on this unique circumstance is limited [21–29]. However, given the increase in gender affirmation surgeries being performed and an aging cohort of initial gender affirmation patients, the incidence can only be expected to rise and it is important for providers to have an understanding of management in these patients.

The 9 reported cases of prostate cancer are shown in Table 14.2. Of these patients, all were on some form of long-term hormone treatment. While low androgen states were previously thought to be protective against the development of prostate cancer, newer research indicates this may not be the case. Recent studies have found that suppressed testosterone is a risk factor for the development of prostate cancer, particularly more aggressive forms [20, 30, 31].

With regard to PSA screening, there are no known studies on PSA thresholds on transgender male patients. Therefore, no specific recommendations for PSA cutoffs may be made. It is our expert opinion that screening commence at age 40 as noted before. Shared decision making must be conducted between the provider and patient. Should a transgender male patient require

Table 14.2 Prostate cancer reports in transgender females

Author, year	Pt Age	Presentation	Diagnosis	Hormone treatment	Treatment	Survival
Markland 1975 [21]	54	Unknown	Prostate cancer	Yes, unknown time	Unknown	Unknown
Thurston 1994 [22]	64	Prostatism	T3 poorly differentiated adenocarcinoma	12 years	Radiation × 6 months, 6400 cGy	Developed metastatic disease 1 year later, died 6 months following metastases
van Haarst 1998 [23]	63	Weight loss, bone pain	Metastatic prostate cancer	10 years	Chemotherapy	Alive at author publication
Miksad 2006 [24]	60	Gross hematuria, mass on neovaginal exam	Localized Gleason 8	41 years	Androgen deprivation and radiation	Alive at author publication
Dorff 2007 [25]	78	Prostate nodule	Gleason 9 (4 + 5)	23 years	Radiation	Developed metastatic disease 7 months later and received chemotherapy. Was started on ketoconazole after treatment. Alive at author publication.
Turo 2013 [26]	75	LUTS	Localized Gleason 7	30 years	Radiation	Developed metastatic disease 5 years later and received chemotherapy. Died 3 years following metastatic disease
Ellent 2016 [27]	65	Difficulty voiding	Gleason 9 (4 + 5)	35 years	Neoadjuvant chemotherapy and open cystoprostatectomy	Biochemical recurrence 1.5 years post surgery
Sharif 2017 [28]	56	Abnormal DRE	Localized Gleason 7	20 years	RALP + BPLND	Alive at author publication
Deebel 2017 [29]	65	Elevated PSA	Localized Gleason 7	20 years	RALP	Alive at author publication

prostate biopsy, we recommend two possible routes. Should the neovagina have adequate length and caliber, the biopsy may be conducted transvaginally. As a reminder, DRE is also to be done transvaginally in this set of patients. Alternatively, a transperineal biopsy may be performed.

Testicular Cancer

In a systematic review by Joint et al. (2018), 43 articles were analyzed with one case report of testicular cancer described [2]. This case report describes a transgender female who had undergone 2 years of gender-affirming hormone treatment. She was found to have intratubular germ cell carcinoma [32]. It is our recommendation that following orchiectomy the tissue undergoes surgical pathology evaluation for underlying carcinoma of the testicle. Additionally, in patients to present with retroperitoneal mass later on in life, consideration should be given for latent metastatic disease.

Breast Cancer

In caring for the transgender female population, it is important to consider the natural breast tissue. As patients retain the normal breast tissues, they are susceptible to breast cancer. Two large cohort studies examined the rates of breast cancer in transgender female patients. In the first, 2307 patients were examined with 1 developing breast cancer, a rate generally expected in the cismale population [33]. For this reason, they concluded that the hormones typically used by these patients do not appear to increase the risk of breast cancer. These findings were supported by a larger cohort study of 3566 transgender female patients in which 2 developed breast cancer [34]. Compared to the SEER database, this rate did not differ significantly from the expected rate in the cisgender male population. Therefore, while not at increased risk, breast cancer remains a concern for transgender females at the same rate and with risk factors seen in the cisgender male population due to retained natural breast tissue. Physicians should be aware of this and screen patients accordingly if family history reveals they are at increased risk of cancer based on inherited genetic mutations.

Neovagina

A unique concern in these patients is the neovagina, which itself is susceptible to malignancy. There have been two documented case reports of squamous cell carcinoma of the neovagina after penile inversion vaginoplasty and a single case of neoplasia development in the neocervix created from residual glans tissue [2, 35–37]. Cytologic examination was found to look like that of the normal cervix in a small percentage of cases [38]. Despite this, environmental risk factors, such as micro-trauma from sexual intercourse and recurrent dilations, exist and may increase the risk of precancerous lesion formation and cancer screening is recommended [38].

Transgender Males

Cervical Cancer

In a systematic review of transgender oncologic literature, there were no reported cases of cervical cancer in patients having undergone gender affirmation surgery [2]. There are however two reports of cervical cancers in transgender men that were discovered during the planning of affirmation surgery [39]. It is estimated that 8% of transgender male patients having affirmation surgery undergo radical hysterectomy and concomitant removal of the cervix [6]. In these patients the surgical specimen should be examined for potential cervical cancers. In most patients, however, the cervix remains in situ and thus remains at risk for the development of cancer.

With retention of the cervix transgender male patients remain at risk for HPV infection, a known cause of cervical cancer. It is for this reason that patients should undergo surveillance with pelvic exam and Papanicolaou (Pap smear) examination. Professional societies recommend that transgender women undergo the same screening as that performed in cisgender women [40]. However, when rates of Pap smears performed in these two populations are compared, transgender men are screened at lower rates [41] than cisgender women with 27% of transgender men receiving screening compared to 43% of cisgender women [6]. In transgender men who are screened, inadequate pathology specimens are frequently found, attributed to prior testosterone use [42]. Additionally, previous testosterone use may make distinguishing atrophy from dysplasia difficult [3]. Therefore, it is not only the clinical provider that must be aware of specific concerns in the transgender patient, but also the pathologist.

Breast Cancer

The incidence of breast cancer in transgender men has been calculated at 4.3–5.9 per 100,000 [33, 34]. This is close to the rate seen in cisgender men (1 in 100,000) [33]. It has therefore been concluded that the cancer risk in these individuals is in line with their gender identity rather than their gender assigned at birth. The lower than expected rate as compared to cisgender females is attributed to mastectomy and testosterone treatment [33]. As of 2018, there are 18 known cases of breast cancer in transgender men. Greater than 75% of these patients were found to have hormone positive cancers. Additionally, in eight of these cases cancer developed in patients who had previously undergone mastectomy, suggesting this is not completely protective and these patients should still receive standard breast cancer screening as is recommended in ciswomen [2].

Ovarian Cancer

There have been a limited number of ovarian cancer cases in transgender males [2]. As not all individuals undergo complete removal of the female reproductive structures, it is important that providers have a complete surgical history and if the ovaries remain that ovarian cancer be a part of the differential diagnosis when appropriate.

Vaginal Cancer

There exists one case report of vaginal cancer in a transgender male patient who had undergone gender affirmation surgery with hysterectomy and phalloplasty [2]. This patient developed stage IV squamous cell carcinoma of the remnant vaginal tissue, which presented as an invasive mass between the vagina and anus 18 years following surgery [43]. This should be considered in patients with similar findings.

Surgical Considerations

Possibly one of the greatest and most unique concerns in transgender oncology care is the surgical considerations in those having undergone gender affirmation surgery. Those patients requiring surgical intervention after affirmation surgery present a challenge because anatomy may differ from that typically encountered during a given operation. Of particular interest is the transgender female patient requiring extirpative prostate surgery. To date, there have been no reported cases of prostate surgery taking place in a transgender female post genital affirmation surgery. In the few reported cases of prostate cancer occurring in this population, patients have undergone non-surgical management of their disease. There are two reports of a robotic-assisted laparoscopic radical prostatectomy performed on transgender female patients; however, both had only undergone hormonal transformation and/or top surgery [28, 29].

Despite the low number of prostate cancer cases reported in the literature thus far, it can only be assumed this number will increase as the rate of transgender surgery continues to increase. It is likely urologists will encounter those patients needing extirpative prostate surgery who have previously undergone gender affirmation surgery. With no available case reports, these first cases will lay the groundwork for future procedures in terms of surgical approach. Unique considerations we expect to be addressed in these patients include dissection in the posterior plane of the prostate, a challenging bladder neck anastomosis, and likely higher rates of post-prostatectomy incontinence and vesicourethral anastomotic fistula to the neovagina.

Due to the creation of the neovagina and its location between the prostate and rectum, we expect the posterior plane to be fused and the dissection difficult. Attention to the location of the neovagina during this dissection would be critical, as to not disrupt the areolar tissue and potentially compromise blood flow to the flap.

Post-operative continence and healing at the vesicourethral anastomosis could be of concern. The urethra has been shortened and likely scarred in place from the previous procedures. Additionally, the blood supply to the urethra may be compromised following proximal division of the urethra, especially if the interval from affirmation surgery is short. In addition to the baseline risks of incontinence following prostatectomy, these individuals may have lost some function of their external sphincter during the genital affirmation surgery.

While a perineal prostatectomy would present a challenge in this population, the positioning and potential robotic port placement would be unchanged for a retropubic prostatectomy. The space of Retzius, bladder, and position of the prostate and seminal vesicles should also be unchanged. The decision of performing a nerve-sparing procedure should also still be considered, as nerve-sparing prostatectomy may be associated with improved continence.

From an oncologic standpoint, prostate surgery presents what is likely the greatest challenge in those having undergone affirmation surgery. However, any reproductive organ-based cancer in transgender individuals represents a new and evolving area of medicine that may present challenges yet unknown. It is critically important that these be reported in the literature to begin establishing a basis for reference going forward.

Conclusion

In conclusion, the oncologic care of transgender patients is an area in need of research. From basic science research that studies hormone use and cancer risk, to epidemiologic studies that more accurately assess the potential cancer burden in this population, there are many areas that need to be explored. Furthermore, as the transgender population grows, it becomes ever more important that standardized screening recommendations be developed to aid in the care of these patients. As discussed in this chapter, the cancer reports in these patients are limited. We encourage those who care for these patients to remember this population is at risk of under screening. Providers should strive to educate themselves in transgender care, particularly preventative medicine, and provide the critical screening needed in these patients. It is our hope that development of the transgender oncology literature will allow for discoveries to facilitate future encounters with patients.

> **Key Points**
> - Patient history, including surgical, is key to oncologic care of the transgender patient.
> - Patients should be screened for malignancy of organs that remain following gender affirmation surgery.
> - Oncologic concerns of the transgender patient is a field of study likely to expand as this cohort of patients expands. Research should be directed toward this area.

References

1. Kiran T, Davie S, Singh D, Hranilovic S, Pinto AD, Abramovich A, et al. Cancer screening rates among transgender adults: Cross-sectional analysis of primary care data. Can Fam Physician. 2019;65(1):e30–e7.
2. Joint R, Chen ZE, Cameron S. Breast and reproductive cancers in the transgender population: a systematic review. BJOG. 2018;125(12):1505–12.
3. Deutsch M. Guidelines for the primary and gender-affirming care of transgender and gender nonbinary people. 2nd ed: University of California San Francisco, Center of Excellence for Transgender Health, Department of Family and Community Medicine; 2016.
4. Ceres M, Quinn GP, Loscalzo M, Rice D. Cancer screening considerations and cancer screening uptake for lesbian, gay, bisexual, and transgender persons. Semin Oncol Nurs. 2018;34(1):37–51.
5. Feldman J, Deutsch M. Primary care of transgender individuals UpToDate2019 [updated October 2018; cited 2018].
6. James SE, Herman JL, Rankin S, Keisling M, Mottet L, Anafi M. The report of the 2015 U.S. transgender survey. National Center for Transgender Equality: Washinton, DC; 2016.
7. Grant JM, Mottet LA, Tanis J, Herman JL, Harrison J, Keisling M. National transgender discrimination survey report on health and health care. Washington, DC: National Center for Transgender Equality and the National Gay and Lesbian Task Force; 2010.
8. Gatos KC. A literature review of cervical cancer screening in transgender men. Nurs Womens Health. 2018;22(1):52–62.
9. Unger CA. Care of the transgender patient: a survey of gynecologists' current knowledge and practice. J Womens Health (Larchmt). 2015;24(2):114–8.
10. Rebbeck TR. Prostate cancer genetics: variation by race, ethnicity, and geography. Semin Radiat Oncol. 2017;27(1):3–10.
11. Siegel RL, Miller KD, Jemal A. Cancer statistics, 2019. CA Cancer J Clin. 2019;69(1):7–34.
12. Grady D, Gebretsadik T, Kerlikowske K, Ernster V, Petitti D. Hormone replacement therapy and endometrial cancer risk: a meta-analysis. Obstet Gynecol. 1995;85(2):304–13.
13. Smith RA, Andrews KS, Brooks D, Fedewa SA, Manassaram-Baptiste D, Saslow D, et al. Cancer screening in the United States, 2019: a review of current American Cancer Society guidelines and current issues in cancer screening. CA Cancer J Clin. 2019;69(3):184–210.
14. Kent MA, Winoker JS, Grotas AB. Effects of feminizing hormones on sperm production and malignant changes: microscopic examination of post orchiectomy specimens in transwomen. Urology. 2018;121:93–6.
15. Bizic M, Kojovic V, Duisin D, Stanojevic D, Vujovic S, Milosevic A, et al. An overview of neovaginal reconstruction options in male to female transsexuals. Sci World J. 2014;2014:638919.
16. Yamada K, Shida D, Kato T, Yoshida H, Yoshinaga S, Kanemitsu Y. Adenocarcinoma arising in sigmoid colon neovagina 53 years after construction. World J Surg Oncol. 2018;16(1):88.
17. Webster T, Appelbaum H, Weinstein TA, Rosen N, Mitchell I, Levine JJ. Simultaneous development of

ulcerative colitis in the colon and sigmoid neovagina. J Pediatr Surg. 2013;48(3):669–72.

18. McEvenue G, Xu FZ, Cai R, McLean H. Female-to-male gender affirming top surgery: a single surgeon's 15-year retrospective review and treatment algorithm. Aesthet Surg J. 2017;38(1):49–57.

19. Deutsch MB, Radix A, Wesp L. Breast Cancer screening, management, and a review of case study literature in transgender populations. Semin Reprod Med. 2017;35(5):434–41.

20. Gooren L, Morgentaler A. Prostate cancer incidence in orchidectomised male-to-female transsexual persons treated with oestrogens. Andrologia. 2014;46(10):1156–60.

21. Markland C. Transexual surgery. Obstet Gynecol Annu. 1975;4:309–30.

22. Thurston AV. Carcinoma of the prostate in a transsexual. Br J Urol. 1994;73(2):217.

23. van Haarst EP, Newling DW, Gooren LJ, Asscheman H, Prenger DM. Metastatic prostatic carcinoma in a male-to-female transsexual. Br J Urol. 1998;81(5):776.

24. Miksad RA, Bubley G, Church P, Sanda M, Rofsky N, Kaplan I, et al. Prostate cancer in a transgender woman 41 years after initiation of feminization. JAMA. 2006;296(19):2316–7.

25. Dorff TB, Shazer RL, Nepomuceno EM, Tucker SJ. Successful treatment of metastatic androgen-independent prostate carcinoma in a transsexual patient. Clin Genitourin Cancer. 2007;5(5):344–6.

26. Turo R, Jallad S, Prescott S, Cross WR. Metastatic prostate cancer in transsexual diagnosed after three decades of estrogen therapy. Can Urol Assoc J. 2013;7(7–8):E544–6.

27. Ellent E, Matrana MR. Metastatic prostate cancer 35 years after sex reassignment surgery. Clin Genitourin Cancer. 2016;14(2):e207–9.

28. Sharif A, Malhotra NR, Acosta AM, Kajdacsy-Balla AA, Bosland M, Guzman G, et al. The development of prostate adenocarcinoma in a transgender male to female patient: could estrogen therapy have played a role? Prostate. 2017;77(8):824–8.

29. Deebel NA, Morin JP, Autorino R, Vince R, Grob B, Hampton LJ. Prostate Cancer in transgender women: incidence, etiopathogenesis, and management challenges. Urology. 2017;110:166–71.

30. Morgentaler A, Rhoden EL. Prevalence of prostate cancer among hypogonadal men with prostate-specific antigen levels of 4.0 ng/mL or less. Urology. 2006;68(6):1263–7.

31. Hoffman MA, DeWolf WC, Morgentaler A. Is low serum free testosterone a marker for high grade prostate cancer? J Urol. 2000;163(3):824–7.

32. Wolf-Gould CS, Wolf-Gould CH. A transgender woman with testicular cancer: a new twist on an old problem. LGBT Health. 2016;3(1):90–5.

33. Gooren LJ, van Trotsenburg MA, Giltay EJ, van Diest PJ. Breast cancer development in transsexual subjects receiving cross-sex hormone treatment. J Sex Med. 2013;10(12):3129–34.

34. Brown GR, Jones KT. Incidence of breast cancer in a cohort of 5,135 transgender veterans. Breast Cancer Res Treat. 2015;149(1):191–8.

35. Harder Y, Erni D, Banic A. Squamous cell carcinoma of the penile skin in a neovagina 20 years after male-to-female reassignment. Br J Plast Surg. 2002;55(5):449–51.

36. Fernandes HM, Manolitsas TP, Jobling TW. Carcinoma of the neovagina after male-to-female reassignment. J Low Genit Tract Dis. 2014;18(2):E43–5.

37. Lawrence A. Vaginal neoplasia in a male-to-female transsexual: case report, review of the literature, and recommendations for cytological screening. Int J Transgender. 2001;5(1).

38. Grosse A, Grosse C, Lenggenhager D, Bode B, Camenisch U, Bode P. Cytology of the neovagina in transgender women and individuals with congenital or acquired absence of a natural vagina. Cytopathology. 2017;28(3):184–91.

39. Braun H, Nash R, Tangpricha V, Brockman J, Ward K, Goodman M. Cancer in transgender people: evidence and methodological considerations. Epidemiol Rev. 2017;39(1):93–107.

40. American College of Obstetricians and Gynecologists. Committee opinion: health care for transgender individuals. Obstet Gynecol. 2011;118(6):1454–8.

41. Peitzmeier SM, Khullar K, Reisner SL, Potter J. Pap test use is lower among female-to-male patients than non-transgender women. Am J Prev Med. 2014;47(6):808–12.

42. Peitzmeier SM, Reisner SL, Harigopal P, Potter J. Female-to-male patients have high prevalence of unsatisfactory Paps compared to non-transgender females: implications for cervical cancer screening. J Gen Intern Med. 2014;29(5):778–84.

43. Schenck TL, Holzbach T, Zantl N, Schuhmacher C, Vogel M, Seidl S, et al. Vaginal carcinoma in a female-to-male transsexual. J Sex Med. 2010;7(8):2899–902.

Care of Transgender Patients: Incontinence

Natasha Ginzburg

Abbreviations

AUA	American Urological Association
BC	Bulbocavernosus
BMI	Body mass index
CHF	Congestive heart failure
EAU	European Association of Urology
ICIQ	International consultation on incontinence questionnaire
ICS	International Continence Society
KHQ	King's Health Questionnaire
NHANES	National Health and Nutrition Examination Survey
NICE	National Institute of Clinical Excellence
OAB	Overactive bladder
OABq	Overactive bladder questionnaire
OAB-SS	Overactive bladder symptoms score
OAB-V8	Overactive bladder 8 questionnaire
PSA	Prostate-specific antigen
PVR	Post-void residual
SUI	Stress urinary incontinence

N. Ginzburg (✉)
Upstate Urology, Syracuse, NY, USA
e-mail: ginzburn@upstate.edu

Incontinence

Background and Epidemiology

Urinary incontinence is a common condition that can have a vast impact on an individual's quality of life. There are no studies focused on rates of urinary incontinence in transgender persons prior to gender affirmation surgery. Due to the sparsity of data, it may be possible to extrapolate some information from cisgender persons in order to understand, evaluate, and treat certain types of incontinence in the transgender individual.

The International Continence Society (ICS) defines various types of urinary incontinence. In general, "urinary incontinence is defined as the complaint of any involuntary leakage of urine" [1]. Incontinence can then be sub-characterized based on other factors, including stress urinary incontinence (SUI), which is defined as involuntary loss of urine associated with physical activity or exertion, or coughing/sneezing. Urge incontinence is incontinence associated temporally with the urge to void. Other types of urinary incontinence may occur immediately after micturition, such as post-void dribbling. Patients may also experience continuous urinary leakage or situational incontinence, as with giggle incontinence, coital incontinence, or functional incontinence [1].

The exact rate and prevalence of urinary incontinence in the general population is a sur-

© Springer Nature Switzerland AG 2021
D. Nikolavsky, S. A. Blakely (eds.), *Urological Care for the Transgender Patient*,
https://doi.org/10.1007/978-3-030-18533-6_15

prisingly elusive figure. The rates reported are dependent on many factors, including type of incontinence studied, patient natal sex, age, and definition of incontinence. The vast majority of epidemiologic studies on incontinence focus on urine loss in presumed cisgender women. When examining the National Health and Nutrition Examination Survey (NHANES), Nygaard et al. identified a prevalence of urinary incontinence in women of 15.7% [2]. The definition focused on the question of urine leakage of "at least weekly or monthly leakage of more than drops." When looking at similar data from NHANES, but defining incontinence as *any* urine leakage, Markland et al. found rates of 51% [3] in women. This large discrepancy is likely related to the definition of incontinence. Certainly, incontinence rates seem to increase with age, with incidence rates increasing from 6.9% to 11% in women less than 55 years of age to 13.8% in women from 54 to 79 years of age [4]. Additionally, urinary incontinence rates can be further divided based on symptom severity (mild, moderate, and severe) as well as by type of incontinence [5], i.e., stress or urge. In cisgender women, rates of urge-predominant incontinence were reported to range from 10% to 20% in the evaluation of the Group Health Cooperative Survey, while rates of stress-predominant incontinence ranged from 16% to 45%. Rates of mixed incontinence were reported ranging from 41% to 57% of all female responders [5].

In the few large studies that examine incontinence in presumed cisgender men, the rates are significantly lower. Markland et al. focused on self-reported urinary incontinence in the NHANES survey, analyzing data for 5297 men over the age of 20. The rate of any urinary incontinence was found to be 12%; however, men over 75 years old had rates of urinary incontinence of 16% [6]. When looking at the subtypes of incontinence, the majority reported urge incontinence (48%), followed by "other incontinence" (23%) and mixed incontinence (15.4%). The percent of those reporting urinary incontinence related to activity (SUI) was 12.5%. These data are consistent with Diokno et al.'s analysis of the National Family Opinion

World Group Panel in the US; again, approximately 12% of cisgender men reported some urinary incontinence [7]. Interestingly, the proportion reporting stress incontinence was higher, a total of 24.5%. When examining a cohort of men with lower urinary tract symptoms, but excluding men with a history of prostate cancer, Helfand et al. found the proportion complaining of stress incontinence to be much lower, at 3.4% [8]. In that cohort, men presenting with any lower urinary tract symptoms were found to have urinary incontinence rates of 50%, including a large proportion of patients with post-void dribbling.

As the scientific literature grows surrounding outcome measures in transgender surgery, we will likely have more data on prevalence and rates of urinary incontinence in patients undergoing genital affirmation procedures. At this time, the vast majority of outcome measures of transgender surgery, both male and female, focus on major post-operative complications, sexual function, and cosmesis rather than urinary quality of life issues [9–12].

There are small series examining urinary dysfunction after gender affirmation surgery. While much of the focus is on major urethral complications, a small series of 52 transgender female patients, rates of urinary urgency were found to be 24.6% and stress incontinence was found to be 23% [13]. A small study of 18 transgender patients by Kuhn et al. demonstrated a significant rate of incontinence of 33%, mostly due to stress urinary incontinence and overactive bladder [14]. Other studies note post-void dribbling rates to be as high as 79% in transgender male patients, with overall incontinence rates in transgender female patients being approximately 16% [15].

Although the exact rates of incontinence vary based on definitions, it is clear that urge incontinence provides a burdensome cost. The National Overactive Bladder Evaluation study examined costs associated with overactive bladder and urge incontinence. In 2007, the costs were estimated at $65.9 billion. Given the increasing age of the US population, this figure is only expected to grow, with a projected cost of $82.6 billion by 2020 [16, 17].

Risk Factors

The discrepancies in prevalence rates may also reflect not only differences in definitions of incontinence, but also, variability in groups analyzed. There are a number of risk factors that have been identified for urinary incontinence in presumed cisgender men and women. The evaluation of the Group Health Cooperative Survey identified several risk factors for urinary incontinence in women; specifically increasing age, more vaginal deliveries, history of hysterectomy, obesity as well as depression [5]. A review published by Almousa et al., excluded parous women and specifically investigated risk factors in younger women with no history of pregnancy or delivery. In this review, higher BMI, childhood enuresis, and high-impact exercise were found to be risk factors for any type of incontinence [18].

In cisgender men, while overall incontinence rates are lower, certain risk factors are consistent. A study conducted in Australia evaluated urinary incontinence after stroke. The study found an increased rate of incontinence after stroke that persisted for over a year in 65% of those with new onset urinary leakage after stroke in both men and women [19]. A population-based study in Taiwan noted a significant increase in rates of incontinence amongst men with diabetes compared to those without [20]. When examining the prevalence of urinary incontinence in the NHANES survey, Markland et al. found hypertension, age as well as depression to be independent risk factors for incontinence in men [6]. Other risk factors identified for bladder overactivity in men include obstructive sleep apnea [21], as well as metabolic syndrome [22]. When specifically examining stress urinary incontinence in cisgender men, the most common risk factor is disruption of the urethral sphincter. This is most likely with prostate surgery such as radical prostatectomy or transurethral resection of prostate. Trauma with injury to the pelvic nerves, radiation, and certain neurological conditions can also predispose men to stress urinary incontinence [23]. In transgender women status post genital affirmation surgery,

disruption of the nerve bundles during dissection to create the neovagina may play a role in future incontinence, as well as the change in anatomic position of the bladder [15]. Even setting aside the complex complications of genital affirmation surgery, it is likely that there is some inherent risk of the procedure itself in increasing risk of urinary incontinence. Certainly, transgender women who have undergone a prior radical prostatectomy or transurethral prostate surgery have a predisposing risk of dysregulation of the bladder neck or neuromuscular control of continence. In our institutional experience, these patients are those more likely to present with stress urinary incontinence or fistula.

Evaluation of Urinary Incontinence

When evaluating any patient with urinary incontinence, it is important to obtain a thorough and thoughtful history. Defining the type of incontinence and any inciting factors is crucial to understanding the potential etiology of the complaint. Whether the incontinence is related to overactive bladder (OAB) type symptoms or to exertion/stress maneuvers is important to evaluate. Specifically, any reversible causes of incontinence should be assessed and addressed (see Table 15.1).

While history alone is not always a reliable method to diagnose a specific type of incontinence, for many patients it can significantly narrow the clinician's differential diagnosis. Key components of the urologic history of the incontinent patient include duration of symptoms and

Table 15.1 Reversible or transient causes of urinary incontinence

D	Delirium
I	Infection (specifically, urinary tract infection)
A	Atrophic vaginitis
P	Pharmaceuticals
P	Psychological disorders
E	Excessive urine output (such as in diabetics, CHF patients)
R	Restricted mobility
S	Stool impaction/constipation

Table adapted from Resnick et al. [24]

any inciting events (surgery, trauma, infection), accounting of events causing leakage (exercise, body positioning, sneeze/cough, urgency), quantification (continuous, daily, weekly, use of pads/liners/diapers), and identifying the impact on the patient. If symptom onset coincided after gender affirmation surgery, the temporal association (immediately after surgery, after packing removal, after initiation of dilation, etc.) should be assessed.

Reviewing the patient's other medical problems, dietary habits, and surgical history is also valuable in assessing incontinence. Optimizing medications while considering their impact on incontinence can be an effective way to decrease incontinence episodes. Special attention should be paid to neurologic diagnoses, depression/anxiety as well as obesity, and metabolic syndrome that can affect incontinence. Surgical history should focus on prior pelvic and spinal surgery as well as pelvic radiation that may impact the neurologic control of voiding. Additionally, transgender male patients should be assessed for prior parity either via vaginal deliveries or cesarean sections. Surgery of the prostate, vagina, or rectum can all impact normal voiding.

The evaluation of the patient's dietary habits is also helpful in assessing incontinence. Caffeine, carbonated beverages, and artificial sweeteners have all been implicated in worsening urinary urgency and detrusor contractions (see Table 15.2). Review and possible elimination of the most common dietary bladder irritants can also impact bladder overactivity symptoms [25].

Table 15.2 Common dietary bladder irritants exacerbating OAB

Most common irritants	Other reported irritants
Caffeine (keep doses <200 mg/day)	Spicy foods
Carbonated beverages	Acidic floods (i.e., tomato, orange juice)
Aspartame/artificial sweeteners	Hidden caffeine sources (chocolate, medications)
Energy drinks	
Alcohol	

Adapted from Wyman et al. [26]

Physical Examination

A physical examination is fundamental in the evaluation of urinary incontinence. General evaluation, obesity, gross neurologic deficits all may influence diagnosis, future testing, and treatment options. An abdominal examination may detect a palpable bladder. Neurologic evaluation, including assessing sensation, upper and lower extremity weakness, as well as bulbocavernosus reflex (BC) can identify neurologic causes of symptoms. In transgender male patients who have not undergone genital affirmation surgery, the examination of the pelvis, vagina, and urethra is important. Vaginal atrophy, common in postmenopausal women, has been shown to effect symptoms of bladder overactivity [27]. Similarly, the assessment of urethral hypermobility, provoking stress incontinence via positive cough stress test, and assessing for pelvic organ prolapse are all central to the examination of the transgender male patient who has not undergone genital surgery. In the transgender female patient who has not undergone genital affirmation surgery, digital rectal examination of the prostate and the assessment of rectal tone are important aspects of the physical examination. The evaluation of the urethral meatus can assess for evidence of meatal stenosis.

In all post-surgical transgender patients, the exact surgical procedure, including any flaps, their blood supply, and current anatomic relationships are crucial to understand. Communication with the original operating surgeon can be extremely helpful as well as obtaining and reviewing original operative and post-operative reports.

For the transgender male who has undergone gender affirmation, the examination of the reconstructed urethral meatus can be valuable, as well as rectal examination to assess for tone. If the patient underwent metoidioplasty, the glans penis may still be utilized to assess bulbocavernosus reflex, although the fraction of neurologically intact transgender patients with an intact BC reflex is unknown.

In the post-surgical transgender female who has undergone genital affirmation surgery, it is important to understand the current anatomic relationships. The vast majority of gender affirmation procedures to construct a neovagina are performed posterior to Denonvillier's fascia, anterior to the rectum. In these patients, examination of the prostate may need to be performed via the examination of the anterior aspect of the neovagina. The urethral meatus should be examined for stenosis, as well as evidence of hypermobility. For patients complaining of stress incontinence, a positive leak with valsalva or cough is important to make the diagnosis of SUI. Careful examination of the neovagina can demonstrate a urogenital fistula, or other structural abnormality (See Figs. 15.1 and 15.2).

Testing

All individuals presenting with urinary incontinence should undergo a urinalysis and post-void residual testing (PVR) [28, 29]. Urinalysis is

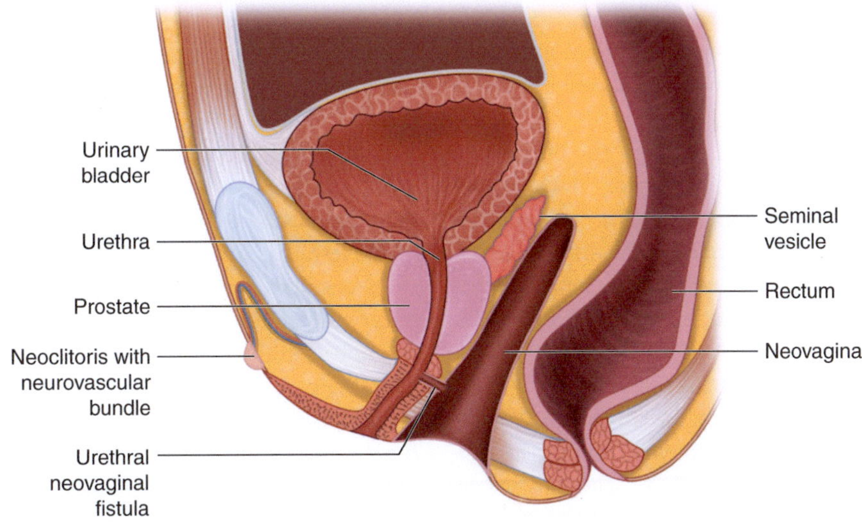

Fig. 15.1 Urethral neovaginal fistula

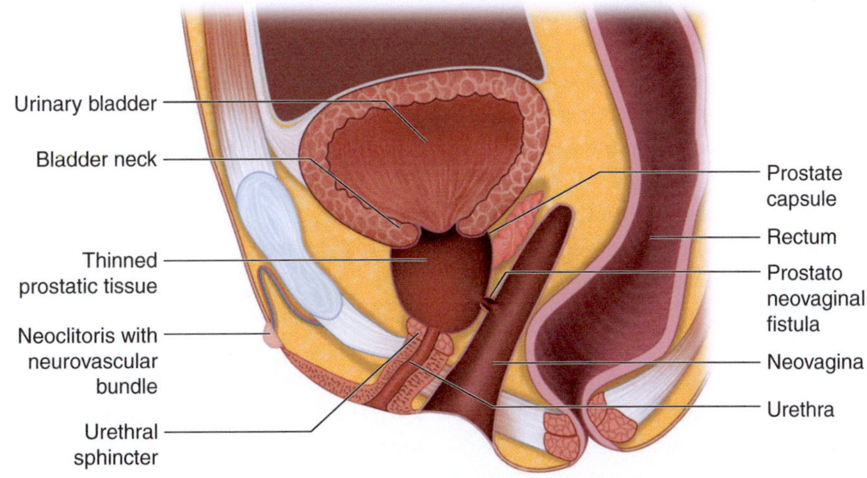

Fig. 15.2 Prostato-negovaginal fistula

important to assess for infection, glucosuria/diabetes as a source of symptoms. PVR can be performed either via ultrasound, or catheterization. Ultrasound examination has been demonstrated to have equivalent accuracy to in-and-out catheterization [30]. The evaluation of post-void residual by either method not only helps to establish evidence of bladder emptying but is also helpful for following baseline bladder emptying after intervention for incontinence.

Patients should also record a voiding or bladder diary. Information obtained should include fluid intake, voiding frequency, volume voided. The length of time has been debated (3–5 days vs 7 days) [31], but finding a compromise between obtaining useful information and patient compliance is important [32].

Pad tests are not necessary for the routine evaluation of urinary incontinence; however, they are an important measure for incontinence research [33]. The volume of a "positive" pad test varies in the cisgender community, and no values exist for transgender patients, but the testing can be useful when following patients through various anti-incontinence treatments.

There are a multitude of questionnaires to assess lower urinary tract symptoms, urinary incontinence, and bladder overactivity. The most useful questionnaires will screen for the amount of incontinence, bother and patient quality of life. The OABq [34], ICIQ [35], and OAB-SS [36], KHQ [37], and OAB-V8 [38] have all been validated in both men and women to assess for incontinence, its impact on quality of life, and symptom bother (see Table 15.3). There are many other questionnaires available that target either cisgender men or women specifically, but none focused on transgender persons. While questionnaires are not a substitute for history, physical exam, and focused testing, they can be useful for following patients.

Uroflowmetry is a useful, noninvasive test to assess certain voiding parameters. There are no accepted normal values in cisgender women, nor in transgender individuals after gender affirmation surgery. Nonetheless, uroflometry can be used to monitor treatment outcomes and to associate treatment outcomes with patient-reported symptoms [39].

Table 15.3 Common questionnaires for the evaluation of lower urinary tract symptoms in both men and women

Questionnaire	Purpose	Length
OABq	Assessing health-related quality of life	33 items
ICIQ	Assessing health-related quality of life	4 items
OAB-SS	Screening for overactivity, incontinence, and symptoms	4 items
OAB-V8	Screening for overactivity and patient awareness	9 items
KHQ	Assessing health-related quality of life	29 items

Urodynamic testing can offer more detailed information on the etiology of urinary complaints, although blind placement of urethral catheters could be challenging in patients after phalloplasty, Routine use of urodynamics is debated; however, most experts agree that urodynamic testing is important prior to invasive surgical procedures, or in patients with failed prior interventions, history of pelvic surgery, difficult diagnostic evaluation or those with a possible neurologic cause of symptoms [40]. The addition of fluoroscopy (video urodynamics) can provide further information of the anatomy at the time of functional evaluation of the bladder.

Routine cystoscopy in the standard OAB or stress incontinence patient is debated [28]. Cystoscopy can provide information on other potential pathologies that can contribute to urinary symptoms such as bladder stones, tumors, strictures, evidence of bladder outlet obstruction. Cystoscopy is important in patients with hematuria or other irritative symptoms, hematuria, prior pelvic or anti-incontinence surgery, or prior to certain transurethral prostate interventions [41].

Prostate-specific antigen (PSA) testing is controversial. Both the European Association of Urology (EAU) and National Institute of Clinical Excellence (NICE) guidelines suggest PSA testing as an option after appropriate counseling [39]. If a diagnosis of prostate cancer will change management, or as the estimate of prostate size and potential disease progression, PSA testing may be clinically useful. The effect of feminizing hormones is still unclear on PSA values; the role of PSA testing in the transgender female population is still to be established.

Treatment of Bladder Overactivity and Urge Incontinence

Once the diagnosis of bladder overactivity and urge incontinence has been made, the first steps in treatment focus on conservative options. Bladder overactivity is defined as urinary urgency, with or without urge incontinence, often with urinary frequency, and/or nocturia in the absence of other pathology [1]. There are no guidelines for the treatment of bladder overactivity that are specific to the transgender community. Assuming a non-neurogenic etiology of the OAB symptoms, treatment can likely follow the OAB guidelines for the general population as developed by the American Urological Association (AUA). All patients can benefit from behavioral modifications, decreasing bladder irritants, and monitoring fluid intake and voiding frequency [26, 28]. Additionally, conservative treatment with pelvic floor physical therapy and deferment techniques can improve outcomes [26, 42]. Interestingly, there is some data that demonstrates up to a third of cis male patients with bladder overactivity will have spontaneous symptom resolution [43].

There is no evidence for the use of topical estrogen in the hormonally treated transgender male patient who has not undergone gender affirmation surgery. There is evidence that topical application of estrogen in low doses does not increase serum estrogen levels above expected post-menopausal levels [44]. It is possible that low-dose vaginal estrogen use may be beneficial for urinary symptoms without impacting the systemic hormones [27].

The majority of pharmacological treatments for OAB are antimuscarinic agents. Various clinical trials have evaluated antimuscarinic use in cisgender male and female populations. In male patients with a prostate, the concern for urinary retention related to bladder outlet obstruction has led to a number of studies specifically evaluating anti-muscarinic use in this population. Fesoterodine, tolterodine with and without additional tamsulosin have been studied in the cisgender male population [45, 46]. Rates of urinary retention due to BPH are low. In the transgender female who still has a prostate, it is unclear what role feminizing hormones will have on bladder obstruction from the remaining prostate. Even in patients with BPH, it appears anti-muscarinics are relatively safe and effective to decrease overactivity symptoms. Mirabegron has been studied specifically in cisgender men in Korea, with good improvement on OAB symptoms and no significant increase in PVR [47].

For patients in whom conservative treatments and medications are not successful in controlling OAB symptoms, third-line treatments may be indicated. The options include sacral neuromodulation, posterior tibial nerve stimulation, and intravesical botulinum toxin administration [28] (see Table 15.4).

Treatment of Stress Urinary Incontinence

Stress incontinence, or stress-predominant mixed incontinence, patients seeking treatment may be offered conservative measures such as pelvic

Table 15.4 Summary of third-line therapies for bladder overactivity [28]

Third-line therapy	Recommendation	Notes
Intradetrusor botulinum Toxin A	100 unit intradetrusor injection for non-neurogenic bladder overactivity	Urinary retention; patient must be willing to self-catheterize if necessary
Sacral neuromodulation	Surgical placement after appropriate response to test stimulation for bladder overactivity symptoms	May require additional surgery; patient must be aware of limitations of device (i.e., MRI compatibility)
Posterior tibial nerve stimulation	May be offered to patients with poor/no response to first-/second-line therapies	Patient must be able to commit to frequent office visits during induction phase as well as follow-up maintenance visits

floor physical therapy and vaginal inserts or pessary. Surgical treatments for stress incontinence in the cisgender female include synthetic or biologic mid-urethral slings, pubovaginal slings, or periurethral bulking [29]. In the transgender male patient who has not undergone gender affirmation surgery, surgical treatments may be offered. In these patients, there should be consideration and discussion of the effects of SUI surgery on future gender affirmation surgery. Phalloplasty in the setting of prior anti-incontinence surgery has not been described; however, patients undergoing phalloplasty often require multiple urethral surgeries [10]. Anti-incontinence surgery may potentially increase the likelihood of devascularization or nerve injury prior to phalloplasty. The AUA SUI surgical guidelines recommend avoidance of mesh for anti-incontinence surgery in patients at risk for poor wound healing or in the presence of significant scarring [29]. For the transgender male who is considering future gender affirmation, surgical treatment of stress incontinence should be weighed against the risks associated with phalloplasty in the setting of prior periurethral surgery.

Surgical treatment of stress, or stress-predominant urinary incontinence, is also a complex endeavor in the postsurgical transgender male patient. In our experience, it is crucial to fully investigate the cause of incontinence in these patients, as there is often an anatomic abnormality underlying as the cause of incontinence (see below). If the patient has true SUI with no other abnormality, surgical correction could be considered once less-invasive options have been exhausted. There is little data on the surgical treatment of de novo SUI in this population. When considering various surgical approaches to treating SUI in the population, one should consider the differences in the histologic architecture in cisgender male vs cisgender female cadavers [48], so the expected support structures may be different at baseline or altered by the genital affirmation surgery (i.e., vaginectomy, lengthening urethroplasty). The dimensions and landmarks of the male and female bony pelvis are not identical, so procedures anchoring to the pubic rami or passing through the obturator foramen would need to be adjusted. Special considerations should be made, accounting for the type of surgical genital affirmation performed. Communication with the original operating surgeon, including evaluation of operative reports, as well as careful planning, is critical. The vascular pedicle of the neophallus should not be compromised during dissection or passage of trocars while placing either biologic or synthetic sling material. Since there is no true bulbar urethra, an artificial urinary sphincter or bulbar male sling may not be feasible. Urethral bulking agents have been attempted with good success in the short term, but long-term data is not available [49].

For the transgender female patient, surgical treatment of pre-gender affirmation stress urinary incontinence is challenging. Stress urinary incontinence in this population would likely be due to prior prostate surgery (such as prostatectomy or anti-BPH procedures), radiation, or urethral surgery. Stress urinary incontinence may be related to injury or devascularitzation to the continence mechanism or its innervation. The cisgender male continence mechanism [50] is related to both membranous urethra and bladder neck (Fig. 15.3). If the bladder neck is compromised (i.e., from prior prostate surgery), the continence is dependent on the membranous urethral sphincter. This may be disrupted during aggressive urethral shortening, or, potentially, from future transurethral procedures (Fig. 15.4). The options for the treatment of stress incontinence in the population of transgender female patients prior to gender affirmation include male sling, artificial urinary sphincter, bladder neck sphincter, and urethral bulking. Bulking agents are no longer recommended in the post-prostatectomy SUI patient; however, they may be useful for those with a neurologic cause of SUI. Additionally, in cisgender males, bladder neck sphincter is thought to be contraindicated after prostatectomy [51]. The position of the bulbourethral male sling, as well as artificial urinary sphincter, would likely result in difficulty during urethral reduction for gender affirmation in these patients.

The post-vaginoplasty transgender female patient who presents with new onset stress urinary incontinence must also be approached

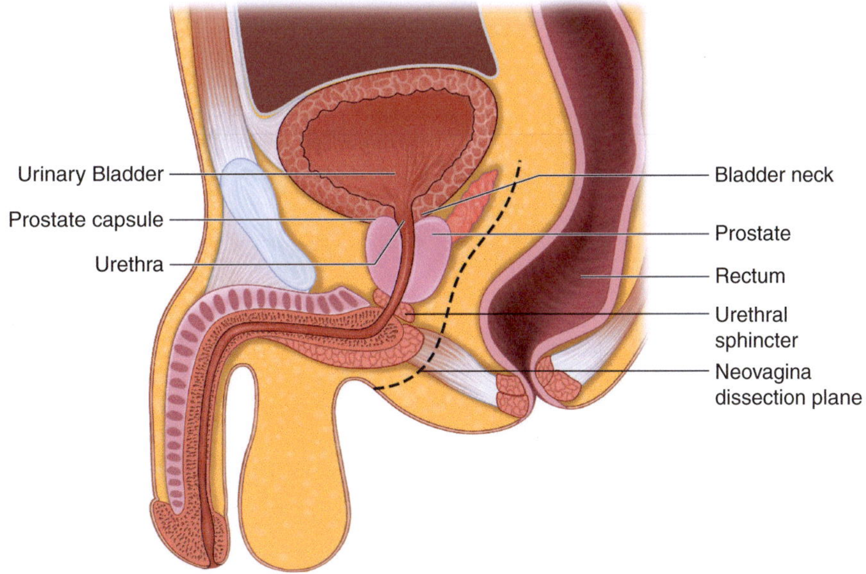

Fig. 15.3 Sagittal view of pre-surgical sagittal anatomy

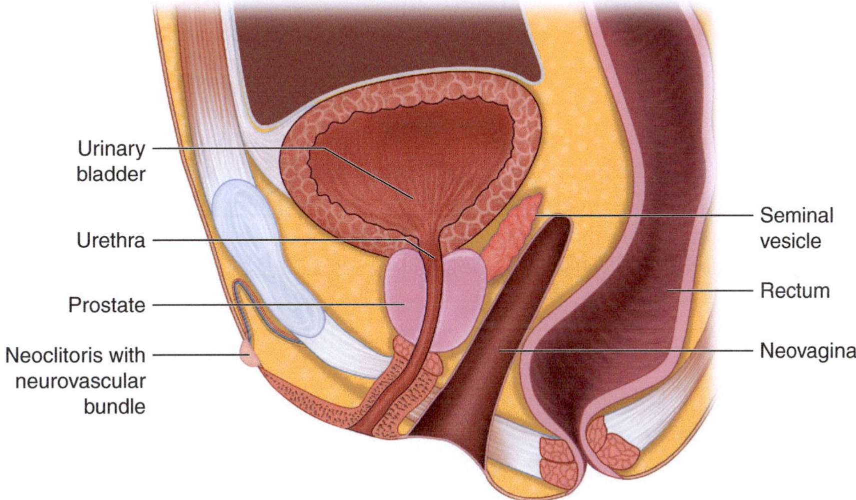

Fig. 15.4 Sagittal view of anatomy after neo-vaginal creation

thoughtfully. For the transgender female patient who has had neovaginal creation, the bulbar urethra has been excised, and the neovagina lies in the created space posterior to Denonvillier's fascia anterior to the rectum (Fig. 15.5). While data on anti-incontinence procedures on post-gender affirmation transgender women is lacking, conceivably, the placement of an autologous fascial sling may be feasible. In our experience, this is a challenging procedure. Dissection must be meticulous to avoid injury of the neovagina. Passage of retropubic instruments should be done with care, particularly in patients with prior retropubic surgery or scarring in the space of Retzius. While data is limited for fascial sling success in the transgender female patient after gender affirmation surgery, case report outcomes in the literature are promising for this approach [52]. While

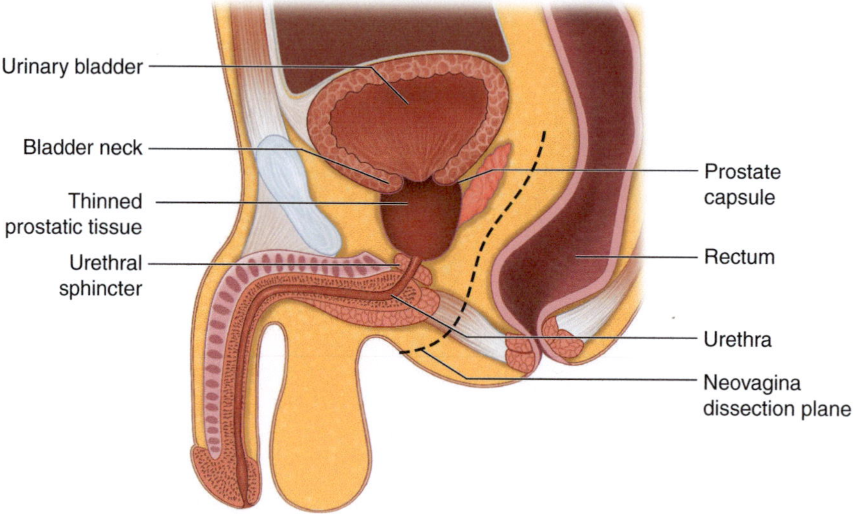

Fig. 15.5 Post-TURP/simple prostatectomy sagittal anatomy

bulking agents have been attempted with reasonable short-term success [49], long-term outcome data is lacking. Conceivably, a bladder neck artificial sphincter may be an option in the absence of prior prostatectomy, as it can provide good outcomes in cisgender females, but does have relatively high complication rates [53].

Knowledge of the most common types of complications of gender affirmation is crucial, as certain causes of incontinence in this population are directly related to complications of surgery (see below).

Types of Incontinence Specific to the Transgender Patient

As discussed earlier, a key component of the evaluation of incontinence in transgender patients is understanding the symptom history. While many transgender patients will present with stress or urge related incontinence, there are a number of incontinence scenarios that are unique to this population, particularly in the patients that have undergone gender affirmation surgery. Both male and female genital affirmation surgeries can result in conditions causing urinary incontinence.

Post-void dribbling is commonly seen in up to 79% of post-operative transgender male patients, thought to be related to pooling in the neo-urethra [15]. To expel this retained urethral urine, it is recommend to educate the patient on compression at the base of the reconstructed scrotum or proximal urethra to help fully empty the urethra [15, 54] in these patients.

Urinary fistulae may occur after neourethra creation or due to dissection too close to the urinary tract. Rates of fistula are variable, but overall suggested to be somewhere between 1% and 6%, including non-urinary tract fistulae (i.e., rectovaginal fistulae) [15, 55].

After genital affirmation surgery in transgender male patients, urinary fistulae may be related to a more distal stricture, obstruction at the anastomosis, or due to remnant vaginal cavity [56, 57]. Some patients after vaginectomy and phalloplasty present with recurrent or remnant vaginal cavity communicating with the anterior urethra via urethra-neovaginal cavity fistula. We suspect that in those patients the colpocleisis/vaginectomy was either incomplete, or the patient's vagina was not fully obliterated. The remnant cavity can then function as a reservoir of urine, particularly in the setting of more distal stricture. In our institutional experience, repair of these fistulae should include repairs of distal

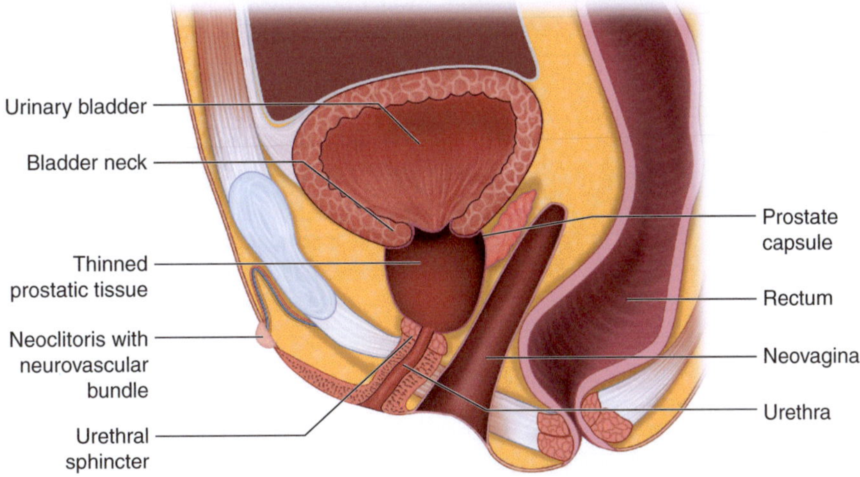

Fig. 15.6 Post-TURP/prostatectomy sagittal anatomy with neovaginal creation

obstruction, and obliteration of the vaginal remnant as well as repairs of fistulae.

Creation of a neovaginal pouch requires pelvic dissection between the rectum and the prostate that can lead to injury of the prostatic urethra, resulting in prostatic or urethral-neovaginal fistula. In patients who have a history of prior transurethral prostate resection or other prostate surgery, the prostate tissue is thinned, and violation of the capsule can predispose to fistula formation (Figs. 15.1, 15.2, and 15.6). Occasionally, several fistulae can occur simultaneously (see Fig. 15.7). Careful examination is crucial to appreciate the patient's anatomy. In our experience, a retrograde urethrogram may be helpful to define anatomy; however, it may be technically difficult to perform and interpret (Fig. 15.8). Examination under anesthesia may be necessary to fully appreciate all defects present. Surgical planning is critical, including review of prior operative reports, and, if possible, discussion with original operating surgeon. Consideration must be made to preserve the neo-vaginal cavity. The use of bulky flaps such as gracilis interposition may obliterate the vaginal space. Additionally, if the defect involves the prostatic capsule or damaged membranous urethra, this tissue may not be suitable for reconstruction. Despite the complexity of repair, we have found that the closure of these fistulae and restoration of

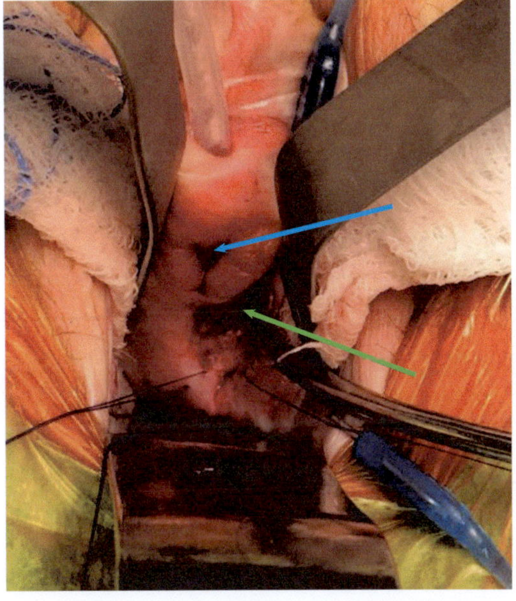

Fig. 15.7 Prostato-neovaginal fistula (green arrow) with distal urethral fistula (blue arrow)

continence is possible by carefully following the tenants of fistula repair, performing a watertight closure without overlapping suture lines and use of appropriate interpositional flaps and/or grafts.

Prolapse of neovagina may potentially contribute to urinary incontinence symptoms in the transgender female patient. The rate of neovaginal

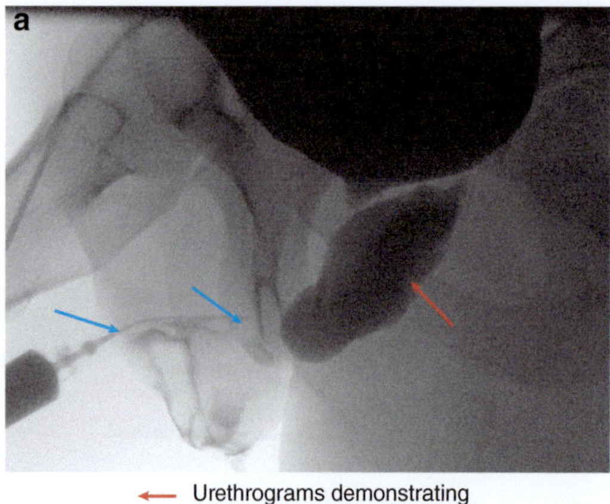

Fig. 15.8 Retrograde (**a**) and antegrade (**b**) urethrograms demonstrating remnant vaginal cavity (red arrows) as well as anastomotic urethral strictures (blue arrows) in neophallus

prolapse reported in the literature varies from 1.9% to 10% [13, 58, 59], largely variable on intraoperative procedures to primarily suspend the apical portion of the neovagina at its creation. In this study by Kuhn et al. [13], the rate of urinary symptoms was recorded at 47%; however, it is unclear if prolapse was investigated independently. For those patients with symptomatic neovaginal prolapse (generally regarded as ICS pelvic organ prolapse quantification as stage 2 or higher with associated symptoms), successful surgical repair has been performed with both sacrospinous fixation and sacrocolpopexy [60–62]. The use of polypropylene mesh graft mate-

rial for sacrocolpopexy was successful in case reports [60], although biologic or autologous fascial material may also be feasible.

These causes of urinary incontinence are unique to the post-gender affirmation transgender patient, and should always be considered. Surgical correction requires careful repair of not only the fistula or remnant cavity, but also any concomitant stricture. Patients must be carefully examined for neovaginal prolapse or other, distinctive causes of incontinence in transgender patients.

Conclusions

Urinary incontinence is a common quality of life issue. Transgender individuals could be expected to have similar rates as the general populace, although large, population-based studies are lacking. The evaluation of urinary incontinence in any person begins with a thorough history and physical examination, with adjuvant testing as needed. In the transgender patient, care must be taken when planning treatment and management strategies, particularly in the light of prior or planned genital surgery.

Take Home Points
- Urinary incontinence rates in transgender individuals should be considered to be similar to the general population.
- Evaluation with thorough history, including detailed surgical history, is critical for understanding the etiology of incontinence in any individual. All attempts should be made to obtain prior operative reports to fully understand the patient's current anatomy.
- Treatment of incontinence requires careful understanding of underlying process as well as attention to potential pitfalls of planned future surgeries.

References

1. Abrams PCL, Fall M, Griffiths D, Rosier P, Ulmsten U, Van Kerrebroeck P, Victor A, Wein A. The standardisation of terminology in lower urinary tract func-

tion: report from the standardisation sub-committee of the international continence society. Urology. 2003;61:37–49.

2. Nygaard I, Barber MD, Burgio KL, Kenton K, Meikle S, Schaffer J, et al. Prevalence of symptomatic pelvic floor disorders in US women. JAMA. 2008;300(11):1311–6.

3. Wu JM, Vaughan CP, Goode PS, Redden DT, Burgio KL, Richter HE, et al. Prevalence and trends of symptomatic pelvic floor disorders in U.S. women. Obstet Gynecol. 2014;123(1):141–8.

4. Minassian VA, Stewart WF, Wood GC. Urinary incontinence in women: variation in prevalence estimates and risk factors. Obstet Gynecol. 2008;111(2 Pt 1):324–31.

5. Melville JKW, Kelaney K. Urinary incontinence in US women, a population-based study. Arch Intern Med. 2005;165(5):537–42.

6. Markland AD, Goode PS, Redden DT, Borrud LG, Burgio KL. Prevalence of urinary incontinence in men: results from the national health and nutrition examination survey. J Urol. 2010;184(3):1022–7.

7. Diokno ACEM, Ibrahim IA, Balasubramaniam M. Prevalence of urinary incontinence in community dwelling men: a cross sectional nationwide epidemiological survey. Int Urol Nephrol. 2006;39(1):129–36.

8. Helfand BT, Smith AR, Lai HH, Yang CC, Gore JL, Erickson BA, et al. Prevalence and characteristics of urinary incontinence in a treatment seeking male prospective cohort: results from the LURN study. J Urol. 2018;200(2):397–404.

9. Raigosa M, Avvedimento S, Yoon TS, Cruz-Gimeno J, Rodriguez G, Fontdevila J. Male-to-female genital reassignment surgery: a retrospective review of surgical technique and complications in 60 patients. J Sexual Med. 2015;12:1837–45.

10. Remington AC, Morrison SD, Massie JP, Crowe CS, Shakir A, Wilson SC, Vyas KS, et al. Outcomes after phalloplasty: do transgender patients and multiple urethral procedures carry a higher rate of complication? Plast Reconstr Surg. 2018;

11. RAA-Ohoo S. Urethral complications after transgender phalloplasty: strategies to treat them and minimize their occurrence. Clin Anat. 2018;31(2):187–90.

12. Lawrence AA. Patient-reported complications and functional outcomes of male-to-female sex reassignment surgery. Arch Sex Behav. 2006;35(6):717–27.

13. Kuhn A, Santi A, Birkhauser M. Vaginal prolapse, pelvic floor function, and related symptoms 16 years after sex reassignment surgery in transsexuals. Fertil Steril. 2011;95(7):2379–82.

14. Kuhn A, Hiltebrand R, Birkhauser M. Do transsexuals have micturition disorders? Eur J Obstet Gynecol Reprod Biol. 2007;131(2):226–30.

15. Hoebeke P, Ceulemans P, De Cuypere G, T'Sjoen G, Weyers S, Decaestecker K, et al. Impact of sex reassignment surgery on lower urinary tract function. Eur Urol. 2005;47:398–402.

16. Milsom I, Coyne KS, Nicholson S, Kvasz M, Chen CI, Wein AJ. Global prevalence and economic burden of urgency urinary incontinence: a systematic review. Eur Urol. 2014;65(1):79–95.

17. Ganz MLSA, Krupski TL, et al. Economic costs of overactive bladder in the Unites States. Urology. 2010;75:526–32.

18. Almousa S, Bandin van Loon A. The prevalence of urinary incontinence in nulliparous adolescent and middle-aged women and the associated risk factors: a systematic review. Maturitas. 2018;107:78–83.

19. Williams MPSV, Bird M, Thrift AG. Urinary symptoms and natural history of uirnary continence after first-ever stroke: a longitudinal population based study. Age Aging. 2012;41:371–6.

20. Lu FPCD, Kuo HK, Wu SC. Sex differences in the impact of diabetes on the risk of geriatric conditions. Geriatr Gerontol Int. 2013;13:116–22.

21. Kemmer H, Mathes AM, Dilk O, Groschel A, Grass C, Stockle M. Obstructive sleep apnea syndrome is associated with overactive bladder and urgency incontinence in men. Sleep. 2009;32(2):271–5.

22. Ohgaki K, Horiuchi K, Kondo Y. Association between metabolic syndrome and male overactive bladder in a Japanese population based on three different sets of criteria for metabolic syndrome and the Overactive Bladder Symptom Score. Urology. 2012;79(6):1372–8.

23. Shamliyan TWJ, Ping R, Wilt T, Kane R. Male urinary incontinence: prevalence, risk factors, and preventative interventions. Rev Urol. 2009;11(3):145–65.

24. Resnick NM, Yalla SV. Management of urinary incontinence in the elderly. N Engl J Med. 1985;313(3):800–5.

25. Dallaso HMMC, Matthews RJ, Donaldson MMD. The association of diet and other lifestyle factors with overactive bladder and stress incontinence: a longitudinal study in women. BJU Int. 2003;92:69–77.

26. Wyman JF, Burgio KL, Newman DK. Practical aspects of lifestyle modifications and behavioural interventions in the treatment of overactive bladder and urgency urinary incontinence. Int J Clin Pract. 2009;63(8):1177–91.

27. Weber MA, Kleijn MH, Langendam M, Limpens J, Heineman MJ, Roovers JP. Local oestrogen for pelvic floor disorders: a systematic review. PLoS One. 2015;10(9)

28. Gormley EA, Lightner DJ, Burgio KL, Chai TC, Clemens JQ, Dj C, Das AK, et al. Diagnosis and treatment of overactive bladder (non-neurogenic) in adults: AUA/SUFU guideline. J Urol. 2012;188(6S):2455–63.

29. Kobashi KC, Albo ME, Dmochowski RR, Ginsberg DA, Goldman HB, Gomelsky A, et al. Surgical treatment of female stress urinary incontinence: AUA/SUFU guideline. J Urol. 2017;198(4):875–83.

30. Al-Shaikh G, Larochelle A, Campbell CE, Schachter J, Baker K, Pascali D. Accuracy of bladder scanning in the assessment of postvoid residual volume. J Obstet Dynaecol Can. 2009;31(6):526–32.

31. Homma Y, Ando T, Yoshida M, Kageyama S, Takei M, Kimoto K, Ishizuka O, et al. Voiding

and incontinence frequencies: variability of diary data and required diary length. Neurourol Urodyn. 2002;21(3):204–9.

32. Ku JH, Jeong IG, Lim DJ, Byun SS, Paick JS, Oh SJ. Voiding diary for the evaluation of urinary incontinence and lower urinary tract symptoms: prospective assessment of patient compliance and burden. Neurourol Urodyn. 2004;23(4):331–5.

33. Abrams PA, Andersson KE, Birder L, Brubaker L, Cardozo L, Chapple C, Cottenden A, Davila W, de Ridder D, Dmochowski R, Drake M, Dubeau C, Dubeau C, Fry C, Hanno P, Hay Smith J, Herschorn S, Hosker G, Kelleher C, Koelbl H, Khoury S, Madoff R, Milsom I, Moore K, Newman D, Nitti V, Norton C, Nygaard I, Payne C, Smith A, Staskin D, Tekgul S, Thuroff J, Tubaro A, Vodusek D, Wein A, Wyndaele JJ. Fourth international consultation on incontinence recommendations of the international scientific committee: evaluation and treatment of urinary incontinence, pelvic organ prolapse, and fecal incontinence. Neurourol Urodyn. 2010;29(1):213–40.

34. Coyne KS, Matza LS, Thompson CL. The responsiveness of the Overactive Bladder Questionnaire (OAB-q). Qual Life Res. 2005;2005(14):3.

35. Avery K, Donovan J, Peters TJ, Shaw C, Gotoh M, Abrams P. ICIQ: a brief and robust measure for evaluating the symptoms and impact of urinary incontinence. Neurourol Urodyn. 2004;23(4):322–30.

36. Blaivas JG, Panagopoulos G, Weiss JP, Somaroo C. Validation of the overactive bladder symptom score. J Urol. 2007;178(2):543–7.

37. Margolis MK, Vats V, Coyne KS, Kelleher C. Establishing the content validity of the King's Health Questionnaire in men and women with overactive bladder in the US. Patient. 2011;4(3):177–87.

38. Coyne KS, Zyczynski T, Margolis MK, Elinoff V, Roberts RG. Validation of an overactive bladder awareness tool for use in primary care settings. Adv Ther. 2005;22(4):381–984.

39. Mangera A, Chapple CR. Application of guidelines to the evaluation of the male patient with urgency and/or incontinence. Curr Opin Urol. 2014;24(6):547–52.

40. Winters JC, Dmochowski RR, Goldman HB, CDA H, Kobashi KC, Kraus SR, Lemack GE, et al. Urodynamic studies in adults: AUA/SUFU guideline. J Urol. 2012;188(6s):2464–72.

41. Gratzke C, Bachmann A, Descazeaud A, Drake MJ, Madersbacher S, Mamoulakis C, et al. EAU guidelines on the assessment of non-neurogenic male lower urinary tract symptoms including benign prostatic obstruction. Eur Urol. 2015;67(6):1099–109.

42. Newman DK, Guzzo T, Lee D, Jayadevappa R. An evidence-based strategy for the conservative management of the male patient with incontinence. Curr Opin Urol. 2014;24(6):553–9.

43. Noguchi N, Chan L, Cumming RG, Blyth FM, Handelsman DJ, Waite LM, et al. Natural history of non-neurogenic overactive bladder and urinary incontinence over 5 years in community-dwelling older men: the concord health and aging in men project. Neurourol Urodyn. 2017;36(2):443–8.

44. Santen RJ. Vaginal administration of estradiol: effects of dose, preparation and timing on plasma estradiol levels. Climacteric. 2015;18(2):121–34.

45. Kaplan SRC, Rovner E, Carlsson M, Bavendam T, Guan Z. Tolterodine and tamsulosin for treatment of men with lower urinary tract symptoms and overactive bladder; a randomized controlled trial. JAMA. 2006;296(19):2319–29.

46. Andersson KE. The use of pharmacotherapy for male patients with urgency and stress incontinence. Curr Opin Urol. 2014;24(6):571–7.

47. Shin DG, Kim HW, Yoon SJ, Song SH, Kim YH, Lee YG, et al. Mirabegron as a treatment for overactive bladder symptoms in men (MIRACLE study): efficacy and safety results from a multicenter, randomized, double-blind, placebo-controlled, parallel comparison phase IV study. Neurourol Urodyn. 2019;38(1):295–304.

48. Hirata E, Fujiwara H, Hayashi S, Ohtsuka A, Abe S-I, Murakami G, Kudo Y, et al. Intergender differences in histological architecture of the fascia pelvis parietalis: a cadaveric study. Clin Anat. 2011;24(4):469–77.

49. Fitzpatrick C, Swierzewski SJ 3rd, McGuire EJ. Periurethral collagen for urinary incontinence after gender reassignment surgery. Urology. 1993;42(4):458–60.

50. TM O. The urethral spincter muscle in the male. Am J Anatomy. 1980;158(2):229–46.

51. Herndon CD, Rink RC, MBK S, Simmons GR, Cain MP, Kaefer M, Casale AJ, et al. The Indiana experience with artificial urinary sphincters in children and young adults. J Urol. 2003;169(2):650–4.

52. Dangle PP, Harrison SC. Stress urinary incontinence after male to female gender reassignment surgery: successful use of a pubo-vaginal sling. Indian J Urol. 2007;23(3):311–3.

53. Peyronnet B, O'Connor E, Khavari R, Capon G, Manunta A, Allue M, et al. AMS-800 Artificial urinary sphincter in female patients with stress urinary incontinence: a systematic review. Neurourol Urodyn. 2019;38 Suppl 4:S28–41.

54. Trum HW, Hoebeke P, Gooren LJ. Sex reassignment of transsexual people from a gynecologist's and urologist's perspective. Acta Obstetrica et Gyn Scand. 2015;94:563–7.

55. Manrique OJ, Adabi K, Martinez-Jorge J, Ciudad P, Nicoli F, Kiranantawat K. Complications and patient-reported outcomes in male-to-female vaginoplasty-where we are today: a systematic review and meta-analysis. Ann Plast Surg. 2018;80(6):684–91.

56. Nikolavsky D, Yamaguchi Y, Levine JP, Zhao LC. Urologic sequelae following phalloplasty in transgendered patients. Urol Clin N Am. 2017;44:113–25.

57. Pan S, Honig SC. Gender-affirming surgery: current concepts. Curr Urol Rep. 2018;19(8):62.

58. Dreher PC, Edwards D, Hager S, Dennis M, Belkoff A, Mora J, et al. Complications of the neovagina in male-to-female transgender surgery: a systematic review and meta-analysis with discussion of management. Clin Anat. 2018;31(2):191–9.

59. Bucci S, Mazzon G, Liguori G, Napoli R, Pavan N, Bormioli S, et al. Neovaginal prolapse in male-to-female transsexuals: an 18-year-long experience. Biomed Res Int. 2014;2014:240761.

60. Kavvadias T, Seifert HH, Ebbing J, Nunez Garcia D, Kind AB. Robotic sacrocolpopexy for recurrent vaginal vault prolapse after sex reassignment surgery in a trans-woman. J Obstet Gynaecol. 2019:1–2.

61. Condous G, Jones R, Lam AM. Male-to-female transsexualism: laparoscopic pelvic floor repair of prolapsed neovagina. Aust N Z J Obstet Gynaecol. 2006;46(3):254–6.

62. Stanojevic DS, Djordjevic ML, Milosevic A, Sansalone S, Slavkovic Z, Ducic S, et al. Sacrospinous ligament fixation for neovaginal prolapse prevention in male-to-female surgery. Urology. 2007;70(4):767–71.

Jillian Cardinali and Darryl Manzer

Introduction

What Is Physical Therapy?

Physical therapists are health care professionals that diagnose and treat individuals who have medical problems or health-related conditions which limit their mobility or ability to perform activities of daily living. Roles of the physical therapist include increasing functional mobility, reducing pain, and restoring function. They also assist in preventing further impairments through the development of individualized home wellness programs and promoting more active lifestyle. The American Physical Therapy Association lists their vision statement in 2019 as "Transforming society by optimizing movement to improve the human experience" [1].

What Is Pelvic Floor Physical Therapy?

Pelvic floor physical therapy is a specialty area of physical therapy which focuses on dysfunctions related to the pelvic floor muscles. The pelvic floor is made up of three muscular and connective-tissue sheets (Fig. 16.1) that function to support the abdominal contents, store and evacuate urine and stool, contribute to lumbopelvic stability and mobility, and aid in sexual arousal and appreciation [2]. Dysfunction of the pelvic floor manifests as bowel, bladder, and sexual symptoms.

Transgender individuals can experience pelvic floor dysfunction both pre- and post-operatively. Recent research indicates that transgender patients have a higher incidence of pelvic floor dysfunction when compared to the cisgender population. Jiang et al. identified a high rate of pre-operative pelvic floor muscle (42%) and bowel dysfunction (37%) in patients scheduled for gender-affirming vaginoplasty [3]. This can be contrasted with the prevalence of 25% identified by Wu et al. for US cisgender women who experience one or more pelvic floor disorders [4]. Jiang et al. also reported that patients who received pre-operative pelvic floor physical therapy experienced less pelvic floor dysfunction post-operatively when compared with patients who did not [3]. However, there is currently a lack of valid patient-reported outcome measures being used to measure the extent of pelvic floor dysfunction post-operatively [5]. Physical therapists who specialize in pelvic floor dysfunction have knowledge regarding anatomy, neuroanatomy, kinesiology, biomechanics, bowel and bladder function, and normal pelvic floor function which makes them uniquely qualified to treat transgender individuals with pelvic floor symptoms.

In our practice, we see patients preoperatively to introduce principles of physical therapy, estab-

J. Cardinali (✉) · D. Manzer
Upstate University Hospital, SUNY Upstate
Medical University, Syracuse, NY, USA
e-mail: cardinaj@upstate.edu; manzerd@upstate.edu

© Springer Nature Switzerland AG 2021
D. Nikolavsky, S. A. Blakely (eds.), *Urological Care for the Transgender Patient*,
https://doi.org/10.1007/978-3-030-18533-6_16

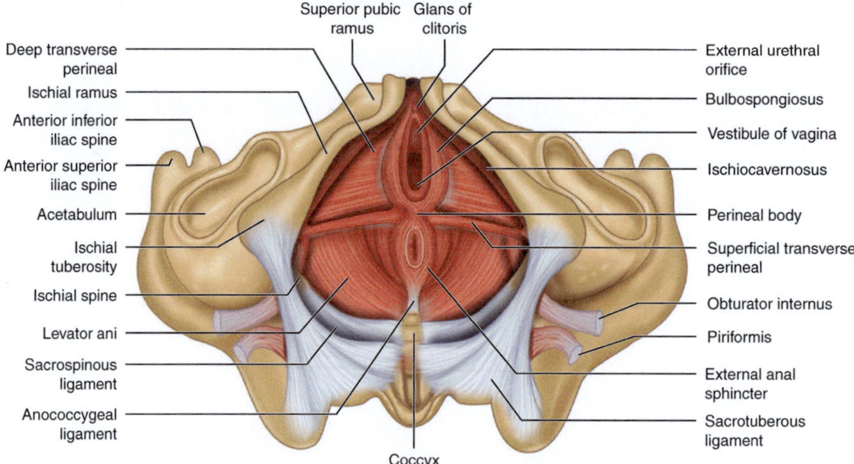

Fig. 16.1 Pelvic floor of a cis-gender female. This figure illustrates the 3 layers of muscle and connective tissue as well as the urethra, the vagina, and the rectum which pass through these layers

lish baseline symptoms, prepare for surgery, and set expectations. One to two weeks post-vaginoplasty, after vaginal packing or a vaginal stent is removed by surgeon, the patient is seen again for evaluation and proper vaginal dilation teaching. We will describe elements of evaluation, treatment, and patient education in subsequent parts of this chapter.

Elements of Patient Management (Table 16.1) [6]

Pelvic floor physical therapists perform an examination that includes an external assessment of the lumbopelvic and hip complex and pelvic floor muscles as well as an internal assessment of the pelvic floor muscles. Findings from this examination drive the physical therapist's evaluation which consists of the diagnosis, prognosis, and plan of care for the patient. The therapist then interacts with the patient to provide procedural interventions, patient-related instruction, and coordination, communication, and documentation. In this chapter, these elements are further broken down as they relate to patient management of transgender individuals.

Table 16.1 Patient management model

I. Examination
(a) History
(b) Systems review
(c)Tests and measures
II. Evaluation
(a) Diagnosis
(b) Prognosis
III. Intervention
(a) Coordination, communication, documentation
(b) Patient-related instruction
(c) Direct intervention

Examination

History

A physical therapy history begins with asking the patient their preferred name and pronoun. During the subjective portion of the history, a patient is asked questions regarding past medical history, past surgical history, allergies, medications, urinary function, bowel function, sexual function, and pain.

Information is gathered from both the patient and the medical record, if available, of the patients past medical and surgical history. Questions should include past surgical procedures including plastic surgery or permanent hair removal. The therapist will also complete a thorough review of current medications and allergies.

During the subjective history, the therapist should gather information regarding urinary function. These questions may include urinary frequency, urinary urgency, incontinence, and difficulty emptying. The patient will be asked to identify specific movements or triggers that are associated with these symptoms. Bowel function is also gathered in the subjective history including the presence of constipation, straining during voiding, and ability to fully evacuate stool.

If the patient is comfortable sharing information on the first visit, the therapist approaches an open conversation on sexual function. Questions should include if they actively participate in sexual intercourse and if they have a preferred partner. If the patient reports pain during sex, they will be asked to identify the possible sources of their pain such as pain with penetration, ejaculation, or positioning.

The final section of the subjective portion of evaluation covers pain. If the patient does experience pain, the patient is asked about their pain in regard to location, onset, intensity, and aggravating and easing factors. Questions may include whether sleep is interrupted or if it is difficult to fall asleep due to their pain.

Systems Review (Table 16.2)

The systems review is a brief or limited examination that serves to screen the patient for systems that may warrant additional examination via tests and measures [6].

Tests and Measures

Tests and measures are the means by which the physical therapist collects data about the patient [6]. Selection of tests and measures are driven by the information obtained during the history and systems review. The clinical examination focuses on the integrity of the lumbopelvic-hip region and related structures, joints, muscles, nerves,

Table 16.2 Physical therapy systems review

System	Assessment
Cardiovascular/pulmonary	Heart rate Respiratory rate Blood pressure Edema
Integumentary	Tissue texture, color, and integrity Post-operative scars Scars from previous abdominal or pelvic surgeries
Musculoskeletal	Symmetry Range of motion Strength Height and weight
Neromuscular	Coordinated movement Gait Mobility Balance Motor control
Communication ability	Affect Cognition Language Learning style

and ligaments. A pelvic floor specialist uses knowledge of anatomy, neuroanatomy, kinesiology, biomechanics, bowel and bladder function, and normal pelvic floor function to choose tests and measures that are sensitive, reliable, and valid [7]. This section describes categories of tests and measures that may be selected in the management of the transgender patient and why.

Posture Postural control supports the breathing mechanism and also the function of the pelvic floor muscles by providing a spatially appropriate and stable base of support for the lower spinal column and pelvis [8]. (Fig. 16.2) The pelvic floor physical therapist looks at sitting and standing posture as well as the patient's pelvic orientation (anterior or posterior pelvic tilt). For example, if the patient sacral sits, there will be increased pressure on the tailbone and posterior pelvic floor muscles which could result in difficulties evacuating stool.

Pain The numeric pain rating scale (NRS) and visual analogue scale (VAS) [9] are commonly used in physical therapy practice to measure baseline pain measures and to track the progress

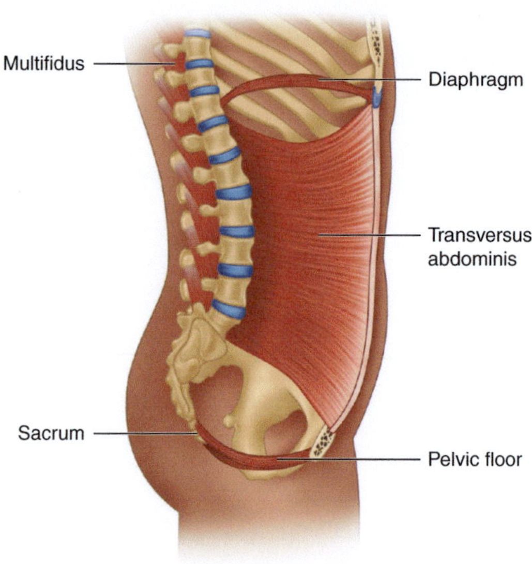

Fig. 16.2 Muscles which support intra-abdominal pressure. Diaphragm – a thin muscle which separates the thoracic cavity from the abdominal cavity. Multifidus – a spinal muscle which stabilizes the vertebral joints. Transverse Abdominis – the deepest of the abdominal muscle which runs horizontally. Pelvic Floor – a group of muscles at the base of the pelvis

of a patient's pain symptoms. These scales can be used to measure the patient's pain both pre-operatively and post-operatively and to monitor the patient's response to physical therapy intervention.

Palpation Gender differences exist in the anatomy of the hips and pelvis. Neuromuscular differences in firing patterns of motor units may arise from these anatomic differences [2]. This can lead to muscle imbalances throughout the pelvis which can contribute to dysfunction. The pelvic floor therapist will perform palpation of the external pelvic musculature (psoas, adductors, superficial PFM) as well as the three layers of the pelvic floor muscles internally. Particular attention is paid to reproduction of symptoms, tenderness, trigger points, tone, and symmetry.

Joint integrity/mobility Gender differences in the anatomy of the pelvis can lead to variation in hip mobility. Also, cisgender female patients are more likely to have mild-to-severe developmen-

tal hip dysplasia which may necessitate balanced muscle strength and length to provide joint stability [2]. Currently there is no evidence to demonstrate whether hormonal replacement therapy could affect joint stability. Physical therapists assess joint integrity and mobility of the lumbar spine, hips, pelvis, and tailbone both actively and passively to determine whether anatomical differences, or imbalances in muscle strength and length could be contributing to the symptoms experienced by the patient.

Motor function An assessment of motor function in regard to the stability of their pelvis is completed. The One Leg Stance Test, also known as the Gillet Test, and the Active Straight Leg Test [10] are utilized to further investigate the motor function of the muscles of the pelvis. These tests can be utilized to assist in prescribing specific stabilization interventions [11]. Postural breathing muscles are also observed. (Fig. 16.2) Pelvic floor function is impacted by both intra-thoracic pressure and intra-abdominal pressure control. Control of the intra-thoracic and intra-abdominal systems are impacted by motor function of the glottis and the diaphragm, as well as the pelvic floor.

Muscle performance Pelvic floor muscle performance is tested via a reliable and validated assessment tool known as the PERFECT [12]. This acronym represents the four measured domains, power, endurance, repetition, and fast contractions. (Table 16.3) The PERFECT is performed with an internal assessment, vaginally or rectally, to allow for the most accurate assessment of muscle performance. This assessment

Table 16.3 PERFECT is an assessment tool proven to be valid and reliable

P = power (or pressure, a measure of strength using a manometric perineometer)
E = endurance
R = repetitions
F = fast contractions
ECT = every contraction timed

Grading is often represented as P/E/R//F, for example, 5/10/10//10

tool is useful in the transgender patient population as the muscle performance may be impaired following surgical intervention.

Integumentary integrity Impairments of the integumentary system may be present during the examination of the transgender patient due to surgical intervention, permanent hair removal procedures, or skin maceration due to incontinence. Observation of skin characteristics, including blistering, continuity of skin color, dermatitis, trophic changes, mobility, sensation, temperature, and turgor are a part of the assessment [7].

Evaluation

Diagnosis

Data gathered from the examination is then organized into recognized clusters, syndromes, or categories to determine a physical therapy diagnosis that is amenable to physical therapy interventions. This diagnosis includes a differential diagnosis based on knowledge of diseases and disorders and a determination of whether there is a need to refer to other health care providers. The patient who has just undergone surgical intervention is likely to have a diagnosis related to neuromusculoskeletal impairments from that surgery. However, both the patient who has undergone surgery and the patient who has not undergone surgery may have underlying neuromusculoskeletal dysfunctions related to the following: Pelvic floor muscle laxity/weakness, incoordination, non-relaxing, contracture, adhesions, or pain syndromes; Musculoskeletal system dysfunction including the joints of the upper extremity, lower extremity, pelvis, and spine; Neurological impairments; Hormonal Influences [7]. All of these factors can impact the bowel, bladder, and sexual function of the patient and are considered in the physical therapy diagnosis.

Prognosis

A prognosis is developed for the patient using evaluative findings to predict recovery and time to achieve the optimal level of function. For the transgender patient, it is especially important to consider the psychosocial and cultural impact on this population. Authors Baiola et al. examined psychological distress and resilience among both transgendered men and women. Their study resulted in 46% of their sample reporting high or very high levels of psychological distress using the Kessler Psychological Distress Scale. They found that factors that are associated with greater psychological distress in transgender individuals include younger age, feeling unable to turn to family for support, and victimization experiences [13]. Factors found to be associated with greater resilience were higher income, identifying as heterosexual, and having frequent contact with lesbian, gay, bisexual, and transgender peers [13]. It is important for the physical therapist to consider psychosocial effects and also to collaborate with patients, family, payors, and other professionals to develop a plan of care that is acceptable, realistic, and culturally competent [7].

Intervention

Coordination, communication, and documentation Intervention provided by the physical therapist begins with effective communication. A multidisciplinary approach to treatment includes communication with the patient, family member, caregivers, practitioners, and payors. This discussion may include a rationale for physical therapy examination or intervention, along with current evidence-based practice. Collaboration with the patient and members of the patient care team will provide for a comprehensive, cohesive, and culturally competent plan of care. Documentation of the examination, procedural intervention, and plan of care allows for continued communication with the team and payors [7].

Patient Related Instruction A behavioral and lifestyle approach to patient treatment allows the physical therapist to provide patient related instructions. Instructions may include education regarding diagnosis, prognosis, anatomy and function, risk reduction/prevention, and wellness strategies. These instructions may include healthy bladder habits, proper fluid intake, constipation management, general education on pelvic floor function and dysfunction, and cleanliness [14].

Direct intervention Direct interventions are selected, applied, or modified based on examination data, the evaluation, the diagnosis, the prognosis, and the anticipated goals and expected outcomes for a particular patient. The interventions selected are specific to each individual patient and are prescribed based on findings from the examination and based on patient response. Examples of direct interventions are provided below.

1. *Therapeutic exercise* – Therapeutic exercise may be used to address musculoskeletal impairments related to strength, power, length, and endurance of the pelvic floor muscles. Examples of exercises to address pelvic floor muscle strength might include activation of the pelvic floor muscles in a gravity-eliminated position (supine). This exercise can then be progressed to be performed in sitting, standing, and with functional activities as the patient's strength improves. Examples of exercises to address pelvic floor muscle length might include diaphragmatic breathing in child's pose (Fig. 16.3) to promote the relaxation of the pelvic floor muscles.

2. *Neuromuscular education* – Neuromuscular education exercises might be used to improve the relaxation or coordination of the pelvic floor muscles. For example, yoga postures combined with diaphragmatic breathing and pelvic floor movement can be utilized to re-train the pelvic floor muscles to contract and relax in a coordinated manner while moving functionally.

3. *Manual therapy techniques* – Manual therapy techniques such as connective tissue and soft tissue mobilization/manipulation might be utilized both internally and externally to manage scar tissue and soft tissue restrictions that might be causing pain or limiting the patient from participating in dilation or exercise interventions. Joint mobilization/manipulation including passive range of motion exercises can be utilized to address any restrictions in joints nearby that may be limiting the ability of the patient to participate in various exercises.

4. *Electrotherapeutic modalities* – Biofeedback, also known as Computerized Visual Feedback, is a procedural intervention which allows for the immediate visual awareness of the targeted muscles [15]. Using either surface EMG or internal sensors, this intervention can be utilized for both up-training and down-training of the pelvic floor muscles. Transcutaneous electrical nerve stimulation (TENS) may be used in the case of pelvic musculoskeletal pain.

5. *Functional training* – Functional training based on the assessment of impairments is beneficial to the patient to address activities of daily living. Training may include proper voiding and defecation techniques such as toileting position, as well as bowel and bladder training techniques. Proper toileting position for improved relaxation of the pelvic floor as well as positioning for decreased pain during intercourse may be reviewed. Functional and transitional mobility techniques as well as proper body mechanics can be reviewed to facilitate proper muscle activation. Within the scope of physical therapy,

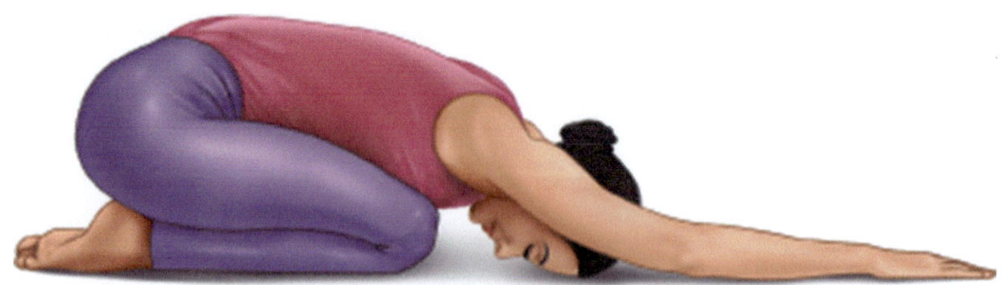

Fig. 16.3 Child's pose. A position that may be used to help facilitate pelvic floor muscle relaxation

Table 16.4 Vaginal dilators are a tool for stretching and maintaining tissue length following surgical procedure

Tips for dilation post-surgically:
Wash hands and dilators pre- and post-dilation each use with mild/gentle soap.
Use water-based lubricant each time one participates in dilation or intercourse.
Positioning is important especially if the patient is in pain:
Lay supine. The head and neck may be propped at about 15 degree angle.
Both legs are propped with pillows supporting knees in abduction and external rotation.
Diaphragmatic breathing can be a useful tool during dilation to allow for pelvic floor relaxation.
Dilation is performed by gently placing the dilator at the vaginal opening and slowly pushing internally at a slight angle toward the low back.
Once the dilator is in the correction position, it should be left in place for about 20 minutes.
Do not push or force the dilator in an effort to create further depth as this may result in a tear or fistula.
Example of post-operative dilation schedule:
Day 1: Dilate 5 times per day
Day 2–30: Dilate 4 times per day
Day 31–90: Dilate 3 times per day
After 3 months: Dilate 2 times per day
After 1 year: Dilate 1 time per day

practice is the prescription, application and, when appropriate, fabrication of supportive devices and equipment. This may include use of pessaries, dilators (Table 16.4), SI joint/maternity belts, and compression garments.

Outcome Measures

Outcome measures are tools that are often used to assess a patient's current status. Data from outcome measures can be used to assist in the creation of a treatment plan of care and measuring progression with physical therapy intervention. Outcome measures that may be used with the transgender population could include, but are not limited to, Incontinence Impact Survey, Pelvic Floor Disability Index, Incontinence Impact Questionnaire Short Form, Prostatitis Symptom Questionnaire, [16] Urogenital Distress Survey, Vulvovaginal Symptoms Questionnaire [17], and Vulvar Pain Functional Questionnaire.

Summary

Physical therapists who specialize in pelvic floor dysfunction have a role in the management of the transgender patient both pre- and post-operatively. These health care professionals can significantly impact the quality of life for transgender patients by addressing bowel, bladder, and sexual dysfunction. The physical therapist performs an evidence-based examination which then drives the development of a diagnosis, prognosis, and plan of care that is specific to each individual patient's needs. This plan of care includes the use of validated and reliable outcome measures to monitor patient response and progress selected interventions. These interventions include direct interventions as well as patient education and coordination, communication, and documentation. Physical therapists are valuable members of the patient care team when managing transgender patients.

Take-Home Points

- Physical therapists are health care professionals who diagnose and treat individuals with limitations in their mobility or ability to perform activities of daily living.
- Pelvic floor physical therapists perform an examination that includes an external assessment of the lumbopelvic and hip complex and the pelvic floor muscles, as well as an internal assessment of the pelvic floor muscles.
- A physical therapy examination will include a history, systems review, tests and measures.
- Physical therapy interventions may include coordination, communication, documentation, patient-related instructions, and direct interventions such as therapeutic exercise, neuromuscular education, manual therapy techniques, electrotherapy modalities, and functional training.

References

1. American Physical Therapy Association. Role of a physical therapist. 2016.; Available at: http://www.apta.org/PTCareers/RoleofaPT/. Accessed 3/7, 2019.
2. Prather H, Spitznagle T, Recognizing DS. Treating pelvic pain and pelvic floor dysfunction. Phys Med Rehabil Clin N Am. 2007;18(3):477–96.
3. Jiang DD, Gallagher S, Burchill L, Berli J, Dugi D. Implementation of a pelvic floor physical therapy program for transgender women undergoing gender-affirming vaginoplasty. Obstet Gynecol. 2019;133(5):1003–11.
4. Wu JM, Vaughan CP, Goode PS, Redden DT, Burgio KL, Richter HE, et al. Prevalence and trends of symptomatic pelvic floor disorders in U.S. women. Obstet Gynecol. 2014;123:141–8.
5. Andreasson M, Georgas K, Elander A, Selvaggi G. Patient-reported outcome measures used in gender confirmation surgery: a systematic review. Plast Reconstr Surg. 2018;141(4):1026–39.
6. American Physical Therapy Association. Guide to physical therapist practice. 2nd ed. Alexandria, Virginia: American Physical Therapy Association; 2003.
7. Specialty Council on Women's Health Physical Therapy American Board of Physical Therapy Specialties. Women's Health Physical Therapy: Description of Specialty Practice Prepublication Draft. 2018:1–48.
8. Key J. The core': understanding it, and retraining its dysfunction. J Bodyw Mov Ther. 2013;17:541–59.
9. Kahl C, Cleland J. Visual analogue scale, numeric pain rating scale and the McGill pain questionnaire: an overview of psychometric properties. Phys The. 2005;10:123–8.
10. Kibsgårda TJ, Röhrla SM, Røisea O, Sturessonb B, Stuge B. Movement of the sacroiliac joint during the Active Straight Leg Raise test in patients with long-lasting severe sacroiliac joint pain. Clin Biomech. 2017;47:40–5.
11. Massery M. Multisystem consequences of impaired breathing mechanics and/or postural control. In: Frownfelter D, Dean E, editors. Cardiovascular and pulmonary physical therapy evidence and practice. 4th ed: Elsevier Health Sciences; 2006. p. 659.
12. Laycock J, Jerwood D. Pelvic floor muscle assessment: the PERFECT scheme. Physiotherapy. 2001;87(12):631.
13. Bariola E, Lyons A, Leonard W, Pitts M, Badcock P, Demographic CM. Psychosocial factors associated with psychological distress and resilience among transgender individuals. Am J Public Health. 2015;105:2108–16.
14. Diokno A, Sampselle C, Herzog R, Raghunathan T, Hines S, Messer K, et al. Prevention of urinary incontinence by behavioral modification program: a randomized, controlled trial among older women in the community. J Urol. 2004;171:1165.
15. Irion J, Irion G. Women's Health in Physical Therapy. Baltimore, MD; Philadelphia, PA: Lippincott Williams & Wilkins; 2010.
16. Litwin M, McNaughton-Collins M, Fowler F Jr, Nickel C, Calhoun E, Pontari M, et al. The National Instities of Health Chronic Prostatitis Symptoms Index: development and validation of a new outcome measure. J Urol. 1999;162:369.
17. Erekson E, Yip S, Webberburn T, Martin D, Li F, Choi J, et al. The VSQ: a questionnaire to measure vulvovaginal symptoms in postmenopausal women. Menopause. 2013;20(9):973.

Part V

Special Topics—Regrets, Robotics, and History

Regrets in Transgender Female: Reversal Phalloplasty

Miroslav L. Djordjevic

Introduction

Transgender surgeons are required by the Standards of Care of the World Professional Association of Transgender Health (WPATH) [1] to follow minimum eligibility criteria for gender affirming surgery. The most recent edition of Standards of Care, version 7, includes the next criteria before surgical transitioniong: (1) 12 months of successful, continuous full-time real-life experience; (2) usually 12 months of continuous appropriate hormonal therapy for those without a medical contraindication; and (3) written recommendations from two mental health professionals for gender affirming surgery that will ensure a high probability of subjectively satisfying outcomes. Surgical transition is the last step in an individual's transition to the preferred gender. It comprises surgical procedures that will reshape the individual's body into a body with the appearance of the desired gender. Since the genital reconstruction represents irreversible step in an individual's transition, the patient must consider the preferred postoperative result they wish to achieve and the surgical options available to them. At this point, it is essential that the patient undergo a detailed preoperative consultation and

M. L. Djordjevic (✉)
Belgrade Center for Urogenital Reconstructive Surgery, School of Medicine, University of Belgrade, Belgrade, Serbia
e-mail: djordjevic@uromiros.com

examination by the surgeon, as well as a discussion with a psychologist/psychiatrist about the surgical outcome, to prevent disappointment or regret following surgery.

In female gender affirmation surgery, the main goal is the creation of a vagina with external genital organs that are as feminine as possible in appearance, with no scars or traumatic postoperative neuromas [2, 3]. Surgical techniques should be classified by the type of flap or graft that will be used for vaginal reconstruction, and include penile/penoscrotal skin grafts, pedicled penile/penoscrotal flaps, free skin grafts, bladder mucosa, or intestinal segments [4, 5]. The aesthetic, sensory, and functional results of vaginoplasty vary greatly. Generally, most authors report that their patients were extremely satisfied with their surgical outcomes overall, with low rate of complications [6–8]. The most commonly performed surgeries in transgender men are bilateral mastectomy with male chest contouring and genital reconstructive surgery, which includes total hysterectomy with bilateral oophorectomy, vaginectomy, reconstruction of the neophallus, urethral reconstruction, and scrotoplasty with the implantation of testicular prostheses. Concerning neophallic reconstruction, two options are available: metoidioplasty and phalloplasty [9].

Despite the successful treatment of early and late surgical complications, regret after gender affirming surgery should be considered as the worst conceivable outcome. Although many

© Springer Nature Switzerland AG 2021
D. Nikolavsky, S. A. Blakely (eds.), *Urological Care for the Transgender Patient*,
https://doi.org/10.1007/978-3-030-18533-6_17

studies have reported psychiatric and psychological problems after hormonal and/or surgical treatment in transgender women, only few have reported on regret. It is not surprising that most previous reports on the regret after gender affirming surgery were based on a small number of cases that were treated non-surgically.

Regret Phenomenon

The treatment of gender dysphoria always raised numerous ethical issues with rapid acknowledgment and recent achievements, and new complex issues in medical management have emerged. With unknown etiology and varying definitions (mental/medical illness, social construct, variation of sex?), who can decide, with 100% certainty, what treatment is in the best interest of a particular patient? The most prominent challenges and ethical questions pertain to the treatment of underage individuals, fertility, and possibility of regret after gender affirming surgery. Main ethical principles are autonomy, beneficence, non-maleficence, and informed consent. The individual must have autonomy of thought and intention when making decisions about medical treatment. This is an especially sensitive field in the treatment of gender dysphoria, because sometimes the individual's desires, hopes, and expectations might not correlate with reality. Medical experts and professionals must be very straightforward regarding specific possibilities, risks, and benefits of medical treatment, especially consideration that the last step in medical transition is irreversible. Beneficence implies doing only good, with the patient's best interest. However, some may consider that mutilation of healthy organs, in case of transitional surgery, is not in line with this principle. Non-maleficence must ensure that the treatment does not harm the individual, either in an emotional, social, or physical sense.

The seventh edition of the Standards of Care of the World Professional Association of Transgender Health (WPATH) offers flexible guidelines for the treatment of people experiencing gender dysphoria and describes the criteria for surgical treatment [1]. Always keeping these principles in mind, WPATH Standards of Care and criteria for diagnosis might not be enough to be certain that we are doing the right thing. Although it may seem that an individual fulfills all these criteria on paper, sometimes we can observe their personal disadvantages, youth, impairment, or desperation. It seems that even with the reassurance and recommendation from a mental health professional, ethical unease cannot be entirely erased because treatment guidelines have preceded the answers to vitally relevant questions [10].

Patients undergoing desired transition are required to provide two recommendation letters from certified psychiatrists and a gender specialist, as well as a confirmation of having been on hormonal therapy prescribed by an endocrinologist for a minimum of one-year period. Gender affirming surgery has been well known for more than 80 years. Previous results from different centers confirm that, in general, most patients were satisfied with the surgical results of their newly formed genitalia [3–6, 8, 11]. In addition to surgical complications, which can always be successfully solved, regret presents one of the worst conceivable outcomes. Several factors are described as a potential risk for regret after transfeminine gender affirmation surgery. Lindemalm et al. [12] defined three categories with different levels of regret: (1) Definite regret – the patient persistently regrets surgery and has applied for transition to original gender; (2) Some regret – indirectly expressed regret and signs of ambivalence about transsexual surgery; and (3) No regret. Additionally, dissatisfaction and regret after transsexual surgery have been reported to be associated with several factors: age over 30 years at first surgery, personality disorders, social instability, secondary transsexualism, heterosexual sexual orientation, dissatisfaction with surgical results, and poor support from the partner or family [13–15]. Despite many studies reporting psychiatric and psychological problems after hormonal and/or surgical treatment, only few have reported on regret and those were usually based on a small number of cases that were treated non-surgically [16]. Interestingly, all data about genital reversal surgery are related to regretful transgender female patients. There are no published reports on reversal surgery in transgender males.

Reversal Surgery

In the past few years, we performed reversal surgery in 12 regretful transgender women who initially underwent gender affirming surgery. All patients were over 30 years old. Generally, they reported their transitions that were characterized with the absence of "real-life experience" prior to surgery, absence or inappropriate hormonal treatment, and/or letters of recommendation that were written by non-experienced professionals. Data about evaluation by mental health professionals before primary transition as well as letters of recommendation were missed. The main factor contributing to regret, in this group, was related to the absence of psychiatric/psychological pretreatment assessment (unstable personality, strong sexual motivation, comorbidity-personality disorders, or underlying psychopathology-borderline or personality disorders) [17, 18]. Motivation for the gender affirming surgery in our regretful patients was not aimed at achieving sexual and gender congruence (e.g., sexually motivated, identity diffusion, emotional and behavioral instability, and the establishment of relationship). Prior to primary transition, they did not fulfill complete diagnostic criteria for gender dysphoria diagnosis (early or late onset), as well as criteria for personality disorder (e.g., borderline). Their hormonal and surgical transitions were characterized with the absence of relief, satisfaction or reduction of anatomic dysphoria and acceptance of body changes, or the absence of real-life experience. It was a reason that three independent well-known WPATH psychiatrists confirmed request for reversal surgery in our regret patients [16].

Phalloplasty in regretful transgender female patients still presents one of the most difficult surgical procedures in genital reconstructive surgery. Phallic reconstruction should, ideally, create an aesthetically pleasing phallus with sufficient length for vaginal penetration as well as tactile and erogenous sensibility enable voiding in standing position, and limit donor site morbidity.

Since total penile reconstruction was first reported, there have been constant endeavors to develop an ideal technique for phalloplasty that can fulfill all the desired objectives. Despite the fact that various phalloplasty techniques were described in recent decades using pedicle or free transfer flaps, the most commonly used flaps in transgender male affirming surgery are radial free forearm and free musculocutaneous latissimus dorsi flap. Recently, the most popular approach is "tube within a tube" forearm flap phalloplasty. Part of the flap along the ulnar border of the forearm, free of hair, is tubed inward around a Foley catheter, creating the neourethra. The remaining part of the flap is wrapped around the neourethra, creating a tube. The pedicle, which consists of radial artery, venae comitantes, lateral cutaneous nerve, and cephalic vein, is dissected carefully and left attached while a second surgical team prepares the recipient groin vessels. Once the recipient site is ready, the radial artery flap is transferred to the groin. End-to-side vascular anastomosis of the radial artery with the femoral artery and end-to-end anastomosis of the cephalic vein with the long saphenous vein are performed. The lateral cutaneous nerve of the forearm is joined to the ilio-ingunal nerve. The neourethra is anastomosed to the advanced female urethra. The clitoris remains undisturbed at the base of the new phallus, retaining its sensation [19, 20]. The advantages of this procedure include the creation of a sensate neophallus with complete urethral lengthening at the same stage. Consistent arterial anatomy and long vascular pedicle with good diameter of the vessels enable easier microsurgical anastomoses. Disadvantages of this technique include the small size and circumference of the neophallus, as well as visible donor site scar. Additionally, smaller volume of the neophallus presents a limitation for the insertion of two cylinders of the penile prostheses.

Due to the personal experience in phalloplasty surgery over the two decades, most of our transgender men undergo musculocutaneous latissimus dorsi flap phalloplasty. The main advantage of this flap is its good surface area, giving an excellent penile size, always sufficient to allow staged urethroplasty and insertion of penile prosthesis. Moreover, the neophallus can be constructed to the size desired by the patient. It was for this reason that we recommend the same type of flap for reversal phalloplasty. Interestingly, none of the patients opted for metoidioplasty as a method of phalloplasty [21]. The Belgrade Center published the first results with this technique in phallic reconstruction in boys with congenital anomalies (epispadias, micropenis and intersex disorders) [22]. In gender affirming surgery, this technique includes the removal of internal female genitalia with vaginectomy, followed by the creation of a neophallus from the latissimus dorsi musculocutaneous flap, fixation at the pubic region, anastomosis with the blood vessels at recipient site and scrotoplasty. Additional stages include neophallic urethral lengthening and penile prosthesis implantation, which could be performed several months after the first stage. Preoperatively, a non-dominant donor site should be treated by a professional massage to improve skin elasticity for easier donor site closure after flap harvesting [21, 23, 24].

Reversal surgery for regretful transgender females included three different steps with total phalloplasty, using the latissimus dorsi flap that was previously described [25]. Good results were obtained in all regretful patients and included good appearance and size of the neophallus, voiding function, and erectile function with penile implants. However, there were disadvantages as well, including lack of tactile sensation of the neophallus and urethral complications that required surgical revision. This issue remains problematic due to the poor sensitivity of the neophallus, with the main sensation restricted to the neoclitoral region.

All patients were interviewed about reasons for the new surgical transition as well as on expectations from the treatment. Also, they were requested to supply letters of recommendation from three independent experienced mental health professionals. Surgery included three steps: (1) removal of the neovagina and other female attributes with scrotoplasty and urethral lengthening; (2) musculocutaneous latissimus dorsi flap total phalloplasty; (3) neophallic urethroplasty with penile prostheses implantation. Preoperatively, the non-dominant donor site was prepared by a professional massage to improve skin elasticity, enabling easier skin closure after harvesting of the flap.

Neovagina is completely removed from the space between rectum and bladder, together with the urethra, except for the part of anterior vaginal wall close to the urethral orifice, which is used for the reconstruction of the bulbar urethra. This flap is joined with all available vascularized hairless tissue of the vulvoclitoral complex to lengthen the neourethra to the maximum extent, creating its pars fixa. In this way, the new urethral opening is usually placed at the mons pubis region, minimizing the requests for urethral reconstruction during the neophalloplasty. The reconstructed urethra is covered with fine surrounding subcutaneous tissue preventing postoperative fistula formation. Vaginal space is closed and perineum fashioned to resemble that of males. Both labia are joined in the midline over the neourethra, creating a one-sac scrotum. Silicone testicle prostheses are inserted into the space completing scrotoplasty (Fig. 17.1a, b).

The patient is placed in the lateral position for harvesting the latissimus dorsi musculocutaneous flap from the non-dominant side. Flap elevation starts with an incision of the anterior skin margin down to the deep fascia, and the plane is developed between the latissimus and anterior serratus muscle, using sharp and blunt dissection. The flap is divided inferiorly and medially, cauterizing the large posterior perforators of the intercostal vessels, and then lifted to expose the neurovascular pedicle. The pedicle, surrounded by fatty tissue, is identified and dissected proximally up to the axillary vessels. The flap is completely elevated except for the neurovascular bundle, which is not transected until the recipient vessels and nerve have been prepared for microanastomosis. Latissimus muscle is fixed at several points to the edges of the skin to prevent layer separation during further dissection. The

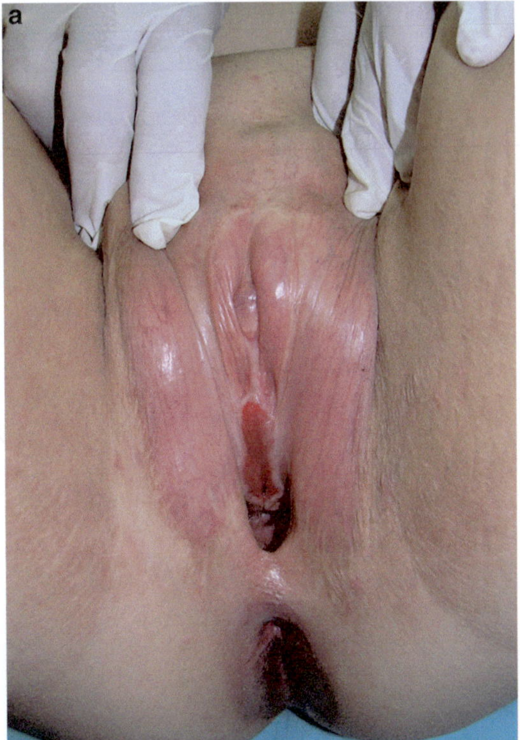

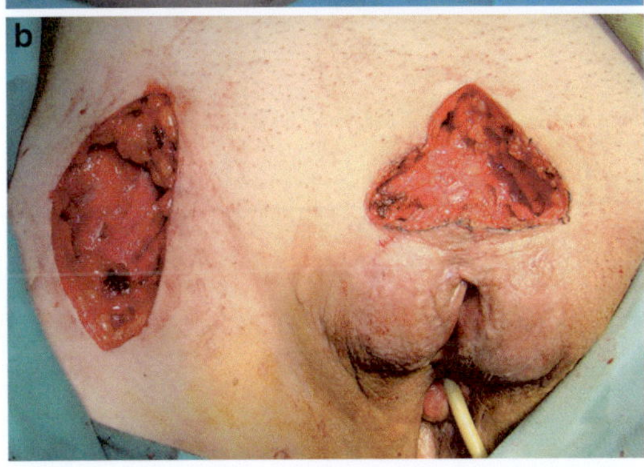

Fig. 17.1 (**a**) Appearance of female genitalia in regretful transgender female. (**b**) Reconstruction of the male genitalia with the insertion of testicle silicone implants

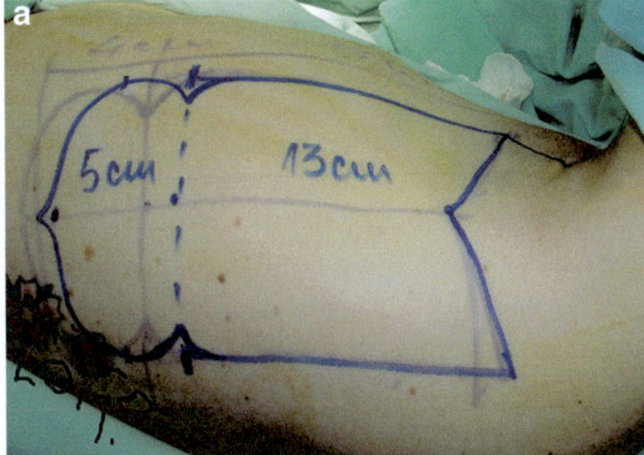

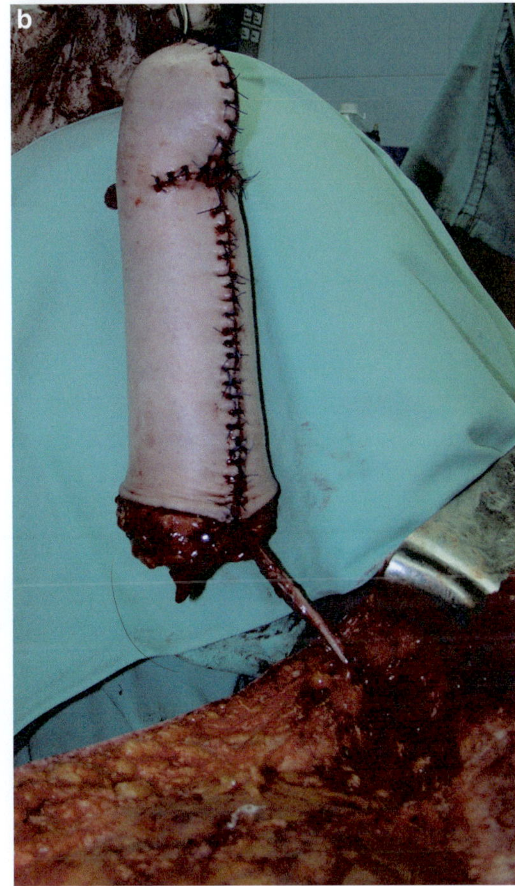

Fig. 17.2 (**a**) Design of the latissimus dorsi musculocutaneous flap. (**b**) Harvesting and tubularization of the flap

flap is tubularized creating the neophallus and closed distally to form the glans (Fig. 17.2a, b). Entirely constructed neophallus is detached from the axillar region after clamping and dividing the subscapular artery, vein and thoracodorsal nerve at their origin, in order to achieve maximal pedicle length. The donor site is approximated and closed directly after adjacent undermining. In the case of significant tension, presented skin defect is covered by split thickness skin grafts [16].

After identifying all neurovascular structures at the recipient site, the thoracodorsal vessels and nerve are divided, the neophallus is transferred to the pelvic region, and a microsurgical vascular anastomosis is performed immediately. The neophallic base is fixed to the skin at the recipient site (Fig. 17.3a, b).

Further stages include urethral lengthening and insertion of penile prosthesis. Staged urethral reconstruction, i.e., neophallic urethroplasty, is performed by using buccal mucosa grafts. The grafts are placed and quilted on the ventral side of the neophallus starting from the advanced urethral meatus to the tip of the glans. Three or more months later, newly created urethral plate is tubularized to form the distal part of the new urethra. Two types of penile prostheses, semirigid or inflatable, can be inserted into the neophallus, enabling penetrative sexual intercourse. A semilunar incision is made at the dorsal side of the neophallus. Hegar dilators are used to create space for the prosthesis to be inserted. Additional fixation to the periostium of the inferior pubic rami is also recommended (Fig 17.4a, b).

Sexual function is an important element of general health, but this is often underexposed by health care professionals dealing with transgender individuals. However, the current literature on postoperative sexual functioning is limited, especially in regretful transgender men and women [16]. In our study, we used International Index of Erectile Function to obtain data about sexual life and satisfaction after reversion surgery. Despite the fact that we reported one of the largest series of regretful patients, a limitation of our study is a lack of statistical analysis due to small sample size. However, we used parts of this questionnaire to estimate some of the reversal functions of individuals electing to transition back to assigned gender at birth. Analyzing the surgical outcome, all of our patients were very satisfied and did not regret their decision to undergo this type of surgery. Finally, strong motivation and good relationship with the partner play a crucial role in achieving a successful sexual life.

Additionally, it is very important to accept that every regret case represents a major clinical and ethical problem. We believe that the need for reversal surgery in regretful patients should be determined individually, considering both preoperative evaluations based on WPATH Standards

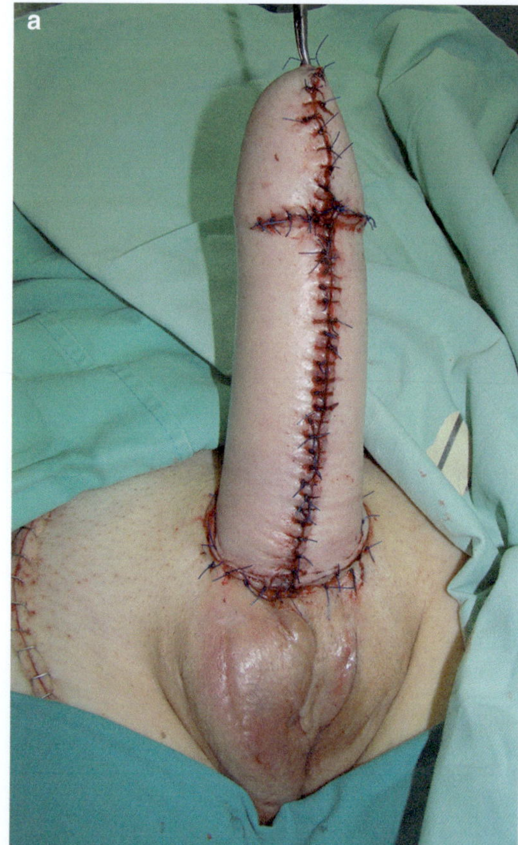

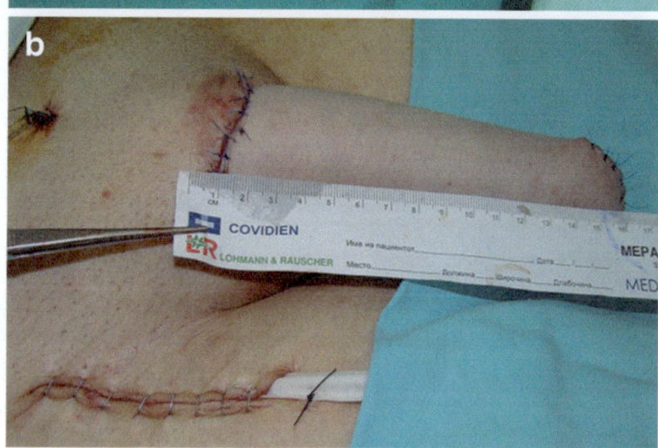

Fig. 17.3 (**a**) Flap transposition in the genital region. Microvascular anastomosis is done. (**b**) Good appearance of the neophallus. Appropriate size and volume are achieved

of Care and patients' expectations from this multistage surgical protocol and possible complications. It is very important to delineate the requests for reversal surgery and surgical procedures used in their management, and to evaluate postoperative outcomes.

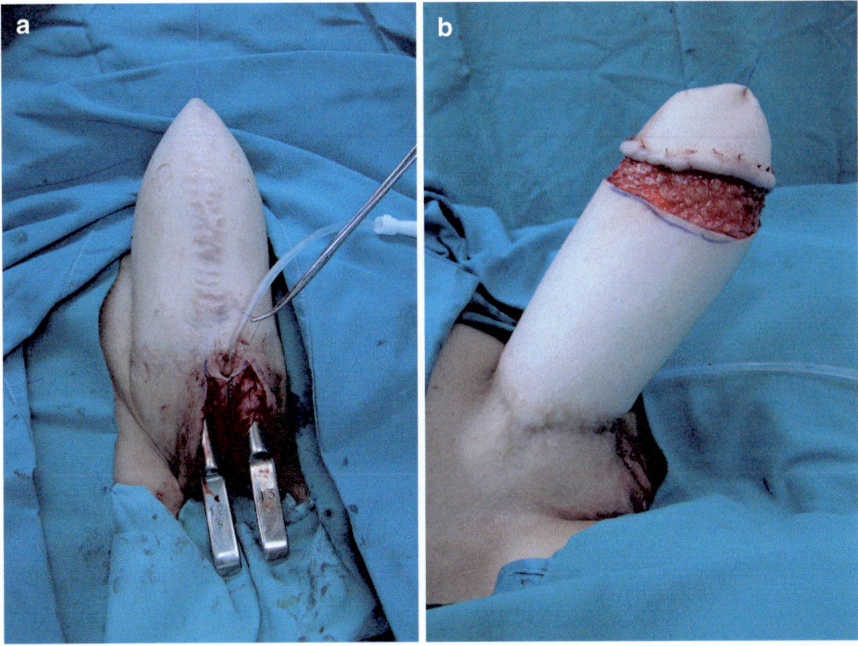

Fig. 17.4 (**a**) Urethral lengthening by hairless genital skin. Hegar dilators are used for the dilation of space for penile prosthesis insertion (ventral approach). (**b**) Appearance in erect state. Glans is reconstructed using Norfolk technique

Conclusions

Health professionals should recognize that not all persons with gender dysphoria need or want all elements of hormonal or surgical therapy. Medical treatment requires a team of experienced experts, and it usually includes mental health professionals, endocrinologists, and surgeons. Psychiatric assessment is the first step and is very complex because it is necessary to exclude other conditions that might mimic gender dysphoria. Following the hormonal treatment and real-life trial, surgery presents the last and usually irreversible step of transition. The vast majority of properly diagnosed transgender patients are satisfied with their decision following gender affirmation surgery, with only a few coming to regret it.

Reversal surgery represents a complex and multistage procedure and is indicated only after a new cycle of thorough preoperative psychiatric and endocrinological treatments. It should be an argument for a strict interpretation of the standards of care in terms of evaluating the patient's mental health, apart from the evaluation of gender dysphoria, and the patient's subsequent need for surgical treatment. We believe that more studies will contribute to increase the experience, resulting in the reduction of wrong choices for gender affirming surgery, as well the number of regret cases.

> **Take Home Points**
> - Gender affirmation surgery presents the main step in transgender transition.
> - Regret after gender affirmation surgery presents the most difficult complication.
> - The number of regret cases is not significant but represent a major clinical and ethical problem.
> - Proper preparation for surgical transition, as well as good support through the process, could prevent or minimize the risk of regret.
> - Reversal surgery is possible and should be determined individually, according to Standards of Care and patients' expectations.

Acknowledgments This work is supported by the Ministry of Science and Technical Development, Republic of Serbia, Project No. 175048.

References

1. Coleman E, Bockting W, Botzer M, et al. Standards of care for the heatlth and transsexuals, transgender, and gender-nonconforming people, version 7. Int J Transgendr. 2011;13:165–232.
2. Karim RB, Hage JJ, Mulder JW. Neovaginoplasty in male transsexuals: review of surgical techniques and recommendations regarding their eligibility. Ann Plast Surg. 1996;37:669–75.
3. Perovic SV, Stanojevic DS, Djordjevic ML. Vaginoplasty in male transsexuals using penile skin and urethral flap. BJU Int. 2000;86:843–50.
4. Krege S, Bex A, Lümmen G, et al. Male-to-female transsexualism: a technique, results and long-term follow-up in 66 patients. BJU Int. 2001;88:396–402.
5. Djordjevic ML, Stanojevic DS, Bizic MR. Rectosigmoid vaginoplasty: clinical experience and outcomes in 86 cases. J Sex Med. 2011;8:3487–94.
6. Selvaggi G, Ceulemans P, de Cuypere G, et al. Gender identity disorder: general overview and surgical treatment for vaginoplasty in male-to-female transsexuals. Plast Recon Surg. 2005;116:135e–45e.
7. Goddard JC, Vickery RM, Qureshi A, et al. Feminizing genitoplasty in adult transsexuals: early and long-term surgical results. BJU Int. 2007;100:607–13.
8. Sohn M, Bosinski HAG. Gender identity disorders: diagnostic and surgical aspects. J Sex Med. 2007;4:1193–208.
9. Bizic MR, Stojanovic B, Djordjevic ML. Genital reconstruction for the transgendered individual. J Pediatr Urol. 2017;13:446–52.
10. Levin SB. Ethical concerns about emerging treatment paradigms for gender dysphoria. J Sex Marital Ther. 2017;23:1–16.
11. Vujovic S, Popovic S, Sbutega-Milosevic G, et al. Transsexualism in Serbia: a twenty-year follow-up study. J Sex Med. 2009;6:1018–23.
12. Lindemalm G, Korlin D, Uddenberg N. Long-term follow-up of "sex change" in 13 male to female transsexuals. Arch Sex Behavior. 1986;15:187–210.
13. Landen M, Walinder J, Hambert G, et al. Factors predictive of regret in sex reassignment. Acta Psychiatrica Scandinavica. 1998;97:284–9.
14. Lawrence AA. Factors associated with satisfaction or regret following male to female sex reassignment surgery. Arch Sex Behavioral. 2003;32:299–315.
15. Olsson SE, Moller A. Regret after sex reassignment surgery in male to female transsexual: a long-term follow-up. Arch Sex Bihavior. 2006;35:501–6.
16. Djordjevic ML, Bizic MR, Duisin D, et al. Reversal surgery in regretful male-to-female transsexuals after sex reassignment surgery. J Sex Med. 2016;13:1000–7.
17. Blanchard R, Steiner BW, Clemmensen LH, et al. Prediction of regrets in postoperative transsexuals. Can J Psychiatr. 1989;34:43–5.
18. Pfafflin F. Regrets after sex reassignment surgery. J Psychol Human Sex. 1992;5:69–85.
19. Selvaggi G, Bellringer J. Gender reassignment surgery: an overview. Nat Rev Urol. 2011;8:274–82.
20. Monstrey S, Houtmeyers P, Lumen N, et al. Radial forearm flap phalloplasty. In: Djordjevic M, Santucci R, editors. Penile reconstructive surgery. Saarbrucken: LAP Lambert Academic Publishing; 2012. p. 254–78.
21. Djordjevic ML, Bizic MR, Stanojevic D. Phalloplasty in female-to-male transsexuals. In: Djordjevic M, Santucci R, editors. Penile reconstructive surgery. Saarbrucken: LAP Lambert Academic Publishing; 2012. p. 279–304.
22. Djordjevic ML, Bumbasirevic MZ, Vukovic PM, et al. Musculocutaneous latissimus dorsi free transfer flap for total phalloplasty in children. J Pediatr Urol. 2006;2:333–9.
23. Ranno R, Veselý J, Hýza P, et al. Neo-phalloplasty with re-innervated latissimus dorsi free flap: a functional study of a novel technique. Acta Chir Plast. 2007;49:3–7.
24. Djordjevic ML, Stojanovic B. Total phalloplasty with latissimus dorsi musculocutaneous flap in female-to-male transgender. In: Tran TA, Panthaki ZJ, Hoballah JJ, Thaller SR, editors. Operative dictations in plastic and reconstructive surgery. Cham, Switzerland: Springer; 2017. p. 577–83.
25. Perovic SV, Djinovic R, Bumbasirevic M, et al. Total phalloplasty using a musculocutaneous latissimus dorsi flap. BJU Int. 2007;100:899–905.

Robotic Applications in Gender Affirming Genital Surgery

Geolani W. Dy, Matthew Katz, Rachel Bluebond-Langner, and Lee C. Zhao

Introduction

Gender confirming vaginoplasty and vaginectomy have traditionally been performed using perineal approaches. The convergence of laparoscopic transabdominal approaches and mainstay perineal techniques in GAS has resulted in a new field of combined robotic-perineal approaches to genital reconstruction [1–4]. Robotic systems are designed to facilitate precise, careful dissection, and suturing in confined spaces, which lends well to reconstruction in the deep pelvis.

Operative Equipment

The da Vinci Robotic System (Intuitive Surgical, Sunnyvale, CA) Xi and SP (Single Port) systems are preferred for robotic genital GAS. The Xi system allows for side docking for concurrent perineal access. Compared with the Xi, the newer da Vinci SP system offers improved ability to work within a narrow space deep within the pelvis in addition to the aesthetic benefits of a single incision.

Robotic Applications in Feminizing Surgery

Feminizing genital GAS may include orchiectomy, penectomy, clitoroplasty, labiaplasty, vulvoplasty, and neovaginal canal creation, typically using penile inversion vaginoplasty (PIV) or intestinal vaginoplasty techniques. PIV is the most common approach for feminizing GAS, repurposing penile shaft and scrotal skin to create the vaginal lining, labia minora, and majora, while the glans penis is modified to become the clitoris [5–7]. PIV using genital tissue alone requires sufficient penoscrotal skin to create neovaginal depth of 12–14 cm. Achieving such depth without additional grafts may be challenging in those with limited genital growth after pubertal blockade, or those who have undergone prior PIV complicated by neovaginal stenosis. Robotic peritoneal flap vaginoplasty with PIV and robotic enteric vaginoplasty are alternatives to traditional penile inversion vaginoplasty for individuals with insufficient genital skin.

Robotic Peritoneal Flap Vaginoplasty

Technique

Jacoby and colleagues describe a robotic technique using peritoneal flap harvest to augment vaginal depth with PIV, minimizing extragenital donor site complications [3]. Here, the surgical

G. W. Dy · R. Bluebond-Langner · L. C. Zhao (✉)
NYU Langone Health, New York, NY, USA
e-mail: lee.zhao@nyumc.org

M. Katz
NYU Langone, New York, NY, USA

© Springer Nature Switzerland AG 2021
D. Nikolavsky, S. A. Blakely (eds.), *Urological Care for the Transgender Patient*,
https://doi.org/10.1007/978-3-030-18533-6_18

technique and early results are summarized. Preoperative preparation includes electrolysis or laser treatment to remove all hair from the redundant scrotal skin along the median raphe, as this skin may be utilized in the construction of the vaginal canal. Prior to surgery, no bowel preparation is performed.

After the induction of general anesthesia, patients are positioned in lithotomy. For venous thromboembolism prophylaxis, sequential compression devices are placed and weight-based subcutaneous heparin is given preoperatively. Preoperative antibiotic prophylaxis is administered.

The operation begins with the reconstruction of the external genitalia, as in traditional perineal PIV. After incising a small rhomboid flap at the perineum and harvesting of medial scrotal skin with preparation for use as a full thickness skin graft, the proximal urethra is exposed. A circumcising incision is made and the penis degloved, then inverted. The corpora cavernosa are opened ventrally, adjacent to the urethra, and the sinusoidal erectile tissue excised. The neurovascular bundle is kept intact with the dorsal aspect of the corpora cavernosa. The glans and preputial tissue are fashioned into a clitoris and clitoral hood. Bilateral orchiectomy is performed.

The perineal dissection involves excision of the bulbospongiosus muscle and ligation of the proximal corpora cavernosa. The ventral bulbar urethra is opened and the corpus spongiosum reduced; its lateral edges oversewn for hemostasis. The central tendon is sharply incised and the perineal dissection carried back along the proximal bulbar urethra. The vulva is created by suturing the neoclitoris to the pubis and attaching it to the urethral mucosa. Labia majora and minora are fashioned from scrotal and penile skin, respectively.

The abdominal portion of the vaginoplasty may commence concurrently if two surgical teams are present (Fig. 18.1). After obtaining intraperitoneal access, the patient is placed in Trendelenburg, the robotic ports are placed inferiorly using the HiDES technique for improved cosmesis [8], and the robot is docked. Figure 18.2 *demonstrates Da Vinci XI Port placement*. If the Da Vinci SP robot is utilized, a circumferential umbilicoplasty incision is made and a 2.7 cm vertical fascial incision made just above the umbilicus, with or without a 5 mm assistant port 2 fingerbreadths above the anterior superior iliac spine on the assistant's side (Fig. 18.3a). Figure 18.3b *demonstrates results of the umbilicoplasty access for the Da Vinci SP at 5 weeks*.

To begin peritoneal flap harvest, the peritoneal ridge is incised at the rectovesical junction, using the vas deferentia as a landmark for initial horizontal incision (Fig. 18.4). Dissection is performed underneath the seminal vesicles. Denonvilliers fascia is then incised to develop a

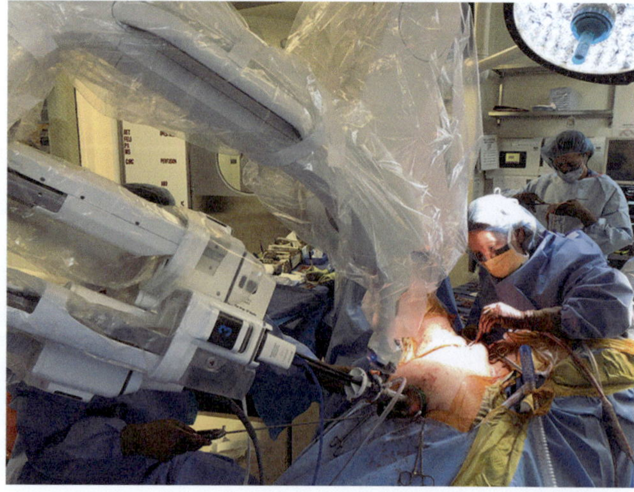

Fig. 18.1 Concurrent robotic dissection and perineal reconstruction during robotic-assisted peritoneal flap vaginoplasty

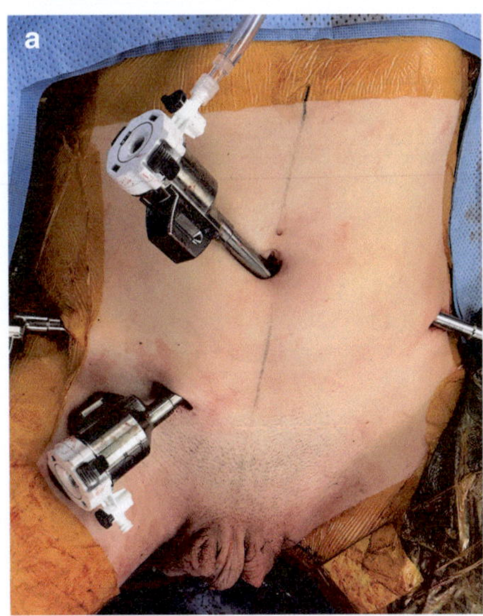
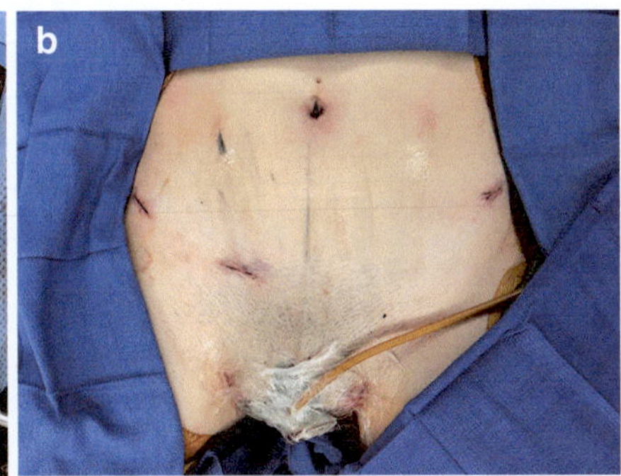

Figs. 18.2 (**a**, **b**) Standard port placement for da Vinci XI robot, vaginoplasty, and vaginectomy

space between the prostate and rectum for the neovaginal canal. The levator ani musculature is partially transected at 3- and 9-o'clock until satisfactory neovaginal width is achieved. The dissection is then continued distally toward the perineum until creating a connection to the external incision. Peritoneal flaps measuring approximately 6 cm × 8 cm are raised from the anterior rectum along the ureters, as well as from the posterior bladder. The prevesical space is opened to lower the bladder and its associated peritoneal flap, reducing tension during the closure of the neovaginal apex.

The skin graft and dilator are introduced into the canal and the outer edge of the skin graft sewn to the free edge of the inverted penile skin and to the perineal flap that was raised at the beginning of the procedure. The inverted skin graft is delivered into the canal and serves as the mid-distal neovaginal lining. Running 3–0 dual barbed, absorbable sutures are used to suture the posterior peritoneal flap to the posterior aspect of the skin graft, and the anterior peritoneal flap to the anterior aspect of the skin graft to create a circumferential canal. The dilator is removed, antibiotic-soaked packing is placed to compress the skin graft portion of the canal (Fig. 18.5a). At the apex of the neovagina, anterior and posterior peritoneal flaps are sutured together using running 3–0 polydiaxone barbed suture to close the vaginal apex (Fig. 18.5b). A vacuum assisted dressing applied over the packing to draw fluid from the wound.

Postoperative Care

On postoperative day 5, the dressing, Foley catheter, and vacuum dressing are removed, and the patient is taught to perform initial dilation using a 32 mm or 35 mm dilator, with the goal of increasing dilator size to 38 mm. Discharge typically occurs on postoperative day 5, with close follow-up in the initial 3–6 months, followed by yearly exams. At these postoperative visits, vaginal canal healing is assessed with direct visualization using a speculum, and depth measured using length-demarcated dilators.

Outcomes

The initial series of peritoneal flap vaginoplasty describes results in 41 transwomen [3]. Preoperatively, 85% of patients were circumcised with an average penile length of 8.7 cm ± 2.5 cm measured from the base of penis to the tip of glans. The length of procedure was 263.0 ± 34.7 minutes. All had an inpatient stay of 5 days. At the mean follow-up of 114 ± 79 days after surgery, vaginal depth and width were 14.2 ± 0.7 cm and 3.6 ± 0.2 cm, respectively. Erogenous sensation was endorsed by all patients postoperatively.

Fig. 18.3 (**a**) Port placement for da Vinci SP robot, (**b**) umbilicoplasty incision at 5 weeks

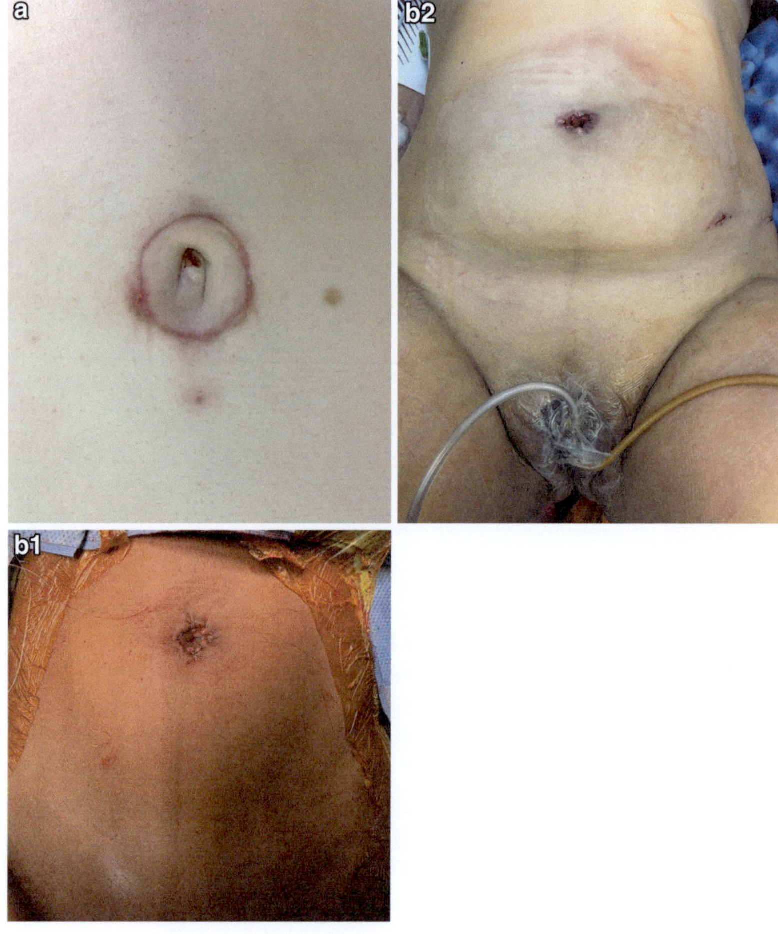

Fig. 18.4 Initial flap development for peritoneal flap vaginoplasty

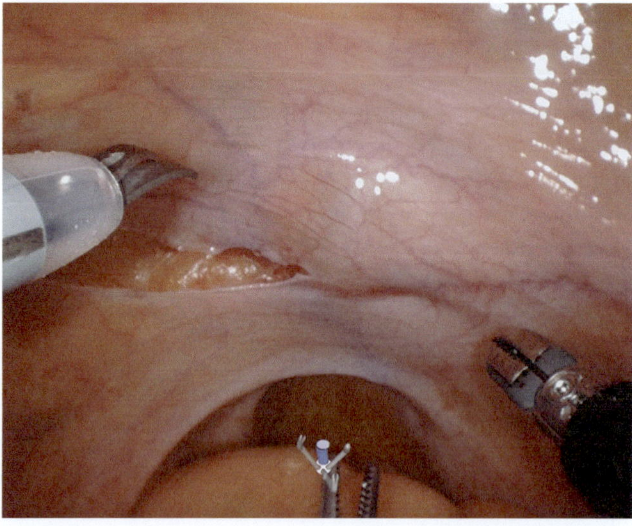

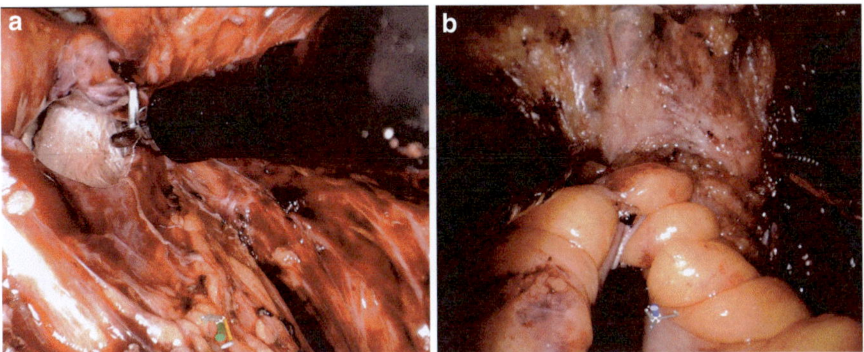

Fig. 18.5 (**a**) Closure of peritoneal flap vaginoplasty with vaginal packing in vault; (**b**) closed apex following peritoneal flap vaginoplasty

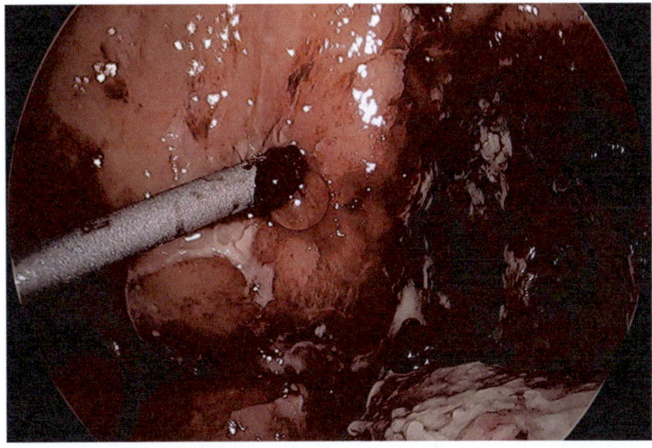

Fig. 18.6 Laparoscopic evacuation of pelvic abscesses 5 weeks after primary peritoneal flap vaginoplasty

The main complications were small areas of delayed wound healing at the introitus, which resolved with local wound care and silver impregnated hydrocolloid dressings. In this approach, the vaginal apex is sutured closed, and excluded from the peritoneal cavity. Since the publication of the initial series, [3] pelvic abscess occurred in one patient at 5 weeks, whose neovagina appeared intact on perineal and laparoscopic assessment. The abscesses were unroofed laparoscopically (Fig. 18.6), and the patient discharged day 1 after the treatment of the abscess on oral antibiotics.

Patients are counseled that they must perform lifelong vaginal dilation. The anastomosis between the inverted penoscrotal skin and the peritoneal flap, which is not present in standard PIV, is theoretically at risk of stenosis, in addition to the introitus and apex as in standard PIV. As in PIV and enteric vaginoplasty, aggressive postoperative dilation of the neovagina can result in perforation, but this risk has not been observed in limited follow-up.

Notably, the peritoneal component of the neovagina does not provide lubrication at the introitus of the vagina. Squamous epithelialization of the peritoneal neovaginal graft has been described at 11 months (range 3–26 months) following the analogous Davydov procedure in patients with vaginal agenesis [4, 9].

Robotic Revision Peritoneal Flap Vaginoplasty

In patients who have vaginal stenosis after prior PIV, or prior penile inversion vulvoplasty without vaginal canal, robotic canal revision may offer satisfactory neovaginal depth without extragenital skin grafts or enteric segments. Port placement and peritoneal flaps harvested as in primary vaginoplasty. A dilator is placed within the stenosed neovagina, and the canal dissection begins with incision onto the vaginal dilator (Fig. 18.7). The intervening scar tissue is excised and incised laterally as needed to accommodate a 38 mm dilator. The peritoneal neovaginal apex is closed over an antibiotic-soaked packing as in primary vaginoplasty. Postoperative care is similar to primary vaginoplasty.

Preliminary results of eight patients who underwent robotic revision peritoneal flap vaginoplasty are promising. In the authors' initial series, the mean operative time was 4 hours and 55 minutes (range 255–400) with no intraoperative complications. Mean length of stay was 5.1 days (range 5–6). Two patients had external wound complications postoperatively, one requiring reoperation for bleeding. With a mean of 120 days' follow-up (18–362), patients had mean depth of 14.5 cm, with a mean depth increase of 4.4 cm (2.4–4.8) from preoperative measurements. Mean width at the follow-up was 3.7 cm (3.5–3.8), representing a mean increase of 0.6 cm (0–0.9) in caliber.

Robotic Enteric Vaginoplasty

For the purposes of this chapter, we will briefly discuss techniques specific to robotic enteric vaginoplasty, as principles and outcomes of enteric vaginoplasty are discussed in Chap. 6. Open and laparoscopic enteric vaginoplasty are well described in transgender women and individuals with vaginal agenesis [8, 10–12]. Kim and colleagues were the first to describe a technique of robotic-perineal sigmoid vaginoplasty in a patient with androgen insensitivity [13]. Robotic approaches have been widely adopted in colorectal surgery with benefits of smaller incisions, increased range of motion, decreased tremor, and ability to suture in small, confined spaces [14]. In vaginoplasty, robotic approaches may also allow for more precise and better visualization of vaginal canal dissection than traditional laparoscopy.

Port placement is performed according to the segment of bowel to be harvested. Pedicled intestinal transfer requires identification of a 12–18 cm intestinal segment, typically sigmoid or ileum, which is then isolated and transferred on its vas-

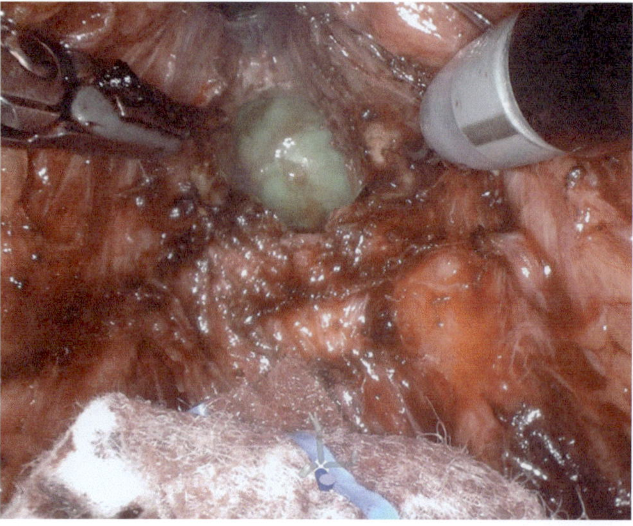

Fig. 18.7 Incision onto vaginal dilator during revision peritoneal flap vaginoplasty in a transwoman with vaginal stenosis

cular pedicle through a canal space dissected between the bladder and rectum [10]. The distal end of the enteric segment is then sutured to skin flaps created from the perineum. To reduce the risk of prolapse, one may affix the lateral portions of the neovagina to the levator ani muscles, [15] or suture the serosa of the bowel to the abdominal wall [13].

Disadvantages include those associated with enteric surgery—diversion colitis, peritonitis, intestinal obstruction, anastomotic leaks and fistulae, injury to adjacent organs and vasculature—as well as introital stenosis, mucocele, constipation, and potentially increased susceptibility to sexually transmitted infections [16].

Robotic Applications in Masculinizing Surgery

Masculinizing genital GAS may include vaginectomy, creation of a neophallus via phalloplasty or metoidioplasty, scrotoplasty, and urethral lengthening, among other procedures. Urethral lengthening allows the patient the ability to stand to void, a common goal for many transgender men who tend to avoid using public restrooms [17, 18]. Vaginectomy, or removal of the vaginal epithelium with closure of the perineum, has been shown to reduce urethral complication rates in patients who undergo urethral lengthening. As such, vaginectomy is now recommended to reduce complications of urethral lengthening in several high-volume centers [19, 20]. The procedure is typically performed transvaginally, similarly to colpocleisis for pelvic organ prolapse in patients assigned female at birth. The major anatomic difference is the widened genital hiatus in patients with prolapse, which allows for vaginal eversion and ample exposure to the mucosa requiring excision. In addition to diminished vaginal caliber and a well-suspended vaginal apex in transgender patients, the bladder may adhere to the vaginal apex following hysterectomy, increasing the risk of bladder injury. Intraoperative risks of the procedure include blood loss requiring transfusion, as well as injury to the rectum or urinary tract leading to vesicovaginal or rectovagi-

nal fistula [20]. Furthermore, incomplete destruction of vaginal tissue with the vaginal introitus can lead to vaginal regrowth and remnant cavity formation. Behind a surgically closed perineum, vaginal mucosal secretions may accumulate, leading to development of a draining vaginal sinus. The presence of a distal urethral stricture and resultant back pressure in the fixed urethra can result in a false passage or urethral diverticulum in the remnant vaginal cavity [21]. Symptoms may include perineal pain, obstructive voiding, urinary leakage, and recurrent urinary tract infections [1].

A robotic-assisted approach to vaginectomy has recently been described, with the potential for a safer and more complete excision due to improved visualization and hemostasis [22]. The authors have further adapted this technique and found several benefits of the robotic approach, including the ability to harvest a vaginal flap from the anterior vaginal wall and vaginal graft from the posterior wall. This otherwise discarded tissue is used for urethral lengthening and limits the need for other donor sites [23]. This technique is in its nascency, with limited follow-up in published studies [22].

Robotic Vaginectomy

Technique
Robotic-assisted vaginectomy begins with perineal dissection. We perform hydro-dissection of the vaginal mucosa circumferentially with a lidocaine and epinephrine mixture, and stain the vaginal mucosa with methylene blue. Initial incision and dissection of the vaginal mucosa is carried distally for 3–4 cm or until visualization is impaired. After obtaining intraperitoneal access, the patient is placed in Trendelenburg, the robotic ports are placed inferiorly using the HiDES technique [8] with the Da Vinci XI, or superior to the umbilicus through an umbilicoplasty incision with the SP robot, with a single 5 mm assistant port 2 fingerbreadths above the anterior superior iliac spine on the assistant's side (Fig. 18.2). The robot is docked. An EEA sizer is placed within the vagina.

If the patient has not yet undergone hysterectomy, this may be performed as an initial step. If no uterus is present, an incision is made through the peritoneum at the vaginal cuff and carried through to the level of the EEA sizer, through the vaginal mucosa (Fig. 18.8). The methylene blue staining assists in identifying mucosal borders. The dissection is then continued circumferentially and may be assisted by an EEA sizer within the rectum, for rectal identification (Fig. 18.9). The posterior vaginal mucosa may be passed off, then thinned for use as a graft in urethral lengthening. The anterior vaginal mucosa is preserved as a flap (Fig. 18.10). The surgeon at the perineum may perform the final dissection close to the urethral meatus, to minimize the creation of a diverticulum inferior to the native urethral meatus. This flap may be sutured at 3 and 9-o'clock to labial tissue to extend the native urethra.

Colpocleisis is then performed transabdominally using circumferential running 3–0 barbed, absorbable sutures to obliterate the vaginal cavity. The authors prefer to use a gracilis flap as an additional measure to reduce vaginal cavity recurrence (Fig. 18.11).

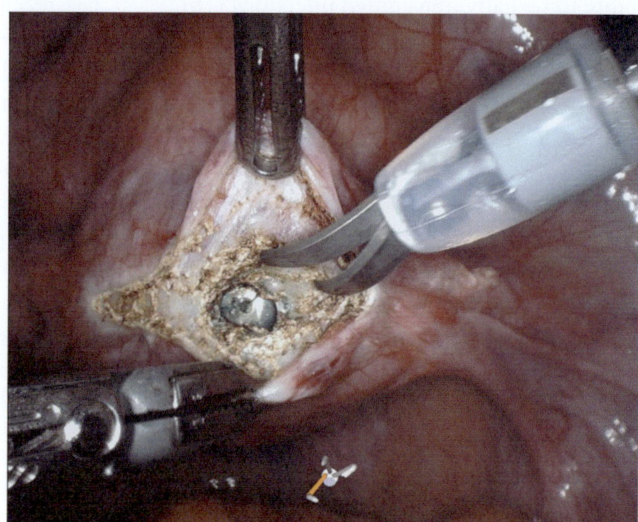

Fig. 18.8 Incision onto vaginal dilator/EEA sizer during robotic vaginectomy in a transmasculine patient

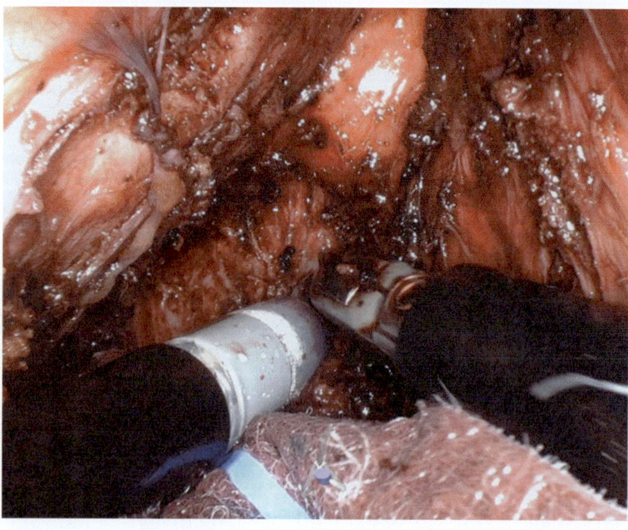

Fig. 18.9 Development of anterior vaginal flap in robotic vaginectomy

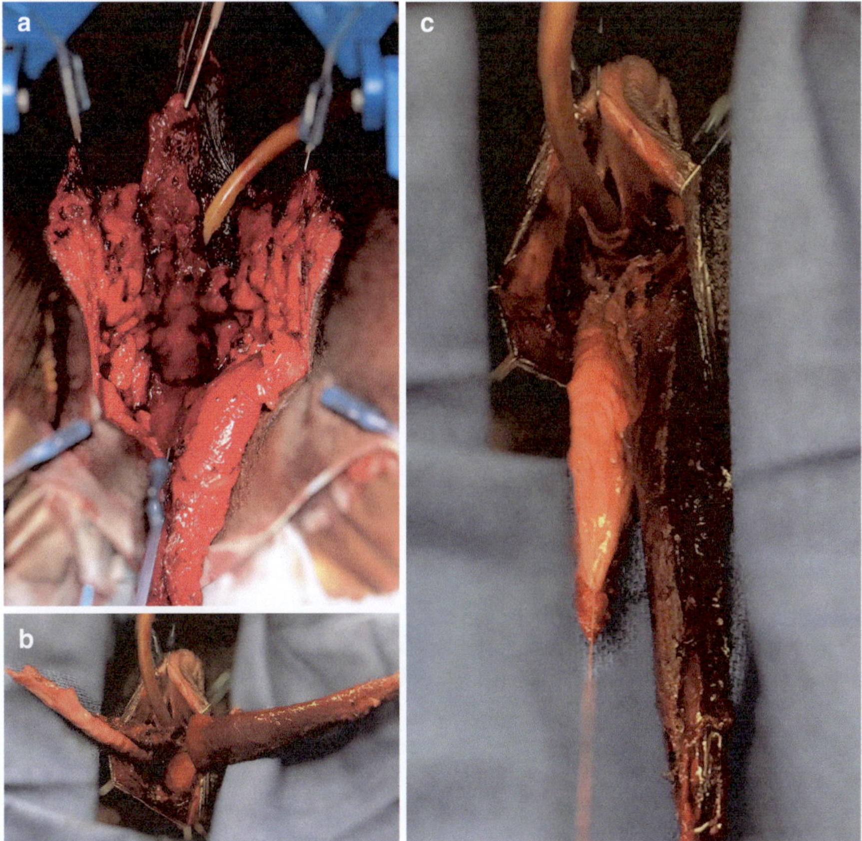

Fig. 18.10 Externalized anterior vaginal flap for urethral lengthening following robotic harvest

Fig. 18.11 Affixing
gracilis flap into vaginal
cavity as adjunct to
colpocleisis

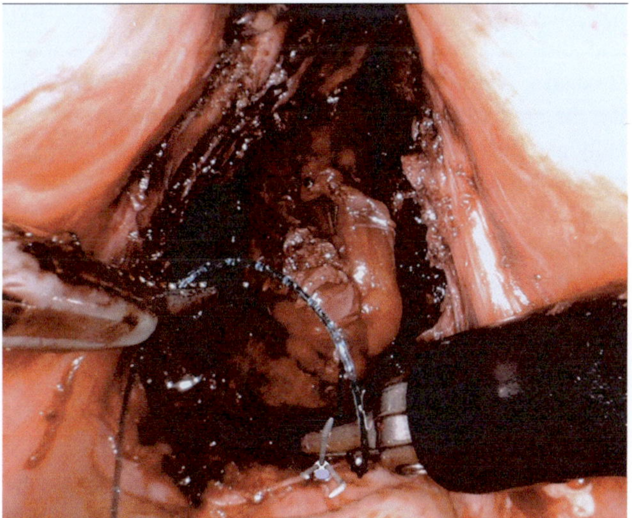

In the authors' initial series of 16 patients who underwent robotic transabdominal primary vaginectomy, the average length of operation was 423.6 ± 84.9 minutes. At 361 ± 176 days' follow-up, there were no major complications. Five patients (31.2%) experienced a minor postoperative complication amenable to conservative management. None developed proximal urethral fistulae, and three presented with distal urethral fistulae after second stage phalloplasty, at mean postoperative day 349 ± 51.4.

Robotic Vaginal Remnant Excision

A transabdominal approach may be used for resection of symptomatic vaginal remnants. Preoperative studies such as a CT cystogram, retrograde urethrogram and voiding cystourethrogram, and cystoscopic exam under anesthesia may assist in delineating the location and size of a re-epithelialized vaginal cavity.

The robotic-assisted repair includes port placement and initial peritoneal incision in the same location as in primary vaginectomy. Under transurethral cystoscopic guidance, the vaginal remnant is examined endoscopically. Using the near-infrared setting on the robotic platform to visualize the light of the cystoscope transabdominally, the vaginal remnant portion can be targeted and dissected free without injury to adjacent structures. After the excision of the remnant cavity, the urethral defect may be oversewn robotically, avoiding any external perineal incisions and minimizing injury to the reconstructed urethra. A foley catheter is left in place for 1–2 weeks postoperatively, and the urethra may be evaluated with a voiding cystourethrogram or peri-catheter retrograde urethrogram at the time of catheter removal.

Potential Complications of Robotic GAS Approaches

Risks of Robotic Canal Dissection

Rectal, bladder, and urethral injury are potential complications of robotic transabdominal canal dissection. This dissection involves the same key steps as a posterior approach to robotic-assisted laparoscopic prostatectomy (RALP). After the incision of Denonvillier's fascia, the inter-fascial plane just beneath the prostatic fascia is identified. All dissection is performed under direct visualization using the robotic camera; monopolar cautery is avoided near the serosa of the rectum. In larger series, rectal injury during RALP was 0.17–0.23% for non-irradiated pelvises, and 0.9% in salvage cases [20–22]. Until longer-term follow-up is available, such surrogate measures from prostatectomy literature may be used to counsel patients regarding the risk of rectal injury. Remaining in an appropriate plane also allows the surgeon to avoid injury to the prostate, urethra, and external urinary sphincter, to minimize risks postoperative urinary incontinence.

General Risks of Transabdominal Robotic Approaches

In addition to the intraoperative risks specific to each procedure, other potential complications are those reported with other robotic pelvic operations: complications from positioning, initial access, bleeding, visceral injury, ureteral injury, equipment malfunction, need for open conversion, and venous thromboembolism, among others. Extended operative and lithotomy time are established risk factors for positioning-related complications (23–24). It is recommended that only surgeons experienced in robotic pelvic surgery perform the pelvic portion of the operation to reduce the risk of complications.

Future Directions

The costs associated with the robotic component warrant consideration. Until such analyses are available to compare robotic and perineal approaches in GCS, the prostatectomy literature may be utilized as a surrogate. Although robotic-assisted prostatectomy is costlier than open approaches, there is potential for moderate long-term cost advantages if a robotic approach produces higher quality outcomes (26–27). Robotic approaches allow for minimal incisions and excellent exposure in cases of enteric vaginoplasty [13]. Peritoneal flap vaginoplasty has potential to lower risk apical stenosis and costly revision procedures in high risk patients.

As demand for GAS grows, a robotic transabdominal approach may be more accessible to urologic trainees than perineal dissection, as RALP is a much more common procedure than perineal prostatectomy or rectourethral fistula repair.

Robotic techniques are in their nascency but have enormous potential for integration into genital GAS, especially in individuals with limited genital skin who seek vaginoplasty, and in transmasculine patients seeking vaginectomy. Standardized clinical outcome measures are lacking, as are longer-term data [7]. As the field of GAS expands, rigorous assessment of clinical and patient-reported outcomes will be essential to understanding the role of robotic approaches in GAS.

Take-Home Points
- Robotic transabdominal approaches to genital gender confirming surgery (GCS), combined with traditional perineal approaches, allow for enhanced visualization and improved access to deep pelvic structures, and potential for new reconstructive techniques.
- Robotic applications in vaginoplasty include bowel vaginoplasty, as well as primary and revision peritoneal flap vaginoplasty.
- Vaginal remnant excision and primary vaginectomy with the harvest of vaginal mucosa for masculinizing urethral lengthening and can be performed using combined robotic and perineal approaches.
- Larger studies are needed to compare the risks and benefits of robotic GCS with perineal approaches.
- Further optimization of emerging techniques, assessment of long-term results, and development of standardized outcome measures are critical future directions for robotic GCS.

References

1. Dy GW, Sun J, Granieri MA, Zhao LC. Reconstructive management pearls for the transgender patient. Curr Urol Rep. 2018;19(6):36.
2. Bianchi S, Berlanda N, Brunetti F, Bulfoni A, Ferrero Caroggio C, Fedele L. Creation of a neovagina by laparoscopic modified davydov vaginoplasty in patients with partial androgen insensitivity syndrome. J Minim Invasive Gynecol. 2017;24(7):1211–7.
3. Jacoby A, Maliha S, Granieri MA, Dy G, Bluebond-Langner R, Zhao LC. Robotic davydov peritoneal flap vaginoplasty for augmentation of vaginal depth in feminizing vaginoplasty. J Urol. 2019;201(6):1171–6.
4. Fedele L, Frontino G, Restelli E, Ciappina N, Motta F, Bianchi S. Creation of a neovagina by Davydov's laparoscopic modified technique in patients with Rokitansky syndrome. Am J Obstet Gynecol. 2010;202(1):33.e1–6.
5. Buncamper ME, van der Sluis WB, van der Pas RS, Ozer M, Smit JM, Witte BI, et al. Surgical outcome after penile inversion vaginoplasty: a retrospective study of 475 transgender women. Plast Reconstr Surg. 2016;138(5):999–1007.
6. Hadj-Moussa M, Ohl DA, Kuzon WM Jr. Feminizing genital gender-confirmation surgery. Sexual Med Rev. 2018;6(3):457–68.e2.
7. Horbach SE, Bouman MB, Smit JM, Ozer M, Buncamper ME, Mullender MG. Outcome of vaginoplasty in male-to-female transgenders: a systematic review of surgical techniques. J Sex Med. 2015;12(6):1499–512.
8. Morrison SD, Satterwhite T, Grant DW, Kirby J, Laub DR Sr, VanMaasdam J. Long-term outcomes of rectosigmoid neocolporrhaphy in male-to-female gender reassignment surgery. Plast Reconstr Surg. 2015;136(2):386–94.
9. Herman CJ, Willemsen WN, Mastboom JL, Vooijs GP. Artificial vaginas: possible sources of epithelialization. Hum Pathol. 1982;13(12):1100–5.
10. Claes KEY, Pattyn P, D'Arpa S, Robbens C, Monstrey SJ. Male-to-female gender confirmation surgery: intestinal vaginoplasty. Clin Plast Surg. 2018;45(3):351–60.
11. Bouman MB, van der Sluis WB, Buncamper ME, Ozer M, Mullender MG, Meijerink WJ. Primary total laparoscopic sigmoid vaginoplasty in transgender women with penoscrotal hypoplasia: a prospective cohort study of surgical outcomes and follow-up of 42 patients. Plast Reconstr Surg. 2016;138(4):614e–23e.
12. Djordjevic ML, Stanojevic DS, Bizic MR. Rectosigmoid vaginoplasty: clinical experience and outcomes in 86 cases. J Sex Med. 2011;8(12):3487–94.
13. Kim C, Campbell B, Ferrer F. Robotic sigmoid vaginoplasty: a novel technique. Urology. 2008;72(4):847–9.
14. Baek SK, Carmichael JC, Pigazzi A. Robotic surgery: colon and rectum. Cancer (Sudbury, Mass). 2013;19(2):140–6.

15. Imparato E, Alfei A, Aspesi G, Meus AL, Spinillo A. Long-term results of sigmoid vaginoplasty in a consecutive series of 62 patients. Int Urogynecol J Pelvic Floor Dysfunct. 2007;18(12):1465–9.

16. Hage JJ, Karim RB, Asscheman H, Bloemena E, Cuesta MA. Unfavorable long-term results of rectosigmoid neocolpopoiesis. Plast Reconstr Surg. 1995;95(5):842–8; discussion 9–50

17. Hage JJ, Bout CA, Bloem JJ, Megens JA. Phalloplasty in female-to-male transsexuals: what do our patients ask for? Ann Plast Surg. 1993;30(4):323–6.

18. James SE, Herman JL, Rankin S, Keisling M, Mottet L, Anafi M. The report of the 2015 U.S. transgender survey. Washington, DC: National Center for Transgender Equality; 2016.

19. Massie JP, Morrison SD, Wilson SC, Crane CN, Chen ML. Phalloplasty with urethral lengthening: addition of a vascularized bulbospongiosus flap from vaginectomy reduces postoperative urethral complications. Plast Reconstr Surg. 2017;140(4):551e–8e.

20. Al-Tamimi M, Pigot GL, van der Sluis WB, van de Grift TC, Mullender MG, Groenman F, et al. Colpectomy significantly reduces the risk of urethral fistula formation after urethral lengthening in transgender men undergoing genital gender affirming surgery. J Urol. 2018;200(6):1315–22.

21. Nikolavsky D, Hughes M, Zhao LC. Urologic complications after phalloplasty or metoidioplasty. Clin Plast Surg. 2018;45(3):425–35.

22. Groenman F, Nikkels C, Huirne J, van Trotsenburg M, Trum H. Robot-assisted laparoscopic colpectomy in female-to-male transgender patients; technique and outcomes of a prospective cohort study. Surg Endosc. 2017;31(8):3363–9.

23. Weinberg A, Granieri M, Cohen O, Bluebond-Langner R, Levine J, Zhao L. 027 robotic-assisted vaginectomy, mobilization of vaginal mucosa for urethral lengthening and a gracilis muscle flap for phalloplasty: a novel technique for female-to-male genital reconstruction. J Sex Med. 2018;15(2):S13–S4.

Jasmine Bhinder and Prashant Upadhyaya

Introduction

Gender dysphoria is the inner conflict and distress caused by a discrepancy between a person's gender identity and that person's sex assigned at birth (and the associated gender role and/or primary and secondary sex characteristics). According to the Diagnostic & Statistical Manual of Mental Disorders (DSM-V), an estimated 1.4% of the population worldwide has been diagnosed with gender dysphoria [1].

A variety of treatments are available to transgender individuals affected by gender dysphoria to transition to the gender with which they identify. Gender affirmation encompasses not only genital surgery, but psychotherapy, hormonal therapy, and non-genital surgical procedures. This holistic and multidisciplinary approach is vital when individuals are transitioning to a specific gender role.

Ancient History and Mythology

The earliest reports of gender identity alteration can be traced back to Egypt, 1500 BC when King Thutmose passed away and Queen Hatshepsut became the pharaoh of Egypt. Queen Hatshepsut was the third woman to become pharaoh during three thousand years of Egyptian history. Knowing that her position as a ruler was highly controversial, she sought out opportunities to portray her image as more masculine. Her images and statues were depicted as a male pharaoh, with large muscles and a beard, wearing men's clothing [2].

In ancient Rome (509 to 27 BC), it was socially acceptable for a freeborn Roman man to have and want sex with both female and male partners. They were free to engage with either gender without fear of perceived loss of their masculinity as long as they took the penetrative role [3]. Male partners were usually slaves, entertainers, or sex workers. Emperor Nero, (37–68 AD) supposedly killed his wife, Poppaea Sabina, and married his young male slave, Sporus, later that year. The young boy was castrated by Nero and appeared in public as his wife wearing feminine clothing that was customary for a Roman empress [3]. Elagabalus (204–222 AD) was another Roman emperor known for his controversial (by the people of Rome) sexual orientation and habits. The emperor routinely attempted to enhance his looks by using cosmetics and was preferred to be called by female roles such as: wife, queen, or mistress. Elagabalus had a secret room in his palace where he committed "acts of indecency," as it was called at the time by biographer Cassius Dio [4]. According to Cassius

J. Bhinder · P. Upadhyaya (✉)
Department of Surgery, SUNY Upstate Medical
University, Syracuse, NY, USA
e-mail: jbhinder@buffalo.edu; upadhyap@upstate.edu

© Springer Nature Switzerland AG 2021
D. Nikolavsky, S. A. Blakely (eds.), *Urological Care for the Transgender Patient*,
https://doi.org/10.1007/978-3-030-18533-6_19

Dio and other historians, Elagabalus would wear female clothing, cosmetics, and wigs, while using the discreet room with men who were instructed to play along with his role. He would also take this female role and prostitute himself in brothels within the city. Elagabalus has been characterized as transgender, as he offered a substantial reward to any doctor that could give him female genitalia. Due to his eccentric and "indecent" behavior, Elagabalus' grandmother had him assassinated [4, 5].

In India, Hindu epics make reference to deities and heroes whose behaviors can be interpreted as transgender [6]. The Mahabharata is an ancient Indian epic, which is thought to have been composed in 400 BC. Shikandi is a character in the Mahabharata who was originally born as a girl named 'Shikhandini" to a king, Drupada. A divine voice told Drupada to raise Shikhandi as a son; and so she was treated like a man and trained in warfare to fight alongside his father [6].

Throughout history and around the world, there are groups of individuals who neither categorize themselves as man or woman. Those who embrace this gender role are referred to as the third gender or third sex. The third gender can represent different things in various cultures around the world. The indigenous Māhū of Hawaii represents those who are present in an intermediary state between man and woman and have an unspecified gender [7]. Māhū played an important role in Hawaiian culture. They were notable teachers, priests, and healers. They performed hula dances and chanted temples and passed along cultural knowledge to future generations [7].

The concept of the third gender has also been used to describe a group of people in India called the Hijra. In ancient India, the Hijras were well respected and held religious authority, important court positions, and administrative roles in India [8]. Numerous people sought out blessings from the Hijras during religious ceremonies. However, after the British colonization of India, the Western concept (at that time) of scrutinizing anyone who was not "straight" became a prominent theme in Indian society. The Hijra community became social outcasts and this exile is responsible for the socioeconomic difficulties and stigmas that they face today. Due to widespread discrimination, they are often forced to beg for money and are employed as prostitutes [8].

Modern History – Europe

During the modern era (twentieth century), there have been numerous accounts of transgender individuals across the globe. However, at this time there was limited aid for transgender people and they often kept their feelings discreet due to fear of rejection. In many countries, even wearing clothing associated with the opposite gender was illegal and individuals displaying what was considered as "acts of homosexuality" were often persecuted. At this time in history homosexual and transgender, people were considered as having a psychological disorder needing a conversion treatment which often consisted of drastic measures such as psychotherapy, electroconvulsive therapy, lobotomy, hypnosis, and involuntary holding in an asylum [9].

Magnus Hirschfeld, a German physician, is considered the father of transgender healthcare. His primary interest in the rights of gay individuals began as he witnessed many of his homosexual patients committing suicide. One particular young patient from the army had a significant impact on Hirschfeld and ignited his interest in being a strong advocate for homosexual and transgender rights. He was a young army officer who Hirschfeld was treating for depression. He committed suicide and left behind a note saying, despite his greatest efforts, he was not able to end his desire for other men and therefore ended his life due to guilt and shame. He also mentioned in his note that he lacked the courage to tell his parents the truth and hoped that Hirschfeld could help the people of Germany understand and accept homosexuality and homosexuals one day [10].

Hirschfeld and his colleagues established the Institute for Sexual Science in Berlin, the world's first institute devoted to sexology. This institute housed all of Hirschfeld's major works and studies on sexuality and also provided medical appointments and educational services. Individuals from all over Europe visited the institute to gain a clearer understanding of their sexuality. Other clinical staff within the institute included psychiatrists, endocrinologists, gynecologists, and a dermatologist. Hirschfeld's institution became a safe haven for transgender people. He offered individuals not only a shelter to avoid abuse, but also provided them with jobs and therapy, and eventually performed surgeries to transition them to the gender they feel is their true self. The first documented gender affirmation surgery was performed on one of the institute's employees, Dora Richter. Dora had an orchiectomy in 1922, and later penectomy and vaginoplasty in 1931 [11]. Although Dora was the first to have surgery at the institute, arguably the most famous patient was Lili Elbe. Her life story has been depicted in the movie *The Danish Girl*. Lili had a total of four surgeries during her transfeminine affirmation and passed away secondary to sepsis after her last procedure, a uterine transplant, in 1931. In 1933, the Nazis took power in Germany and ordered the police to enforce book burnings on topics they considered "sexually immoral." Within 4 months of Nazi ruling, the Hirschfeld institute was destroyed and all of his works from the library were burned [11]. In history, this institute remains the first of its kind to accept and provide support and medical options for transgender individuals.

Another notable physician who is credited for the innovation of gender affirmation surgery for transwomen is Dr. Georges Burou. Burou was a French gynecologist who independently pioneered the anterior pedicled penile skin flap inversion vaginoplasty. He performed over 800 vaginoplasties for individuals from all over the world in his sex reassignment clinic, "Clinique du Parc" in Casablanca. His first case was reported in 1956 and his technique is still the predominant surgical approach used today [12].

Sir Harold Gillies, also known as the "father of modern plastic surgery," pioneered numerous procedures on wounded soldiers during World War I and II [13]. The foundations of his work and techniques established are still used until this day including the basic principles of facial recon-struction, bone/cartilage grafting, and tissue transfer for burns. He is specially credited with devising a technique – which he'd first encountered in a Russian textbook – called the "Tubed Pedicle" [13]. Prior to the war, Gillies routinely performed surgery to correct hypospadias in children. He applied this experience during the war for genital reconstruction in wounded soldiers. Following WWII, Gillies and his colleague, Ralph Millard, in 1946 performed the world's first transmasculine gender affirmation surgery. The first patient was Michael Dillon who had heard stories about the work Gillies had done to reconstruct wounded soldiers and sought him out to conduct a genital affirmation operation. He is also considered to be the first female-assigned individual known to have taken testosterone for the purpose of transforming his body. Michael Dillon was a doctor from an aristocratic British family, who had entered medicine in order to better understand his own masculine identity and how he could change his body to be like other men. Between 1946 and 1949, Gillies performed over 13 operations on him, using skin from his legs and stomach. To conceal that he was performing gender affirmation procedures, Dr. Gillies falsely diagnosed his patient with hypospadias [14].

Modern History (Twentieth Century Onwards) – United States

Up until this point in history, there was not much attention on transgender individuals in the United States, nor had any documented case of gender affirmation surgery taken place until 1951. This had changed when Christine Jorgensen became be the first American to undergo gender affirmation surgery. At an early age, Jorgensen felt like a "woman stuck within a man's body" and stated she was more envious of females than interested in them [15]. At this time, the only existing treatment was available in Denmark. This consisted of both hormonal therapy and several surgical procedures. Upon returning to the United States, she was very open about her gender identity and the procedures she had undergone. Due to her to public disclosure, this event brought significant attention to the transgender movement in America when her story was published in the *New York Times* and *New York Daily News* in 1952 [15].

Dr. Harry Benjamin was a German-born endocrinologist who had a keen interested in sexology. He became close friends with Magnus Hirschfeld and gained a deeper understanding of transgender individuals [16]. Benjamin moved to New York City in 1913 and was the first in America to actively prescribe hormones to transgender individuals. His initial case was a young boy who came to see him because "he wanted to become a girl." His mother who was looking for anything to help his situation accompanied him. Eventually, Benjamin decided to treat the boy with estrogen and arranged for them to visit Germany for surgery [17]. Benjamin continued to help hundreds of transgender patients by prescribing hormones and suggested they visit surgeons abroad due to the fact that no physician at the time was openly performing gender-affirming operations in the United States. Benjamin supported the use of hormonal therapy and affirmation surgeries, and opposed psychotherapy as a treatment for gender dysphoria. Psychotherapy at the time was aimed at adjusting the mind to fit the body. Dr. Benjamin was not convinced that this approach was effective and believed in altering the body to fit the mind instead. He persistently argued that psychotherapy did not decrease an individual's desire to alter their sex, but forced them to keep their feelings hidden which lead to "depression and misery" [16].

During the 1970s, Benjamin along with a group of therapists and psychologists formed the Harry Benjamin International Gender Dysphoria Association (HBIGDA). This association used Benjamin's case studies to outline standards of care for transgender individuals who desired medical and surgical treatment [16]. In 2007 HBIGDA was renamed as the World Professional Association for Transgender Health (WPATH).

In 1966, The John Hopkins Gender Identity Clinic became the first institution in the United States to perform gender affirmation procedures. The clinic was comprised of two plastic surgeons, two psychiatrists, two psychologists, a urologist, and a pediatrician. Initially, the clinic was experimental and operated under secrecy until the doctors were confident they could perform the procedures. However, the news was out when a reporter from the *New York Daily News* interviewed a female that admitted to having undergone a gender affirming operation at Johns Hopkins [18]. Between 1966 and 1979, only 30 surgeries had been performed at Hopkins [18]. Although short-lived, this clinic was a major movement in transgender history as it took transgender individuals and their concerns seriously during a time when they were often disregarded as having mental illness.

The founder of the Gender Identity Clinic, John Money, surprisingly believed that gender was learned rather than innate. He claimed that gender identity could be created socially with "nurture over nature" and his idea was enforced when Dr. Money published the "John/Joan case". The John/Joan case refers to an experiment that occurred when two twin boys had routine circumcision, but due to error during the procedure, one of the boy's genitalia was mutilated. Dr. Money counseled the parents and encouraged them to raise the son with mutilated genitalia as a daughter [19]. He assured them that by making their son appear feminine, treating him as a daughter, and with the use of hormones, they could successfully raise the child as a girl. Dr. Money published this experiment as a great success; however, years later a man named David Reimer identified himself as the object of this case, which revealed its major flaws and skewed results. David states he grew up as a troubled and depressed girl and immediately reassumed his male identity as soon as his parents revealed the truth of his past. In his early twenties he attempted to commit suicide twice in relation to the distress and emotional suffering experienced throughout his childhood. After suffering from years of depression, he unfortunately committed suicide late in his 30s [19].

Notable mention must also be made of Dr. Stanley H. Biber who was among the first surgeons to offer transgender surgery in the United States. He started performing gender affirmation surgeries in 1969 and is credited with performing over 4000 operations. He practiced in a small town called Trinidad, CO until 2003 [20]. He became so famous and prolific that the town earned the reputation as "the sex-change capital of the world." His first patient to undergo gender affirmation surgery was a friend and social worker from the only hospital in the town. Dr. Bieber consulted his colleagues at Johns Hopkins University hospital and went ahead with the procedure. His practice has since been taken over by a protégée, Dr. Marci Bowers, who herself underwent affirmation surgery and is widely considered an authority in the field [20].

Transgender Individuals Today

After many years of struggling for acceptance, transgender individuals are now entering a more hopeful era in the United States. In 2011, Chaz Bono, a transgender male author, actor, and musician, was the focus of an Emmy-nominated documentary *Becoming Chaz* which chronicled his transition. He was then widely supported as a contestant on the popular reality television show, *Dancing with the Stars*. In April of 2015, Caitlyn Jenner, previously Bruce Jenner, winner of the men's decathlon event at the 1976 Summer Olympics in Montreal and reality television personality, revealed herself as a transgender woman. She publicly disclosed her inner frustrations and gender dysphoria from a young age and published a book in 2017, which speaks on her struggles and transition to a public life as a female [21].

Every transgender person has unique needs, and while many elect to undergo physical transformation, not all chose to do so. For those that wish to pursue physical transition numerous options exist including cross-sex hormone therapy and gender affirmation surgery. At the time of this writing, nearly all insurance carriers recognize transgender care as necessary have policy statements on coverage. Although transgender people still face various forms of discrimination and have a far way to go, we are gradually moving toward a more acceptable community for all.

> **Take Home Points**
> - Gender dysphoria is the inner conflict and distress caused by a discrepancy between a person's gender identity and that person's sex assigned at birth (and the associated gender role and/or primary and secondary sex characteristics).
> - The earliest reports of gender identity alteration can be traced back to Egypt (1500 BC), ancient Rome and from Hindu epics.
> - Magnus Hirschfeld established the Institute for Sexual Science in Berlin, the world's first institute devoted to sexology. This institution was a safe haven for transgender people. It offered individuals shelter to avoid abuse, provided them with jobs, therapy, and eventually surgery to transition them to the gender they feel is their true self.
> - Dr. Georges Burou was a French gynecologist who pioneered the anterior pedicled penile skin flap inversion vaginoplasty and his technique is still the predominant approach used today.
> - Christine Jorgensen is the first American to undergo gender affirmation surgery.
> - After many years of struggling for acceptance, transgender individuals are now entering a more hopeful era in the United States.
> - Gender reassignment affirmation encompasses not only genital surgery, but psychotherapy, hormonal therapy, and non-genital surgical procedures.

References

1. Byne W, Karasic DH, Coleman E, Eyler AE, Kidd JD, Meyer-Bahlburg HFL, Pleak RR, Pula J. Gender dysphoria in adults: an overview and primer for psychiatrists. Transgend Health. 2018;3(1):57–70.
2. History.com Editors. Hatshepsut. History [Internet]. 2009 [updated 2018; cited 2019 March 2]. Available from: https://www.history.com/topics/ancient-history/hatshepsut

3. C. Rolfe, ed., Suetonius, 2 Vols., The Loeb Classical Library (London: William Heinemann, and New York: The MacMillan Co., 1914), II.87-187.

4. N. Sheldon. 11 Remarkable Transgender People from History [Internet]. 2019 [cited 2019 August 11]. Available from: https://historycollection.co/11-remarkable-transgender-people-history/

5. Benjamin H, Green R. The Transsexual Phenomenon, Appendix C: Transsexualism: Mythological, Historical, and Cross-Cultural Aspects. New York: The Julian Press, Inc.; 1966.

6. Martini F. The Legend of Shikhandi, the Transgendered Warrior Who Paid the Price of Opposing Powerful Men [Internet]. 2018 [cited 2019 August 11]. Available from: https://www.ancient-origins.net/history/legend-shikhandi-transgendered-warrior-who-paid-price-opposing-powerful-men-009369

7. Odo C, Hawelu A. Eon a Mahu o Hawa'i: the extraordinary health needs of Hawai'I'sMahu. Pac Health Dialog. 2001;8(2):327–34.

8. Gandikota I. India's Relationship With the Third Gender [Internet]. 2018 [cited 2019 August 20]. Available from: https://cas.uab.edu/humanrights/2018/10/29/indias-relationship-with-the-third-gender/

9. Stekel W. Is homosexuality curable? Psychoanal Rev. 1930;17(443):447–8.

10. Bauer H. The hirschfeld archives: violence, death, and modern queer culture. Philadelphia, USA: Temple University Press; 2017.

11. Ralf Dose, Magnus Hirschfeld: The Origins of the Gay Liberation Movement (New York City: Monthly Review Press, 2014).

12. Hage JJ, Karim RB, Laub DR. On the origin of pedicled skin inversion vaginoplasty: life and work of Dr. Georges Burou of Casablanca. Ann Plast Surg. 2007;59(6):723–9.

13. David F. The Kiwi war surgeon who helped pioneer modern facial surgery [Internet]. 2018 [cited 2019 March 2]. Available from: https://www.noted.co.nz/currently/history/sir-harold-gillies-kiwi-war-surgeon-pioneer-modern-facial-surgery/

14. 1129 Sir Harold Gillies: Pioneer of Phalloplasty and the Birth of Uroplastic Surgery. The Journal of Urology, 183(4s), p.e437.

15. Jorgensen C. Christine Jorgensen: a personal autobiography. New York. New York: Bantam Books; 1967. p. 105.

16. Kristen S. Harry Benjamin [Internet]. 2019. [cited 2019 March 2]. Available from: https://www.britannica.com/biography/Harry-Benjamin

17. Meyerowitz J. How sex changed: a history of transsexuality in the United States. Cambridge. Mass: Harvard University; 2002. p. 143.

18. Meagan D. How one of America's best medical schools started a secret transgender surgery clinic [Internet]. 2016. [cited 2019 March 2]. Available from: https://timeline.com/americas-first-transgender-clinic-b56928e20f5f

19. Colapinto J. As nature made him: the boy who was raised as a girl. New York: HarperCollins Publishers; 2000.

20. Stanley H. Biber, 82, Surgeon Among First to Do Sex Changes, Dies. https://www.nytimes.com/2006/01/21/us/stanley-h-biber-82-surgeon-among-first-to-do-sex-changes-dies.html

21. Eve G. Transgender Today [Internet]. 2013 [cited 2019 March 2]. Available from: https://www.apa.org/monitor/2013/04/transgender

Index

© Springer Nature Switzerland AG 2021
D. Nikolavsky, S. A. Blakely (eds.), *Urological Care for the Transgender Patient*,
https://doi.org/10.1007/978-3-030-18533-6

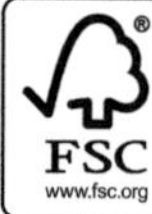

MIX
Papier aus verantwortungsvollen Quellen
Paper from responsible sources
FSC® C105338

If you have any concerns about our products,
you can contact us on
ProductSafety@springernature.com

In case Publisher is established outside the EU,
the EU authorized representative is:
Springer Nature Customer Service Center GmbH
Europaplatz 3, 69115 Heidelberg, Germany

Printed by Libri Plureos GmbH
in Hamburg, Germany